Everything
You Need to
Know about
Medical
Tests

Everything
You Need to
Know about
Medical
Tests

Springhouse Corporation
Springhouse, PA

STAFF

Senior Publisher
Matthew Cahill

Clinical Manager
Cindy Tryniszewski, RN, MSN

Art Director
John Hubbard

Senior Editor
Michael Shaw

Editors
Marcia Andrews, Peter H. Johnson, Pat Wittig

Copy Editors
Cynthia C. Breuninger (manager), Priscilla
DeWitt, Mary Durkin, Lynette High, Kathryn A.
Marino, Christina P. Ponczek, Doris Weinstock

Designers
Stephanie Peters (senior associate art director),
Lesley Weissman-Cook (book designer), Elaine
K. Ezrow, Donald G. Knauss, Amy Litz, Mary
Ludwicki, Kaaren Mitchel, Mary Stangl

Typography
Diane Paluba (manager), Elizabeth Bergman,
Joyce Rossi Biletz, Phyllis Marron, Valerie
Rosenberger

Manufacturing
Deborah Meiris (director), Pat Dorshaw, T.A. Landis

Production Coordinator
Margaret A. Rastiello

Editorial Assistants
Mary Madden, Beverly Lane

EYNMT-060997

R A member of the Reed Elsevier plc group

Library of Congress Cataloging-in-Publication Data
Everything you need to know about medical tests.
    p. cm.
    Includes index.
    1. Medicine, Popular. 2. Diagnosis. 3. Function
tests (Medicine)   I. Springhouse Corporation.
RC81.E9155 1996
616.07′5 — dc20   95-10232
    ISBN 0-87434-933-8   CIP

CONTENTS

ADVISORY BOARD

CONTRIBUTORS & CONSULTANTS

Charol Abrams, MS, MT (ASCP) SH, CLS (NCA), CLSp (H), CLS Consultant, Philadelphia

Barbara A. Ankenbrand, RN, BS, MA, Professor of Nursing, Mt. Mercy College, Cedar Rapids, Iowa

Wendy L. Baker, RN, BSN, MS, Staff, Critical Care Medicine Unit, University of Michigan Hospitals, Ann Arbor

Debra C. Broadwell, RN, PhD, ET, Associate Professor of Nursing, Emory University, Atlanta

Lillian S. Brunner, MSN, ScD, LittD, FAAN, Nurse-Author, Brunner Associates, Inc., Berwyn, Pa.

Judith Byrne, BS, MT (ASCP), Affiliate Member, American Society of Clinical Pathologists

Ricardo L. Camponovo, MD, Consultant in Anatomic and Clinical Pathology, Scottsdale (Ariz.) Community Hospital

Luther Christman, RN, PhD, FAAN, Former Dean, College of Nursing, and Former Vice President, Nursing Affairs, Rush-Presbyterian-St. Luke's Medical Center, Chicago

James Robert Cronmiller, BS, MA, MS, Medical Technologist, Genesee Hospital, Rochester, N.Y.

Ellen Digan, MA, MT (ASCP), Professor of Biology and Coordinator, MLT Program, Manchester Community Technical College, Manchester, Conn.

Stanley J. Dudrick, MD, FACS, Program Director and Associate Chairman, Department of Surgery, St. Mary's Hospital, Waterbury, Conn.

Barbara Boyd Egoville, RN, MSN, Former Instructor, Critical Care Nursing, Lankenau Hospital School of Nursing, Philadelphia

John J. Fenton, PhD, DABcc, FNACB, Director of Chemistry, Crozer-Chester Medical Center, Chester, Pa., and Associate Professor of Clinical Chemistry, West Chester University of Pennsylvania

Sr. Rebecca Fidler, MT (ASCP), PhD, Former Chairperson, Health Sciences, Salem (W. Va.) College

Ruth Ann Fitzpatrick, MD, Director, Division of Endocrinology, Crozer-Chester Medical Center, Chester, Pa.; and Clinical Assistant Professor of Medicine, Hahnemann Medical College, Philadelphia

Nancy Flynn, RN,C, MSN, Clinical Educator, Bryn Mawr (Pa.) Hospital

Pamela W. Gitschier, MT, MS, Technical Chemistry Supervisor, St. Luke's Hospital, Bethlehem, Pa.

Sandra K. Goodnough Hanheman, RN, MSN, PhD, Clinical Professor, Graduate Program, Texas Woman's University College of Nursing, Houston

Mary Chapman Gyetvan, RN, BSEd, MSN, Independent Clinical Consultant, Springhouse Corporation, Springhouse, Pa.

John J. Hagarty, MD, Surgical Pathologist, Emeritus Director of Laboratories, and Attending Pathologist, Holy Redeemer Hospital, Meadowbrook, Pa.

Annette L. Harmon, RN, MSN, CEN, Assistant Director of Nursing, Newton-Wellesley Hospital, Newton-Lower Falls, Mass.

Connie S. Heflin, RN, MSN, Associate Professor of Nursing, Paducah Community College, Paducah, Ky.

Richard Edward Honigman, MD, FAAP, Pediatrician, Levittown, N.Y.

Joyce LeFever Kee, RN, MSN, Associate Professor, College of Nursing, University of Delaware, Newark

Mary Frances Keen, RN, DNSc, Associate Professor, University of Miami School of Nursing, Coral Gables, Fla.

Rose M. Kenny, MD, Associate Pathologist, Doylestown (Pa.) Hospital

Catherine E. Kirby, RN, MSN, Nurse Consultant, Nursing Technomics, National Technomics, West Chester, Pa.

Paul M. Kirschenfeld, MD, FACP, FCCP, Medical Director, Intensive Care Unit, and Program Director, Internal Medicine Residency Program, Atlantic City (N.J.) Medical Center

William E. Kline, MS, MT (ASCP), SBB, Director, Technical Services, St. Paul (Minn.) Red Cross

Marc S. Lapayowker, MD, Chairman, Department of Radiology, Abington (Pa.) Memorial Hospital

Gizell Maria Rossetti Larson, MD, Staff Neurologist, Nicolet Clinic, Neenah, Wis.

Peter G. Lavine, MD, Director, Coronary Care Unit, Crozer-Chester Medical Center, Chester, Pa.

Dennis E. Leavelle, MD, Associate Professor and Consultant, Mayo Medical Laboratories, Mayo Clinic, Rochester, Minn.

Michél E. Lloyd, MT (ASCP), SBB, Senior Technologist, St. Luke's Hospital, Bethlehem, Pa.

Thomas E. Mackell, MD, FAAOS, Orthopedic Surgeon, Doylestown (Pa.) Hospital

Lillian Madden, RN, MSN, CCRN, Clinical Educator, Misericordia Hospital, Philadelphia

Elizabeth Anne Mallon, MS, MT (ASCP), Transplant Coordinator, Thomas Jefferson University Hospital, Philadelphia

Marylou K. McHugh, RN, EDd, Director of Graduate Program, Department of Nursing, LaSalle University, Philadelphia

Joan C. McManus, RN, MA, Assistant Professor of Nursing, Bergen Community College, Paramus, N.J.

S. Breanndan Moore, MB, BCh, FRCPI, Chairman, Division of Transfusion Medicine, and Professor of Laboratory Medicine, Mayo Clinic and Mayo Medical School, Rochester, Minn.

Barbara A. Moyer, RN, MSN, Education Nurse Specialist, Lehigh Valley Hospital, Allentown, Pa.; and Assistant Professor, Allentown College of St. Francis de Sales, Center Valley, Pa.

John E. Nestler, MD, Fellow in Endocrinology, University of Pennsylvania, Philadelphia

Patricia J. Noone, RN, BSN, MEd, Senior Associate Professor of Nursing, Bucks County Community College, Newtown, Pa.

Gary M. Oderda, PharmD, MPH, Professor and Chairman, Department of Pharmacy Practice, College of Pharmacy, University of Utah, Salt Lake City

John J. O'Shea, MD, Chief, Leukocyte Cell Biology Section, Arthritis and Rheumatism Branch, National Institute of Arthritis and Musculoskeletal and Skin Diseases, National Institutes of Health, Frederick, Md.

Catherine Paradiso, RN, CCRN, MS, Clinical Nurse Specialist, St. Vincent's Medical Center of Richmond, Staten Island, N.Y.

Ara G. Paul, BS, MS, PhD, Dean and Professor, College of Pharmacy, University of Michigan, Ann Arbor

Mae E. Paulfrey, RN, MN, Assistant Professor, University of San Francisco School of Nursing

Barbara Madigan Preston, RN, MSN, Vascular Nurse Clinical Specialist and Consultant, Hospital of the University of Pennsylvania, Philadelphia

Frances W. Quinless, RN, PhD, CCRN, Assistant Professor, Rutgers University College of Nursing, Newark, N.J.

Linda T. Raichle, PhD, MT (ASCP), Laboratory Training Advisor, National Laboratory Training Network, Exton, Pa.

Teresa A. Richardson, MT, MLT (AMT), Medical Laboratory Technologist, Quakertown (Pa.) Community Hospital

Carolyn Robertson, RN, MSN, Diabetes Nurse Specialist, New York University School of Medicine

Thomas E. Rubbert, BSL, LLB, JD, Attorney, Pasadena, Calif.

Harrison J. Shull, Jr., MD, FACP, Assistant Professor of Medicine, Vanderbilt University, Nashville, Tenn.

Joan Simpson, MS, MT (ASCP), Consultant, Mansfield Center, Conn.

Marian J. Hoffman Sperk, RN, MSN, CNSN, Clinical Nurse Specialist-Nutrition, Lehigh Valley Hospital, Allentown, Pa.

Johanna K. Stiesmeyer, RN, MS, CCRN, Critical Care Clinical Educator, El Camino Hospital, Mountain View, Calif.

Basia Belza Tack, RN, MSN, ANP, Professor, School of Nursing, University of Washington, Seattle

Deborah Porter Thornton, MEd, MT (ASCP), SC, Assistant Professor, Medical Laboratory Science Program, Department of Molecular and Microbiology, University of Central Florida, Orlando

Richard W. Tureck, MD, Professor of Obstetrics and Gynecology; Director, In Vitro Fertilization and Embryo Transfer Program, University of Pennsylvania School of Medicine, Philadelphia

Cheryl A. Walker, RN, MN, CFNP, CANP, MBA, Assistant Professor, School of Nursing, University of Colorado Health Science Center, Denver

Ronald J. Wapner, MD, Director, Division of Maternal and Fetal Medicine, Thomas Jefferson University Hospital, Philadelphia

Martin Weisberg, MD, FACOG, Assistant Professor of Obstetrics-Gynecology, Psychiatry, and Human Behavior, Jefferson Medical College of Thomas Jefferson University, Philadelphia

Elaine Gilligan Whelan, RN, MSN, MA, Associate Professor of Nursing, Bergen Community College, Paramus, N.J.

Jay W. Wilborn, CLS, MEd, Program Director, MLT-AD, Corland County Community College, Hot Springs, Ark.

Beverly A. Zenk Wheat, RN, MA, Oncology Nurse Consultant, Stanford (Calif.) University Hospital

FOREWORD

High-tech tests, such as CAT scans and MRI scans, capture the headlines. But these are just some of the literally hundreds of tests performed every day to help doctors diagnose illnesses.

Some tests, such as those performed on blood samples, may seem commonplace and, except for the jab of a needle, uneventful to the person whose blood is being drawn. However, just as our blood replenishes all of our body's cells, this vital substance yields a bounty of clues to illnesses throughout the body. Testing the blood's enzymes, for instance, helps us diagnose heart attacks, diseases of the liver and pancreas, and certain inherited illnesses. Testing the blood's hormones helps us spot thyroid problems, infertility in men and women, and certain cancers. Testing the blood's sugars helps us detect diabetes and keep tabs on therapy for this potentially damaging disease.

Beyond blood tests, there are tests of urine, tests of tiny samples of tissue from the breast and internal organs, and tests of the fluids in the spine, around the lungs, and in the abdomen. There are also X-rays, vision and hearing tests, exercise tests, and scans of the heart, lungs, bones, and brain that use mildly radioactive substances to detect illness. In all, there are well over 400 tests. And this book tells you about each one in a clear, accurate, and readily understandable way.

Everything You Need to Know about Medical Tests helps you become informed and prepared for virtually any test that you or a loved one may undergo.

Prepared with the help of more than 70 doctors and medical authorities, this comprehensive reference offers information and advice that can't be found in any other reference for concerned consumers. To be understood appropriately, the tests in this book must be viewed as one part of the medical evaluation performed by your doctor, who will interpret the results in light of your medical history and physical exam. Of course, medical tests alone cannot provide the whole picture of an illness. But the more you know about them, the more you'll be able to participate in decisions about your health care.

For each test in the book, you'll find clear answers, usually in a page or two, to these essential questions:

- Why is this test done?
- What should you know before the test?
- What happens during the test?
- What happens after the test?
- Does the test have risks?
- What are the normal results?
- If the results are abnormal, what do they mean?

Besides this core information, you'll find many special features, each of them marked by a small picture. For instance, you'll find:

- *Self-Help:* what you can do to feel better or care for yourself
- *How Your Body Works:* easy-to-understand explanations and illustrations of how the eyes allow us to see, what the thyroid gland does, how sound travels through the ear to the brain, and many other fascinating body functions
- *Insight into Illness:* why an illness occurs and how it progresses — all clearly spelled out in words and illustrations

With all of these features, *Everything You Need to Know about Medical Tests* will prove informative and indispensable time and time again.

Dr. S. Breanndan Moore
Chairman, Division of Transfusion Medicine
Professor of Laboratory Medicine
Mayo Clinic and Mayo Medical School
Rochester, Minn.

1

X-RAYS:
Screening for Illness or Injury

NERVOUS SYSTEM

SKULL X-RAYS

Although of limited value in evaluating head injuries, skull X-rays are extremely valuable for studying abnormalities of the base of the skull and the cranial vault. They also allow doctors to study skull problems present at birth as well as to evaluate bone defects of the skull caused by other diseases.

Skull X-rays evaluate the three groups of bones that make up the skull: the calvaria (called the vault of the skull), the mandible (known as the jaw bone), and the facial bones. The vault and the facial bones are connected by immovable joints that have irregular serrated edges called sutures.

Taken together, the bones of the skull are so complex that a complete exam requires several X-rays of each area.

> *Taken together, the bones of the skull are so complex that a complete exam requires several X-rays of each area.*

Why is this test done?
Skull X-rays may be performed for the following reasons:
- To help detect fractures after a head injury
- To help diagnose tumors of the pituitary gland, a tiny oval-shaped organ attached to the brain
- To detect skull problems present at birth or caused by other diseases.

What should you know before the test?
- An X-ray technician will perform the test, usually in the radiology department. The test takes about 15 minutes and doesn't cause discomfort.
- You won't need to fast or avoid fluids before the test. But you'll need to take off your glasses or any jewelry that would be in the X-ray field. If you wear dentures, you'll have to remove them.

What happens during the test?
- You lie on an X-ray table or sit in a chair and are asked to stay perfectly still. Foam pads, sandbags, or a headband may be used to keep your head still and increase your comfort.

- The technician usually takes five different X-rays of your head. The X-ray films are developed and checked for quality before you leave the area.

What are the normal results?

A radiologist interprets the X-rays. This special doctor evaluates the size, shape, thickness, and position of bones in your head, the blood vessels, and other structures. All should be normal for your age.

What do abnormal results mean?

Skull X-rays can often show fractures of the vault or base of the skull. However, they won't be able to show fractures of the base if the bone is dense there.

Skull X-rays can also show skull problems that are present at birth. In addition, they can show areas of the brain where too much calcium is present. Certain brain tumors, such as oligodendrogliomas or meningiomas, contain calcium.

Skull X-rays may reveal changes in skull structure caused by other illnesses, such as Paget's disease.

ANGIOGRAM OF THE BRAIN'S BLOOD VESSELS

Called *cerebral angiography* by doctors, this test involves X-rays of the brain's blood vessels after injection of a special dye into an artery in the neck, inner thigh, or other area. This dye shows up on X-rays once it reaches the brain and circulates through its blood vessels.

Usually, this test is performed when the doctor suspects an abnormality in the brain's blood vessels. The abnormality may have been suggested first by the results of a computed tomography (CAT) scan of the brain or a spinal tap.

Why is this test done?

The angiogram may be performed for the following reasons:
- To detect problems in the blood vessels within or leading to the brain (for example, aneurysms, malformation of blood vessels, thrombosis, narrowing, or blockage)
- To study any blood vessel in the brain that is positioned unusually (because of a tumor, a blood clot, swelling, a spasm, increased pressure within the brain, or hydrocephalus)
- To locate clips applied to blood vessels during surgery and to check the condition of these blood vessels.

What should you know before the test?

- You'll learn about the test, including who will perform it, where it will take place, and how long it will last (usually 2 to 4 hours, depending on the tests ordered). You'll be positioned on an X-ray table, with your head immobilized, and you should remain still when asked.
- Tell the doctor or nurse if you have allergies to iodine, iodine-containing substances (such as shrimp or scallops), or injected dyes used in other tests. You'll be told about possible side effects from the dye injected for the test.
- You'll need to fast for 8 to 10 hours before the test.
- You'll put on a hospital gown and remove all jewelry, dentures, and hairpins. Be sure to urinate before leaving the room.
- You may receive a sedative and another drug 30 to 45 minutes before the test. You'll also receive a local anesthetic. (Some people — especially children — will receive a general anesthetic.)
- You'll need to sign a form that gives your consent to perform the test. Be sure to read this form carefully and ask questions if you don't understand any portion of it.

What happens during the test?

- You lie on an X-ray table while the site for the injection is shaved. You need to lie still with your arms at your sides.
- A local anesthetic is injected. Then the artery is entered with a needle.
- After X-rays verify the placement of the needle, the doctor injects the special dye. You may feel a brief burning sensation as the dye is injected. After the injection, you may feel warm and flushed, have a brief headache, or have a salty taste in your mouth. You may even feel nauseated and vomit.

- After the injection, X-rays are taken, developed, and reviewed. Depending on the results, more dye may be injected and another series of X-rays taken.
- When a satisfactory series of X-rays is obtained, the doctor removes the needle. A nurse checks for any bleeding and applies a bandage.

What happens after the test?

- Typically, you'll rest in bed for 12 to 24 hours and receive pain medications. A nurse will check you hourly for the first 4 hours and then every 4 hours.
- You'll have an ice bag over the injection area to ease discomfort and minimize swelling.
- If the injection was made in the inner thigh area, keep your leg straight for 12 hours or longer. If it was made in the neck area, the nurse will check your swallowing and breathing.
- After the test, you may resume your usual diet. Drink fluids to help pass the special dye.

Does the test have risks?

- This test shouldn't be done if a person has liver, kidney, or thyroid disease.
- It also shouldn't be done if a person is allergic to iodine or the test dye.

What are the normal results?

The test should show normal circulation through the brain's blood vessels.

What do abnormal results mean?

Changes inside the brain's blood vessels suggest a disorder, such as spasms, plaque, fistulas, arteriovenous malformation, or arteriosclerosis. Reduced blood flow to the brain's blood vessels may be related to increased pressure inside the brain.

If any blood vessels in the brain aren't in their usual position, this change may indicate a tumor, an area of swelling, or blocked flow of spinal fluid. If a tumor is present, the test can show blood vessels within a tumor, which can tell the doctor about the tumor's position and nature.

After the test, most people rest in bed for 12 to 24 hours and receive pain medications. An ice bag over the injection area helps ease discomfort and minimize swelling.

MYELOGRAPHY

This test evaluates an area of the spine called the *subarachnoid space.* It requires injection of a special dye. Because the dye weighs more than spinal fluid, it flows through the subarachnoid space to the dependent area when the person, lying face down on a special table, is tilted up or down. The test allows the doctor to see the flow of the dye and the outline of the subarachnoid space. X-rays are taken to provide a permanent record.

Why is this test done?
Myelography may be performed for the following reasons:
- To find tumors and herniated disks that partially or totally block the flow of spinal fluid
- To help detect arachnoiditis, spinal nerve root injury, or tumors.

What should you know before the test?
- You'll need to fast and avoid fluids for 8 hours before the test. If the test is scheduled for the afternoon and hospital policy permits, you may have clear fluids before the test.
- You'll be told about the test, including who will do it, where it will take place, and how long it will last (usually an hour or more). You'll need to stay overnight in the hospital.
- Tell the doctor or nurse if you have allergies to iodine, iodine-containing substances (such as shrimp or scallops), or injected dyes used in other tests. You'll be told about the possible side effects from the dye injected for the test. You may feel some pain caused by your positioning during the test and the insertion of the needle.
- Tell the doctor if you've ever had a seizure.
- Just before the test, remove any jewelry or other metal objects that would obscure the X-rays.
- You may receive some medication, such as an enema, a sedative to relax you, and a drug to reduce swallowing during the test.
- You'll need to sign a form that gives your consent to perform the test. Be sure to read this form carefully and ask questions if you don't understand any portion of it.

The test can locate problems within or surrounding the spinal cord, such as herniated disks and tumors.

What happens during the test?

- You lie on your side at the edge of a table, with your chin on your chest and your knees drawn up to your abdomen.
- The doctor inserts a needle into your lower back, in an area between two disks. Some spinal fluid may be removed for routine tests.
- A nurse turns you onto your stomach and secures you with straps across your upper back, under your arms, and across your ankles. You'll need to extend your chin to prevent the dye from flowing beyond the test area.
- The doctor injects the dye and tilts the table so that the dye flows through the spinal area. You may feel a brief burning sensation as the dye is injected. After the injection, you may feel warm and flushed, have a brief headache, or have a salty taste in your mouth. You may even feel nauseated and vomit.
- Tell the nurse or doctor if you get a headache or have trouble swallowing or breathing deeply enough. You'll be able to rest periodically during the test.
- The doctor observes the flow of the dye and takes X-rays. After satisfactory X-rays are obtained, the doctor removes the needle. The nurse then cleans the needle site with an antiseptic solution and applies a small bandage.

The doctor injects the dye and tilts the table so that the dye flows through the spinal area.

What happens after the test?

- Typically, you'll rest in a hospital bed for 6 to 24 hours and receive pain medications. A nurse will check you every half-hour for the first 4 hours and then every 4 hours.
- Drink extra fluids. The nurse will want you to urinate at least once within 8 hours of the test.
- Tell the nurse if you have any back pain, headache, or stiff neck. If there are no complications, you may go home and resume your usual diet and activities the day after the test.

Does the test have risks?

Generally, myelography shouldn't be performed if a person has increased pressure inside the brain, allergies to iodine or the special dye, or infection at the puncture site.

What are the normal results?

Normally, the dye flows freely through the spinal area, showing no blockages or structural abnormalities.

What do abnormal results mean?

The test can locate problems within or surrounding the spinal cord, such as herniated disks and tumors. If the test confirms a spinal tumor, the person may be taken directly to the operating room.

Myelography may help locate or confirm a ruptured disk, spinal narrowing, or an abscess and may occasionally confirm the need for surgery. This test may also detect syringomyelia (an abnormality marked by fluid-filled cavities within the spinal cord and widening of the cord itself), arachnoiditis, and spinal nerve root injury.

EYE

X-RAYS OF THE EYE'S ORBIT

The orbit is the cavity that houses the eye and the lacrimal glands as well as blood vessels, nerves, muscles, and fat. (See *Structures revealed by X-rays of the eye's orbit.*) Because portions of the orbit have thin bones that break easily, X-rays of this area are commonly taken after a facial injury. They're also useful in diagnosing eye and orbit diseases.

Special X-ray techniques can reveal foreign bodies in the orbit or eye that are otherwise invisible. In some cases, X-rays are used with computed tomography (CAT) scans and an ultrasound test to better define an abnormality.

Why is this test done?

X-rays of the eye's orbit may be performed for the following reasons:
- To help detect fractures and diseases of the orbit
- To help locate foreign objects in the eye.

What should you know before the test?

- You'll learn about the test, including who will perform it, where it will be performed, and the expected duration (about 15 minutes). The test is painless unless you've suffered a facial injury, in which case positioning may cause some discomfort. You'll be asked to turn your head from side to side and to flex or extend your neck.

Structures revealed by X-rays of the eye's orbit

X-rays of the eye's orbit reveal many small structures in the surrounding area. This illustration shows some of the common reference points.

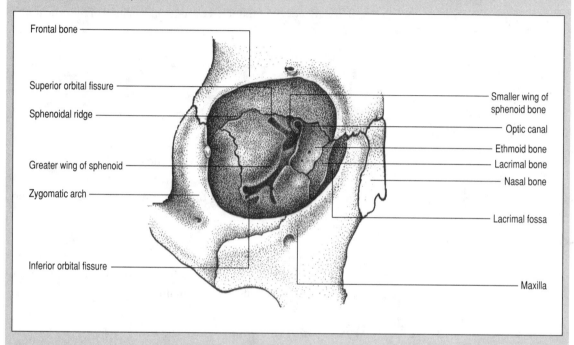

Frontal bone

Superior orbital fissure

Sphenoidal ridge

Greater wing of sphenoid

Zygomatic arch

Inferior orbital fissure

Smaller wing of sphenoid bone

Optic canal

Ethmoid bone

Lacrimal bone

Nasal bone

Lacrimal fossa

Maxilla

What happens during the test?

- You lie on the X-ray table or sit in a chair. While the X-rays are taken, you have to remain still.
- Usually, a series of X-rays is taken from different angles. These X-rays must be developed and inspected before you can leave.

What are the normal results?

The eye's orbit has a roof, a floor, and walls. The bones of the roof and floor are very thin. The floor bones, in fact, can be less than 1 millimeter thick. The walls are thicker. The X-rays should show no broken bones in the orbit or other problems.

What do abnormal results mean?

Broken bones from a facial injury are most common in the thin structures of the floor and ethmoid bone. Generally, enlargement of the orbit indicates a problem, such as a growing tumor. Destruction of the orbit's walls may indicate a malignant tumor or an infection. A benign tumor or cyst produces a clear-cut indentation of the orbital wall.

ANGIOGRAM OF THE EYE

In this test, called *fluorescein angiography* by doctors, a special camera takes rapid-sequence photographs of the eye. The photographs are taken after the injection of a special dye called *sodium fluorescein* into a vein in the arm. The dye lets the doctor see the appearance of blood vessels within the eye.

Why is this test done?

An angiogram of the eye may be performed to help find retinal problems, tumors, and circulatory or inflammatory disorders.

What should you know before the test?

■ You'll be told about the test, including who will do it, where it will take place, and that it usually about lasts about 30 minutes.
■ Tell the doctor or nurse if you have glaucoma or have ever had a bad reaction to dilating eyedrops. During the test, eyedrops will be instilled to dilate your pupils and a dye will be injected into your arm. Your eyes will be photographed with a special camera before and after the injection.
■ You'll need to sign a form that gives your consent to perform the test. Be sure to read this form carefully and ask questions if you don't understand any portion of it.

What happens during the test?

■ The nurse gives you eyedrops. Then you sit in the examining chair, facing the camera. You should loosen or remove any restrictive clothing around your neck.
■ You place your chin in the chin rest and your forehead against the bar. Then you open your eyes wide and stare straight ahead, while

keeping your teeth together and maintaining normal breathing and blinking.

- The nurse cleans your inner forearm with an antiseptic solution; then the dye is injected rapidly. You should maintain your position and continue to stare straight ahead.
- You may experience nausea and a feeling of warmth. Tell the doctor or nurse how you feel, especially if the eyedrops or the dye makes you feel like vomiting, if you have a dry mouth or metallic taste, if you feel light-headed or faint, or if you start to itch.
- As the dye is injected, 25 to 30 photographs are taken in rapid sequence. Each photograph is taken 1 second after the other.
- The needle and syringe are removed carefully. Pressure and a dressing are applied to the injection site.
- If late-phase photographs are needed, you'll sit and relax for 20 minutes. Then another 5 to 10 photographs may be taken.

What happens after the test?

- Your skin and urine will be slightly discolored for a day or two afterward.
- Your near vision will be blurred for up to 12 hours. During this period, you should avoid direct sunlight. You also shouldn't drive.

Does the test have risks?

- The dye used in the test can cause nausea, vomiting, sneezing, numbness of the tongue, and dizziness. These sensations will go away shortly.
- The dye rarely causes severe problems, such as breathing difficulty. The doctor will give an injection if this complication occurs.

What are the normal results?

After rapid injection, the dye reaches the retina in 15 seconds and fills its blood vessels. After filling the vessels, the dye recirculates through them about 30 to 60 minutes after the injection. Normally, there is no leakage of the dye from the retina's blood vessels.

What do abnormal results mean?

The test can detect tiny aneurysms, arteriovenous shunts, and formation of new blood vessels. It can also find eye diseases caused by high blood pressure. The test can reveal tumors and swelling or inflammation of the retina.

After the test, your near vision will be blurred for up to 12 hours. You should avoid direct sunlight and let someone else drive.

LUNGS & SINUSES

CHEST X-RAY

In this test, X-rays penetrate the chest and produce a black-and-white image on specially treated film. Normal areas of the lung let X-rays pass through them with little or no change. These normal areas look dark on X-ray film. In contrast, abnormal areas of the lung, such as foreign bodies, fluids, and tumors, change the X-rays. These abnormal areas look dense on X-ray film.

A chest X-ray is most useful when it's compared with previous X-rays. This comparison allows the doctor to detect changes.

Why is this test done?

A chest X-ray may be performed for the following reasons:
- To detect lung diseases, such as pneumonia, a collapsed lung, and lung cancer
- To detect problems in the chest area, such as cancer and heart disease
- To determine the location and size of a tumor
- To help evaluate lung condition and breathing.

What should you know before the test?

- You won't need to fast or limit fluids beforehand.
- You'll be given a gown without snaps to put on. And you'll need to remove any jewelry, such as a necklace, that may be in the X-ray field.
- You'll receive directions on how to breathe during the test.

What happens during the test?

- If a stationary X-ray machine is used, you stand or sit in front of it.
- If you're in a bed, a portable X-ray machine is used. The head of your bed will be raised.
- The nurse or technician tells you to take a deep breath and to hold it momentarily while each X-ray is being taken. Doing this provides the clearest view of your lungs.

Chest X-rays aren't usually done during the first 3 months of pregnancy because of the risk of birth defects.

Does the test have risks?

Chest X-rays aren't usually done during the first 3 months of pregnancy because of the risk of birth defects. However, when they're absolutely necessary, a lead apron will be placed over the mother's abdomen to shield the fetus from the X-rays.

What are the normal results?

To make an accurate diagnosis, the doctor reviews the results of the X-rays as part of a battery of tests. The doctor, for instance, might also look at the results of breathing tests and the physical exam.

What do abnormal results mean?

Chest X-rays can reveal dozens of different disorders. (See *Disorders revealed by chest X-ray.*)

SINUS X-RAY

The sinuses — air-filled cavities lined with mucous membranes — lie within the maxillary, ethmoid, sphenoid, and frontal bones of the face. In this test, X-rays pass through the sinuses and react on specially sensitized film, forming an image that allows a doctor to study the sinuses.

Why is this test done?

A sinus X-ray may be performed for the following reasons:
- To detect injury or illness in the sinus area
- To confirm cancer or inflammation in the sinus area
- To determine the location and size of a malignant tumor.

What should you know before the test?

- You'll find out about the test, including who will perform it, where it will take place, and its expected duration (usually 10 to 15 minutes). You'll be asked to sit upright and to avoid moving while the X-rays are being taken to prevent blurring of the image.
- Your head may be immobilized in a foam vise during the test to help maintain the correct position. The vise doesn't hurt.

Disorders revealed by chest X-ray

Chest X-rays can help detect disorders of the heart, lungs, ribs, and other structures. Some of the chief disorders they can help doctors find are:
- atherosclerosis
- bronchitis
- collapsed lung
- congestive heart failure
- cystic fibrosis
- emphysema
- fractures of the ribs or spine
- lung cancer
- pneumonia
- tuberculosis.

- You'll remove any dentures, all jewelry, and metal objects that could obscure the X-rays.

What happens during the test?

- You sit upright (with your head in a foam vise) between the X-ray tube and a film cassette.
- The X-ray tube is positioned at different angles and your head is placed in various standard positions while the sinuses are filmed.

Does the test have risks?

Sinus X-rays aren't usually done during pregnancy because of the risk of birth defects. However, when they're absolutely necessary, a lead-lined apron placed over the mother's stomach can shield the fetus.

What are the normal results?

Normal sinuses allow X-rays to pass through them. The sinuses are filled with air, which appears black on X-ray film.

What do abnormal results mean?

Sinus X-rays can detect sinus injury or fracture, sinus infections, and benign and malignant tumors.

CHEST FLUOROSCOPY

In this test, a continuous stream of X-rays passes through the chest and casts shadows of the heart, lungs, and diaphragm on a fluorescent screen. Because fluoroscopy reveals less detail than chest X-rays, it's used only when the doctor needs to look within the chest to detect or rule out a problem.

Why is this test done?

Fluoroscopy may be performed for the following reasons:

- To assess lung expansion and contraction during quiet breathing, deep breathing, and coughing
- To evaluate movement and paralysis of the diaphragm
- To detect blockages in the bronchi (the airways leading to the lungs) and lung disease.

What should you know before the test?

- You'll learn about the test, including who will perform it, where it will take place, and its expected duration (usually 5 minutes).
- During the test, you'll be asked to follow specific instructions — for example, to breathe deeply and to cough — while X-ray images are taken.
- You'll remove all jewelry within the X-ray field.

What happens during the test?

During the test, the motion of your lungs and heart is observed on a screen. Special equipment may be used to intensify the images, or a videotape recording may be made for later study.

Does the test have risks?

Fluoroscopy should not be performed during pregnancy because of the risk of birth defects.

What are the normal results?

The normal diaphragmatic movement is synchronous and symmetrical.

What do abnormal results mean?

Diminished diaphragmatic movement may indicate lung disease. Diminished or paradoxical diaphragmatic movement may indicate paralysis of the diaphragm.

During fluoroscopy, the motion of your lungs and heart is observed on a screen. A videotape recording may be made for later study.

CHEST TOMOGRAPHY

This test provides clear X-rays of chest areas that are otherwise in the shadows of overlying or underlying structures. In this test, an X-ray tube and film swing around the person in opposite directions, creating a sharply defined X-ray picture of a specific area the doctor wishes to study. Because tomography exposes a person to high levels of radiation, it's used only to evaluate significant chest problems.

Why is this test done?

Chest tomography may be performed for the following reasons:
- To identify calcified or fatty deposits in dense lung tissue
- To locate tumors, especially those blocking a bronchus, one of the main breathing passages
- To find lesions, especially those located deep within the chest.

What should you know before the test?

- You won't need to fast or limit fluids beforehand. The test itself takes 30 to 60 minutes.
- You'll probably be warned that the test equipment is noisy because of rapidly moving metal-on-metal parts and that the X-ray tube swings overhead.
- You'll receive directions on breathing and movement during the test. You may be advised to close your eyes to prevent unintended movement.
- Just before the test, you'll need to remove all jewelry, such as a necklace, that's within the X-ray field.

What happens during the test?

- You lie on an X-ray table on your back and your side. The X-ray tube swings over you, taking many pictures from different angles.
- You need to breathe normally during the test but remain perfectly still. Foam wedges help you remain motionless.

Does the test have risks?

Because the test exposes a person to high levels of radiation, it's never performed during pregnancy.

What are the normal results?

A normal tomogram resembles a normal chest X-ray and shows no abnormalities.

What do abnormal results mean?

A radiologist interprets the X-ray films. A finding of calcium accumulation in the center of a lung nodule suggests a benign tumor. However, a nodule with an irregular border suggests a malignant tumor. A sharply defined nodule suggests a persistent inflammation called a *granuloma*.

Because tomography exposes a person to high levels of radiation, it's used only to evaluate significant chest problems.

The test can identify widening or narrowing of a bronchus and the extension of a tumor to the ribs or spine.

BRONCHOGRAPHY

This type of X-ray examines the breathing passages after a special dye is passed through a tube (called a *catheter*) into the trachea and bronchi. The dye coats the bronchial tree, permitting the doctor to see any anatomic deviations. Since the development of the computed tomography (CAT) scan, bronchography is used less frequently.

Why is this test done?
Bronchography may be performed for the following reasons:
- To help detect bronchiectasis, bronchial blockages, lung cancer, cysts, and cavities
- To help pinpoint the cause of a bloody cough.

What should you know before the test?
- You'll find out about the test, including who will perform it, where it will take place, and its expected duration.
- You'll need to fast for 12 hours before the test.
- Tell the doctor or nurse if you have allergies to anesthetics, iodine, or the dyes used in any tests.
- If you have a cough, you may be given an expectorant before the test.
- If the test will be performed under local anesthesia, you'll receive a sedative to help you relax and to suppress the gag reflex. The anesthetic itself will have an unpleasant taste. During the test, you may experience some difficulty breathing. Be assured that your breathing passages won't be blocked and that you'll get enough oxygen. The catheter will pass more easily if you relax.
- If the test will be performed under general anesthesia, you'll receive a sedative before the test to help you relax.
- If you wear dentures, you'll need to remove them just before the test.
- You'll need to sign a form that gives your consent to perform the test. Be sure to read this form carefully and ask questions if you don't understand any portion of it.

If the test is to be performed under local anesthesia, you'll receive a sedative to help you relax and to suppress the gag reflex. The catheter will pass more easily if you relax.

What happens during the test?

- After a local anesthetic is sprayed into your mouth and throat, a bronchoscope or catheter is passed into the trachea, and the anesthetic and dye are given through it.
- You are placed in various positions during the test to move the dye into different areas of the bronchial tree.
- If you received a local anesthetic for the test, tell the doctor or nurse if you have trouble breathing, start to itch, or feel your heart pounding or fluttering. These are signs of an allergic reaction to the anesthetic or dye, which must be treated with medication.

What happens after the test?

- You won't be able to eat or drink until your gag reflex returns. It usually comes back in about 2 hours.
- You'll be asked to cough gently to help clear any remaining dye from your breathing passages. Another X-ray of your cleared breathing passages is usually done in 24 to 48 hours.
- If you have a sore throat, tell the nurse. You can have throat lozenges or a liquid gargle once your gag reflex returns.
- Don't resume your usual activities until the next day.

Does the test have risks?

- Bronchography shouldn't be done if you are pregnant, if you have allergies to iodine or the test dye, or if you have difficulty breathing.
- A person with asthma may have a spasm in the airway when the dye is given.
- A person with chronic bronchitis or emphysema may have a breathing passage blocked by the dye.
- Pneumonia can occur if the dye isn't cleared by coughing from your breathing passages.

What are the normal results?

The right bronchus is shorter, wider, and more vertical than the left bronchus. Successive branches of the bronchi become smaller in diameter and are free of any blockages or problems.

What do abnormal results mean?

Bronchography may show bronchiectasis or bronchial blockages due to tumors, cysts, cavities, or foreign objects. Findings must be correlated with the person's physical exam, medical history, and perhaps other tests.

ANGIOGRAM OF THE LUNGS

Also called *pulmonary arteriography* or *angiography* by doctors, this test evaluates the lungs' blood vessels to help identify the cause of a person's symptoms. In this test, X-rays are taken after the injection of a special dye into the pulmonary artery or one of its branches.

Why is this test done?

An angiogram of the lungs may be performed for the following reasons:
- To detect pulmonary embolism in a person who has symptoms but whose lung scan is inconclusive or normal
- To evaluate lung circulation before surgery in a person who was born with heart disease.

What should you know before the test?

- You'll learn who will perform the test and where and that it will take approximately 1 hour.
- You'll be told about the possible side effects from the dye injected for the test. Your heart rate will be monitored continuously during the procedure.
- Tell the doctor or nurse if you have allergies to anesthetics, iodine, shellfish (such as shrimp or scallops), or the dyes used in any tests.
- You'll need to fast for 8 hours.
- You'll receive a form that asks your consent to perform the test. Be sure to read this form carefully before signing it. Ask questions if you don't understand any portion of it.

The doctor injects a special dye that circulates through the blood vessels of your lungs as X-rays are taken.

What happens during the test?

- You lie on your back, the local anesthetic is injected, and a heart monitor is attached to you.
- The doctor makes a small incision in a vein in your forearm or groin area. Then the doctor inserts a small tube called a *catheter* into the vein and slowly moves it through the vein all the way to an artery in your lung.
- Next, the doctor injects the special dye, which circulates through your lungs' blood vessels while X-rays are taken. You may experience an urge to cough, a flushed feeling, nausea, or a salty taste for 5 minutes after the injection.
- After the X-rays are taken, the doctor slowly pulls the catheter back and removes it. The nurse applies a dressing over the catheter insertion site.

What happens after the test?

- You'll rest in bed for about 6 hours. A nurse will check your condition regularly during this time.
- The nurse will tell you about any restriction of activity. You may resume your usual diet after the test. Be sure to drink plenty of fluids.

Does the test have risks?

- The test can cause complications, such as a blockage of an artery, a tear in the heart, an irregular heartbeat from irritation of the heart, and kidney failure from a severe allergy to the test dye.
- The test shouldn't be done during pregnancy and in people who are allergic to iodine, shellfish, or the dyes used in medical tests.

What are the normal results?

Normally, the dye flows symmetrically and without interruption through the blood vessels of the lungs.

What do abnormal results mean?

Interruption of blood flow may be caused by an embolism (a clot that obstructs circulation), vascular filling defects, or stenosis.

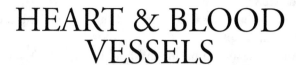

HEART & BLOOD VESSELS

CARDIAC X-RAYS

These X-rays are among the most frequently used tests for evaluating heart disease and its effects on the blood vessels of the lungs. (See *The cardiac series,* page 24.) They show images of the thorax, mediastinum, heart, and lungs. In a routine evaluation, two different views are taken.

Why is this test done?
Cardiac X-rays may be performed for the following reasons:
- To help detect heart disease and abnormalities that change the size, shape, or appearance of the heart and lungs
- To check for the correct position of pulmonary artery and cardiac catheters and of pacemaker wires.

What should you know before the test?
- You'll learn about the test, including who will perform it and where. The test exposes you to little radiation and is harmless.
- You'll remove jewelry, other metal objects, and clothing above your waist and put on a hospital gown.

What happens during the test?
The procedure depends on how the X-rays are taken.

Front and back views
- You stand up about 6 feet (2 meters) from the X-ray machine with your back to the machine and your chin resting on top of the film cassette holder.
- The holder is adjusted to slightly extend your neck. You then place your hands on your hips, with your shoulders touching the holder, and center your chest against it.
- You take a deep breath and hold it while the X-ray film is exposed.

The cardiac series

The cardiac series uses X-rays to provide a constant image of the heart in motion on a fluoroscope screen. This allows the doctor to view the heart's chambers in motion from four directions, allowing a full study of the heart's action.

High radiation exposure

The cardiac series exposes a person to 15 to 20 times more radiation than conventional cardiac X-rays. It usually isn't performed on pregnant women and may be restricted in other people as well. In many cases, an echocardiogram is done instead. This test uses ultra-high-frequency sound waves to create an image of heart structures.

Left side view

- You extend your arms over your head and put your left side flush against the cassette.
- You then take a deep breath and hold it while the X-ray film is exposed.

Does the test have risks?

Cardiac X-rays usually aren't done during the first 3 months of pregnancy. However, when they're absolutely necessary, a lead shield or apron should cover the mother's stomach and pelvic area during the X-ray exposure.

What are the normal results?

The heart and lungs should have a normal size, shape, and condition on the X-rays.

What do abnormal results mean?

Cardiac X-rays must be evaluated in light of a person's medical history, physical exam, and the results of previous X-rays and electrocardiograms. An abnormal silhouette of the heart usually indicates enlargement of the left or right ventricle or the left atrium. The test can also show the first signs of congestion in the lungs' blood vessels.

X-RAYS OF THE LEG VEINS

Called *venography* or *ascending contrast phlebography* by doctors, this test checks the condition of the deep leg veins. It's the definitive test for detecting a condition called *deep vein thrombosis*.

Venography is expensive. A combination of three noninvasive tests — Doppler ultrasound, impedance plethysmography, and a nuclear scan with a radioisotope — provides an acceptable, but less accurate, alternative to X-rays of the leg veins.

Why is this test done?

X-rays of the leg veins may be performed for the following reasons:
- To confirm a diagnosis of deep venous thrombosis
- To distinguish blood clots from vein obstructions (such as a large tumor of the pelvis pressing on the leg veins)
- To evaluate vein problems present at birth
- To check how the valves within the deep leg veins work (especially helpful in identifying the cause of leg swelling)
- To locate a suitable vein for arterial bypass grafting.

What should you know before the test?

- You'll learn about the test, including who will perform it, where it will take place, and that it will last 30 to 45 minutes. You may feel a burning sensation in your leg during injection of the dye and some discomfort during the test. Complications from the dye are rare, but be sure to tell the doctor or nurse if you feel nauseated, have trouble breathing, or other problems.
- Tell the doctor or nurse if you have allergies to anesthetics, iodine, shellfish (such as shrimp or scallops), or the dyes used in any tests.
- You'll need to fast and to drink only clear liquids for 4 hours before the test.
- Just before the test, you should urinate, remove all clothing below the waist, and put on a hospital gown.
- You may receive a sedative if you're tense just before the test.
- You'll receive a form that asks your consent to perform the test. Be sure to read this form carefully before signing it. Ask questions if you don't understand any portion of it.

After the X-rays of your leg veins, you receive an injection of fluids to clear the dye from your veins.

What happens during the test?

- You lie on a tilting X-ray table so that the leg being tested doesn't bear any weight. You are told to relax this leg and keep it still. A tourniquet may be tied around your ankle.
- The doctor slowly injects the dye into a surface vein in your foot. Be sure to tell the doctor or nurse if you have nausea, severe burning or itching, tightness in the throat or chest, or trouble breathing.
- Using a fluoroscope, the doctor watches the movement of the dye through your leg veins and takes X-rays.
- After the X-rays, you receive an injection of fluids to clear the dye from your veins. Then the needle is removed and a bandage applied.

What happens after the test?

- The nurse will check your condition regularly. You'll receive pain medication to counteract the irritating effects of the dye.
- If the test indicates deep vein thrombosis, you'll receive medication and have to rest in bed with your leg supported or elevated.
- You'll be able to resume your usual diet.

Does the test have risks?

- The test isn't used routinely, because it exposes a person to relatively high doses of radiation and can cause complications, such as phlebitis, local tissue damage and, occasionally, deep vein thrombosis itself.
- Rarely, the dye used in the test causes a severe allergic reaction. Such reactions usually occur within a half-hour of the injection and require medication.

What are the normal results?

A normal test shows no problems in the leg veins.

What do abnormal results mean?

A test that shows consistent filling defects, an abrupt termination of a column of the test dye, unfilled major deep veins, or diversion of flow confirms a diagnosis of deep vein thrombosis.

DIGESTIVE SYSTEM

BARIUM SWALLOW

A barium swallow allows a doctor to examine the upper part of the digestive tract. When undergoing this test, a person drinks thick and thin mixtures of barium sulfate, a chalky drink with the consistency (but not the flavor) of a milk shake. The barium can be seen on an X-ray as it passes through the digestive tract.

This test is most commonly done as part of the upper GI series. It's usually performed when a person has a history of swallowing difficulty or vomiting.

Why is this test done?

A barium swallow may be performed for the following reasons:

- To diagnose hiatal hernia, a condition in which the stomach slides upward into the esophagus or along side it
- To diagnose pouches or sacs called *diverticula,* which may form in the upper digestive tract
- To diagnose esophageal varices, which are abnormal enlarged veins
- To detect narrowing of the upper digestive tract
- To identify ulcers, tumors, and polyps.

What should you know before the test?

- You'll need to fast after midnight the night before the test. (If an infant is being tested, feeding must be delayed to ensure full digestion of barium.)
- You'll learn about the test, including who will perform it, where it will take place, and its expected duration (about 30 minutes).
- You'll be asked to drink a barium preparation during the test. First, you'll receive a thick mixture, then a thin one. Altogether, you'll drink 12 to 14 ounces (about 350 to 400 milliliters) during the test.
- You'll be placed in various positions on a tilting X-ray table and X-ray films will be taken.
- Just before the test, you'll put on a hospital gown and remove any jewelry, dentures, hair clips, or other objects from the X-ray field.
- You'll receive a form that asks your consent to perform the test. Be sure to read this form carefully before signing it. Ask questions if you don't understand any portion of it.

A barium swallow may reveal problems in the pharynx, esophagus, or stomach.

What happens during the test?

- After you're secured on your back on the X-ray table, the table is tilted until you're upright. Then your heart, lungs, and abdomen are examined.
- Next, you take one swallow of the thick barium mixture, and X-rays are taken as the mixture moves through the pharynx, the uppermost part of your digestive tract.
- Then you're asked to take several swallows of the thin barium mixture. This part of the test examines your esophagus, which lies just downstream from your pharynx. During this portion of the test, you may be asked to swallow a "barium marshmallow" (a piece of soft white bread that has been soaked in barium).

■ As the test continues, you're secured to the X-ray table, which is tilted so that the movement of any barium through your esophagus can be seen.

■ Next, you take several more swallows of barium while your esophagus is examined and X-rayed. After the table is moved to a horizontal position, you take yet a few more swallows of barium and are X-rayed.

What happens after the test?

■ You'll be able to resume your normal diet. However, because you drank barium, your stools will be chalky and light-colored for 1 to 3 days.

■ If you don't have a bowel movement in 2 or 3 days, let your doctor know.

Does the test have risks?

A barium swallow shouldn't be done on any person who has a blocked intestine.

What are the normal results?

After the barium is swallowed, it pours over the base of the tongue into the pharynx. It's propelled by the normal digestive wave (which is called *peristalsis*) through the entire length of the esophagus in about 2 seconds. When it reaches the base of the esophagus, a sphincter opens and allows the barium to enter the stomach. After the barium passes, the sphincter closes. Normally, the barium evenly fills the pharynx and esophagus, and their linings look smooth and regular.

What do abnormal results mean?

A barium swallow may reveal problems in the pharynx, esophagus, or stomach. These problems include hiatal hernia, diverticula, and varices.

The test may detect narrowing, tumors, polyps, ulcers, and motility disorders, such as pharyngeal muscle disorders, spasms in the esophagus, and achalasia. However, a definite diagnosis commonly requires a biopsy or other tests.

UPPER G.I. AND SMALL-BOWEL SERIES

This test examines the upper and middle portions of the digestive tract (the esophagus, stomach, and small intestine). It requires ingestion of barium sulfate, a chalky drink with the consistency (but not the flavor) of a milk shake. Barium can be seen on X-rays as it passes through the digestive tract.

This test is performed when a person has:
- upper GI symptoms, such as difficulty in swallowing, vomiting, or burning or gnawing pain in the center of the stomach
- signs of small-bowel disease, such as diarrhea and unexplained weight loss
- signs of bleeding in the digestive tract, such as blood in vomit or dark, tarry stools.

Why is this test done?

The upper GI and small-bowel series may be performed for the following reasons:
- To diagnose hiatal hernia, a condition in which the stomach slides upward into the esophagus or alongside it
- To diagnose diverticula, which resemble pouches, in the upper digestive tract
- To diagnose esophageal varices, which are abnormal enlarged veins
- To help detect narrowing of the upper digestive tract
- To help diagnose ulcers, tumors, regional enteritis, and malabsorption syndrome
- To help detect motility disorders.

What should you know before the test?

- You'll need to follow a low-fiber diet for 2 or 3 days before the test. After midnight on the night before the test, you'll need to fast. If you smoke, you must stop after midnight.
- You'll learn about the test, including who will perform it, where it will take place, and its expected duration (up to 6 hours). Be sure to bring a good book along to pass the time.
- You'll be told about the barium preparation that you must drink during the test. First, you'll receive a thick mixture, then a thin one. Altogether, you'll drink 16 to 20 ounces (about 500 to 700 milliliters) during the test.

- You'll be placed in different positions on a tilting X-ray table and X-ray films will be taken. During the test, your abdomen may be compressed to ensure proper coating of the stomach or intestinal walls with barium or to separate overlapping loops of your small intestine.
- Just before the test, you'll put on a hospital gown and remove any jewelry, dentures, hair clips, or other objects from the X-ray field.
- You'll receive a form that asks your consent to perform the test. Be sure to read this form carefully before signing it. Ask questions if you don't understand any portion of it.

What happens during the test?

- After you're secured on your back on the X-ray table, the table is tilted until you're upright. Then your heart, lungs, and abdomen are examined.
- You're asked to take several swallows of barium, and its passage through your esophagus is observed. Then X-rays are taken from many angles.
- When barium enters your stomach, the doctor or an assistant may press your stomach inward to make sure that the barium coats it thoroughly.
- You may be asked to sip barium through a perforated straw. As you do, a small amount of air also enters your stomach. This allows detailed examination and X-rays of the folds of your stomach. Next, you drink the remaining barium as the doctor observes the filling of the stomach and emptying into the duodenum, the first part of the small intestine.
- Two series of X-rays of the stomach and duodenum are taken from different angles.
- The passage of barium into the remainder of the small intestine is then observed, and X-rays are taken at 30- to 60-minute intervals.

During the test, you're asked to take several swallows of barium, and its passage through your esophagus is observed. X-rays are taken from many angles.

What happens after the test?

- You'll receive a cathartic or enema.
- Your stools will be lightly-colored for 1 to 3 days. However, if you don't have a bowel movement in 2 or 3 days, let your doctor know.

Does the test have risks?

The upper GI and small-bowel series shouldn't be done if a person has a blockage or tear of the digestive tract. Barium may worsen the blockage or seep into the abdominal cavity.

What are the normal results?

After the barium is swallowed, it pours over the base of the tongue into the pharynx. It's propelled by contractions of the digestive tract (which is called *peristalsis*) through the entire length of the esophagus in about 2 seconds. When it reaches the base of the esophagus, a sphincter opens and allows the barium to enter the stomach. After the barium passes, the sphincter closes. Normally, the barium evenly fills the pharynx and esophagus, and their linings look smooth and regular.

As barium enters the stomach, it outlines the characteristic folds called *rugae.* When the stomach is completely filled with barium, its outer contour appears smooth and regular without evidence of flattened, rigid areas.

After barium enters the stomach, it quickly empties into the duodenum and reveals circular folds. These folds deepen and become more numerous in the next portion of the small intestine, the jejunum. The barium temporarily lodges between these folds, producing a speckled pattern on X-rays. As barium enters the ileum, the circular folds become less prominent and, except for their broadness, resemble those in the duodenum. The X-rays also show that the diameter of the small intestine tapers gradually from the duodenum to the ileum.

Normally, when the stomach is completely filled with barium, its outer contour appears smooth and regular without evidence of flattened, rigid areas.

What do abnormal results mean?

X-rays of the esophagus may reveal strictures, tumors, hiatal hernia, diverticula, varices, and ulcers. Benign strictures usually dilate the esophagus, whereas malignant ones cause erosive changes. Tumors produce filling defects in the column of barium, but only malignant ones change the mucosal contour. Nevertheless, biopsy is necessary for a definite diagnosis of both esophageal strictures and tumors.

Motility disorders, such as esophageal spasm, are usually difficult to detect because spasms are erratic and transient. Another test, called *manometry,* is generally performed to detect these disorders.

X-rays of the stomach may reveal tumors and ulcers. Malignant tumors appear as filling defects on the X-ray film and usually disrupt peristalsis. Benign tumors appear as outpouchings of the gastric mucosa and generally don't affect peristalsis. Ulcers occur most commonly in the stomach and duodenum, and these two areas are thus examined together. Benign ulcers usually show evidence of partial or complete healing and are characterized by radiating folds extending to the edge of the ulcer crater. Malignant ulcers, usually associated with a suspicious mass, generally have radiating folds that extend beyond the ulcer crater to the edge of the mass. However, biopsy is necessary for a definite diagnosis of both tumors and ulcers.

X-rays of the small intestine may reveal regional enteritis, malabsorption syndrome, and tumors.

BARIUM ENEMA

Also called a *lower GI exam,* this test involves X-ray examination of the large intestine. It's done for people with a history of altered bowel habits, lower abdominal pain, or the passage of blood, mucus, or pus in the stools.

In the single-contrast technique, barium sulfate is inserted into the rectum. In the double-contrast technique, barium sulfate and air are inserted into the rectum. The single-contrast technique shows a profile view of the large intestine. The double-contrast technique shows profile and frontal views. The latter technique best detects small tumors (especially polyps), early inflammatory disease, and the subtle bleeding caused by ulcers.

Why is this test done?
A barium enema may be performed for the following reasons:
- To help diagnose colon cancer, rectal cancer, and inflammatory disease
- To detect polyps, diverticula, and structural changes in the large intestine.

What should you know before the test?
- You'll learn about the test, including who will perform it, where it will take place, and its expected duration (30 to 45 minutes).
- You'll learn that the accuracy of the test depends on your cooperation with the prescribed diet and bowel preparation. A common bowel preparation technique includes restricted intake of dairy products and maintenance of a liquid diet for 24 hours before the test. You'll be encouraged to drink five 8-ounce (250-milliliter) glasses of water or clear liquids 12 to 24 hours before the test.
- You'll receive an enema or repeat enemas until no stools remain in your large intestine to obscure the X-rays.

- You'll be placed on a tilting X-ray table and adequately draped. During the test, you'll be secured to the table and assisted to various positions.
- You'll learn that you may experience cramping pains or the urge to defecate as the barium or air is introduced into the intestine. If so, breathe deeply and slowly through your mouth to ease this discomfort.
- During the test, you must keep your anus tightly contracted against the rectal tube to hold the tube in position and help prevent leakage of barium. If the barium leaks out, the intestinal walls won't be adequately coated and the test results may be inaccurate.
- You'll receive a form that asks your consent to perform the test. Be sure to read this form carefully before signing it. Ask questions if you don't understand any portion of it.

What happens during the test?

- You lie on your back on a tilting radiographic table as X-rays of your abdomen are taken.
- You are helped to a different position, and a well-lubricated rectal tube is inserted through the anus.
- The doctor or assistant slowly delivers the barium enema through the tube, and the filling process is monitored. To aid filling, the table may be tilted or you may be assisted to a different position.
- As the flow of barium is observed, X-rays are taken of significant findings. When the barium fills the intestine, overhead X-rays of the abdomen are taken. Then the rectal tube is removed. You're escorted to the toilet or provided with a bedpan and asked to expel as much barium as possible.
- Afterward, an additional X-ray is taken.
- A double-contrast barium enema may directly follow this examination or may be performed separately. If it's performed immediately, a thin film of barium remains in your intestine, coating the mucosa, and air is carefully injected to distend the bowel lumen.

What happens after the test?

- You'll need to drink extra fluids because bowel preparation and the test itself can cause dehydration.
- You should rest. This test and the bowel preparation exhaust most people.
- You'll receive a cleansing enema to remove any remaining barium. Your stools will be lightly colored for 24 to 72 hours.

The accuracy of a barium enema test depends on your cooperation in following the prescribed diet and bowel preparation.

Does the test have risks?

■ A barium enema shouldn't be done if a person has a rapid heart rate, severe ulcerative colitis, toxic megacolon, or a suspected perforation in the intestine.

■ This test should be performed cautiously if a person has a blocked intestine, ulcerative colitis, diverticulitis, or severe bloody diarrhea.

■ The test can cause complications, such as a perforation of the colon, water intoxication, and barium granulomas.

What are the normal results?

In the single-contrast enema, the intestine uniformly fills with barium, and the colon's markings are apparent. The intestinal walls collapse as the barium is expelled, and the intestinal lining has a regular, feathery appearance on the X-ray.

In the double-contrast enema, the intestine uniformly expands with air and has a thin layer of barium providing excellent detail of the mucosal pattern. As the person is assisted to various positions, the barium collects on the dependent walls of the intestine by the force of gravity.

What do abnormal results mean?

Most colon cancers occur in the rectosigmoid region and are best detected by a different test called *proctosigmoidoscopy.* However, this test may reveal cancer located higher in the intestine.

X-rays also demonstrate and define the extent of inflammatory disease, such as diverticulitis and ulcerative colitis. Ulcerative colitis usually originates in the anal region and ascends through the intestine.

X-ray films may also reveal polyps, structural changes in the intestine (such as telescoping of the bowel), gastroenteritis, irritable colon, and some cases of acute appendicitis.

X-RAYS OF THE DUODENUM

X-ray examination of the duodenum, the first portion of the small intestine, is called *hypotonic duodenography.* It's performed after barium sulfate and air are delivered into the intestine by a catheter.

This test is done for people who have symptoms of duodenal or pancreatic disease, such as persistent upper abdominal pain. However, it requires other follow-up tests to confirm a diagnosis.

Why is this test done?

Hypotonic duodenography may be performed for the following reasons:

- To detect small duodenal lesions and cancer of the pancreas
- To help diagnose chronic pancreatitis.

What should you know before the test?

- You'll learn about the test, including who will perform it, where it will take place, and its expected duration (approximately an hour). During the test, a tube will be passed through your nose into your duodenum to serve as a channel for the barium and air. As the air is introduced, you may experience a cramping pain. If you do, breathe deeply and slowly through your mouth to help relax the abdominal muscles.
- The drug glucagon or an anticholinergic drug may be given during the test. Glucagon can cause nausea, vomiting, hives, and flushing. The anticholinergic drug can cause dry mouth, thirst, a rapid heartbeat, difficulty urinating, and blurred vision. If you'll be receiving an anticholinergic drug, someone should accompany you home.
- You'll receive a form that asks your consent to perform the test. Be sure to read this form carefully before signing it. Ask questions if you don't understand any portion of it.
- Fast after midnight the night before the test.
- Just before the test, remove any dentures, glasses, necklaces, hairpins, combs, and constricting undergarments. Also, you should urinate.

After the test, you may burp the air the doctor introduced or pass gas. Because of the barium, your stools will look chalky white for 24 to 72 hours.

What happens during the test?

- While you're seated, a catheter is passed through your nose into the stomach. You then lie down on the X-ray table, and the catheter is advanced into the duodenum.
- The drug glucagon may be given through an arm vein. Or an anticholinergic drug may be injected into a muscle.
- The barium is instilled through the catheter, and X-rays are taken of the duodenum. Some of the barium is then withdrawn and air is instilled. Then additional X-rays are taken.
- When the required films have been obtained, the catheter is removed.

What happens after the test?

- If an anticholinergic drug was given, you'll need to urinate within a few hours after the test. If you're alone, you'll need to rest in a waiting area until your vision clears (in about 2 hours).

- You may burp instilled air or pass gas. Because of the barium, your stools will look chalky white for 24 to 72 hours.

Does the test have risks?

- Anticholinergic drugs shouldn't be given to anyone with severe heart disease or glaucoma.
- Glucagon shouldn't be given to anyone who has severe diabetes.
- A person with strictures in the upper digestive tract shouldn't undergo this procedure.
- Elderly or very ill people may vomit from the test or may have heartburn.

What are the normal results?

When barium and air expand the duodenum, the mucosa normally appears smooth and even. The regular contour of the head of the pancreas also appears on the duodenal wall.

What do abnormal results mean?

Irregular nodules or masses on the duodenal wall could mean duodenal lesions, tumors of the pancreas, or chronic pancreatitis. Diagnosis requires further tests, such as endoscopic retrograde cholangiopancreatography, blood and urine tests, and ultrasound and computed tomography (CAT) scans of the pancreas.

X-RAYS OF THE GALLBLADDER

Called *oral cholecystography* by doctors, this X-ray test examines the gallbladder after pills containing a special dye are swallowed. It's performed when a person has symptoms of gallbladder disease, such as pain on the upper right side of the abdomen, fat intolerance, and jaundice.

Why is this test done?

X-rays of the gallbladder may be performed for the following reasons:
- To detect gallstones
- To help diagnose inflammatory disease and tumors of the gallbladder.

What should you know before the test?

■ You'll find out about the test, including who will perform it, where it will take place, and its expected duration (usually 30 to 45 minutes, but a longer test may be necessary). You'll eat a meal containing fat at noon the day before the test and a fat-free meal in the evening. After the evening meal, you can only have water.

■ You'll receive several tablets that contain the special dye used in the test. Swallow the tablets one at a time at 5-minute intervals, with one or two mouthfuls of water. The tablets often cause diarrhea but rarely produce other problems, such as nausea, vomiting, stomach cramps, and painful urination. Tell the nurse immediately if you get any of these symptoms.

■ Tell the doctor or nurse if you have allergies to anesthetics, iodine, shellfish (such as shrimp or scallops), or the dyes used in any tests.

■ You may receive a cleansing enema the morning of the test. This clears the digestive tract for the test.

■ You'll receive a form that asks your consent to perform the test. Be sure to read this form carefully before signing it. Ask questions if you don't understand any portion of it.

What happens during the test?

■ You lie face down on the X-ray table, and the doctor takes and looks at X-rays of your abdomen.

■ You change positions and additional X-rays are taken.

■ You may then be given a fat stimulus, such as a high-fat meal or a synthetic fat-containing agent. The doctor will then observe the emptying of your gallbladder and take X-rays every 15 to 30 minutes. If the gallbladder empties slowly or not at all, these X-rays are also taken at 60 minutes.

What happens after the test?

■ If the results are normal, you can resume your usual diet. If they're abnormal, you may need to stay on a low-fat diet until a definite diagnosis can be made.

■ If gallstones are discovered, you'll need an appropriate diet — usually one that restricts fat — to help prevent attacks.

Does the test have risks?

The test shouldn't be done on a person with severe kidney or liver disease or with allergies to iodine, shellfish, or the dyes used for other diagnostic tests.

The gallbladder normally appears pear-shaped, with smooth, thin walls. Its size varies.

What are the normal results?

The gallbladder normally appears pear-shaped, with smooth, thin walls. Although its size varies, its basic structure — neck, infundibulum, body, and fundus — is clearly outlined on X-rays.

What do abnormal results mean?

The test can detect gallstones, the presence of cholesterol, polyps, and benign tumors. It also can show inflammatory disease such as cholecystitis — with or without gallstone formation.

When the gallbladder fails to contract following consumption of a fatty meal, it may indicate cholecystitis or common bile duct obstruction. If the X-rays are inconclusive, the test will have to be repeated the following day.

EXAMINATION OF THE BILE DUCTS

This test, which doctors call *percutaneous transhepatic cholangiography*, allows the doctor to examine the bile ducts (ducts that carry bile through the liver to the digestive system). It requires injection of a contrast dye directly into the ducts. The test is especially useful for evaluating a person with persistent upper abdominal pain after gallbladder removal and for evaluating a person with severe jaundice.

Why is this test done?

Percutaneous transhepatic cholangiography may be performed for the following reasons:

- To determine the cause of upper abdominal pain following gallbladder removal
- To distinguish between obstructive and nonobstructive jaundice
- To determine the location, the extent and, in many cases, the cause of gallbladder obstruction.

What should you know before the test?

- You'll learn about the test, including who will perform it, where it will take place, and its duration (about 30 minutes). During the test, you'll lie on a tilting X-ray table that rotates into vertical and horizontal positions. You'll be adequately secured to the table and assisted to different positions.

- Tell the doctor or nurse if you have allergies to anesthetics, iodine, shellfish (such as shrimp or scallops), or the dyes used in any tests. Injection of the dye may produce a sensation of pressure and fullness and may cause brief upper back pain on the right side. The injection of the local anesthetic may sting the skin and produce transient pain when it punctures the liver capsule.
- You may receive an antibiotic intravenously every 4 to 6 hours for 24 hours before the procedure.
- You'll need to fast for 8 hours before the test. Just before the procedure, you may receive a sedative.
- You'll receive a form that asks your consent to perform the test. Be sure to read this form carefully before signing it. Ask questions if you don't understand any portion of it.

The bile ducts should have a normal diameter and appear as regular channels, evenly filled with the dye.

What happens during the test?

- You lie on your back on the X-ray table and are adequately secured. Then you'll receive an injection of the local anesthetic.
- While you hold your breath at the end of expiration, the doctor guides a needle into the liver and slowly removes it while injecting the test dye. (See *How dye is injected directly into the liver*, page 40.)
- Using a fluoroscope and monitor, the doctor checks the opacification of the bile ducts and takes X-rays as you're assisted into different positions. When the required X-rays have been taken, the needle is removed.
- The nurse applies a dressing to the puncture site.

What happens after the test?

- A nurse will check your condition regularly.
- You should stay in bed for at least 6 hours after the test, preferably lying on your right side. This will help to prevent bleeding.
- You can resume your usual diet.

Does the test have risks?

- The test shouldn't be done on a person with cholangitis, massive ascites, an uncorrectable blood clotting disorder, or an allergy to iodine.
- It carries the potential risk of bleeding, septicemia, bile peritonitis, and leakage of the dye into the peritoneal cavity.

What are the normal results?

The bile ducts should have a normal diameter and appear as regular channels evenly filled with the dye.

How dye is injected directly into the liver

To obtain a view of the bile ducts, the doctor performs a procedure called *percutaneous transhepatic cholangiography*. In this procedure, the doctor injects a special dye directly into the liver. This illustration shows the path of the needle through the liver into a structure called the *biliary radicle*, the primary root of the bile ducts.

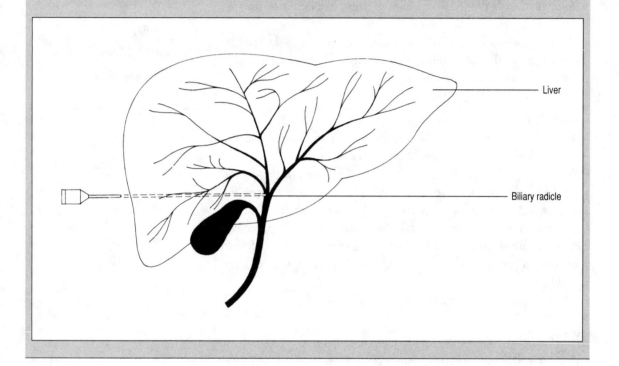

What do abnormal results mean?

What do abnormal results mean?

Distinguishing between obstructive and nonobstructive jaundice hinges on whether bile ducts are dilated or of normal size. Obstructive jaundice is linked to dilated ducts. Nonobstructive jaundice is linked to normal-sized ducts. The obstruction may be caused by cholelithiasis, cancer of the bile ducts, or pancreatic cancer.

When ducts are of normal size and cholestasis is indicated, liver biopsy may be performed to distinguish among hepatitis, cirrhosis, and granulomatous disease.

EXAMINATION OF THE PANCREATIC DUCTS, LIVER, AND BILE DUCTS

A test called *endoscopic retrograde cholangiopancreatography* allows the doctor to examine the pancreatic ducts, liver, and bile ducts. This test uses X-rays and a special instrument called an *endoscope*. The X-rays are taken after the injection of a special dye through one of the endoscope's channels.

The test is performed when a person has confirmed or suspected pancreatic disease or obstructive jaundice of an unknown cause.

Why is this test done?

This test may be performed for the following reasons:
- To evaluate obstructive jaundice
- To diagnose cancer of the duodenum, the pancreas, and the bile ducts
- To locate stones and narrowing in the pancreatic ducts and hepatobiliary tree (the liver and bile ducts).

What should you know before the test?

- You'll learn about the test, including who will perform it, where it will take place, and its expected duration (30 to 60 minutes). At the start of the test, a local anesthetic will be sprayed into your mouth to calm the gag reflex. The spray has an unpleasant taste and makes the tongue and throat feel swollen, causing difficulty in swallowing. You'll also have an intravenous line inserted.
- You'll be told to let saliva drain from the side of your mouth during the test and that suction may be used to remove the saliva. A mouth guard will be inserted to protect your teeth and the endoscope. It won't interfere with your breathing.
- You'll be given a sedative before the insertion of the endoscope to help you relax, but you'll remain conscious during the test. You'll also receive an anticholinergic drug or the drug glucagon after insertion of the scope. The anticholinergic drug can cause dry mouth, thirst, a rapid heartbeat, difficult urination, and blurred vision. The glucagon can cause nausea, vomiting, hives, and flushing.
- When the doctor injects the dye for the test, be prepared to feel warm or flushed. Tell the doctor or nurse if you have allergies to anesthetics, iodine, shellfish (such as shrimp or scallops), or the dyes used in any tests.

- You'll need to fast after midnight before the test.
- Just before the test, remove any jewelry or constricting undergarments. You should urinate to minimize the discomfort of urine retention that may follow the test.
- You'll receive a form that asks your consent to perform the test. Be sure to read this form carefully before signing it. Ask questions if you don't understand any portion of it.

What happens during the test?

- After the nurse inserts an intravenous line, you get a local anesthetic that usually takes effect in about 10 minutes. If a spray is used, hold your breath while your mouth and throat are sprayed.
- You're given a basin to spit into. Because the anesthetic causes drooling, let the saliva drain from the side of your mouth.
- The nurse then inserts the mouth guard. While you're lying on your side, you receive a drug to help you relax.
- After you're relaxed, you bend your head forward and open your mouth. The doctor then guides the endoscope slowly into your stomach.
- You are then helped into a face-down position and are given an anticholinergic drug or glucagon. The doctor passes a small amount of air and the dye through one of the channels of the endoscope and examines the pancreas and the hepatobiliary tree. The doctor also takes X-rays, has them developed, and reviews them.
- When the required X-rays have been taken, the doctor may obtain a small biopsy specimen. Then the doctor removes the endoscope.

What happens after the test?

- The nurse will check your condition often: roughly every 15 minutes for 4 hours, then every hour for 4 hours, and then every 4 hours for 48 hours.
- You won't be able to eat or drink until your gag reflex returns. When it does, you can have fluids and a light meal.
- At the appropriate time, the nurse will remove the intravenous line.
- Tell the nurse if you have a sore throat. Soothing lozenges and warm saline gargles can ease discomfort.

Does the test have risks?

- The test shouldn't be performed on a person with infectious disease, pancreatic pseudocysts, stricture or obstruction of the esophagus or duodenum, and acute pancreatitis, cholangitis, or heart or lung disease.
- The test can cause cholangitis and pancreatitis.
- The test can also cause breathing difficulty, low blood pressure, excessive sweating, a slow heartbeat, and laryngospasm.

What are the normal results?

The dye should uniformly fill the pancreatic duct, the hepatobiliary tree, and the gallbladder.

What do abnormal results mean?

The test may demonstrate obstructive jaundice. Examination of the hepatobiliary tree may reveal stones, strictures, or irregular deviations that suggest bile duct cirrhosis, primary sclerosing cholangitis, or cancer of the bile ducts.

Examination of the pancreatic ducts may also show stones, strictures, and irregular deviations that may indicate pancreatic cysts and pseudocysts, cancer, chronic pancreatitis, pancreatic fibrosis, and papillary stenosis.

Depending on test findings, a definite diagnosis may require further studies.

After you're relaxed, you bend your head forward and open your mouth. The doctor then guides the endoscope slowly into your stomach.

X-RAYS OF THE SPLEEN

This test, called *splenoportography,* consists of X-rays of the spleen's veins and portal system after the injection of a dye into the spleen itself. The test begins with measurement of splenic pressure and continues with X-rays that record the filling of the splenic and portal veins.

Why is this test done?

X-rays of the spleen may be taken for the following reasons:
- To diagnose or evaluate portal hypertension (high blood pressure in the vein leading from the liver to the spleen)
- To discover what stage of cirrhosis the person has.

What should you know before the test?

- You'll learn about the test, including who will perform it and where and that it takes 30 to 45 minutes. You may feel a brief stinging sensation on injection of the local anesthetic and a brief warm or flushed feeling on injection of the test dye. You'll be alerted to report pain on your left upper side immediately.

- Tell the doctor or nurse if you have allergies to anesthetics, iodine, shellfish (such as shrimp or scallops), or the dyes used in any tests. The dye used in this test can cause nausea, vomiting, excessive salivation, flushing, hives, sweating and, rarely, a severe life-threatening allergic reaction. These reactions usually occur 5 to 10 minutes after the injection.

- Fast after the evening meal the day before the procedure.

- About 30 minutes before the procedure, you'll receive a mild sedative and pain medication.

- You'll receive a form that asks your consent to perform the test. Be sure to read this form carefully before signing it. Ask questions if you don't understand any portion of it.

What happens during the test?

- You lie on your back on the X-ray table, with your left hand under your head. The left side of your chest and stomach are cleaned with antiseptics.

- The doctor locates your spleen, takes an X-ray, and injects a local anesthetic.

- You are directed to hold your breath as the doctor inserts the needle into the spleen. Breathe shallowly as the doctor connects a device to the needle to measure spleen pressure.

- After measuring pressure, the doctor removes the device and injects the test dye. X-rays are then taken. When they're completed, the doctor removes the needle and applies a dressing.

What happens after the test?

- The nurse will check you often: roughly every 15 minutes for 1 hour, then every 30 minutes for 2 hours, and then every hour for 4 hours.

- Lie on your left side for 24 hours to minimize the risk of bleeding. Stay in bed for another 24 hours after that.

- You can resume your usual diet. Drink fluids to promote excretion of the dye.

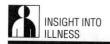

INSIGHT INTO
ILLNESS

Understanding portal hypertension: Its causes and complications

Portal hypertension refers to high blood pressure in the vein leading from the liver to the spleen (the portal vein). It occurs because of increased resistance to blood flow, which may stem from a cause above, within, or below the liver. It may lead to a variety of complications, including an enlarged liver, an enlarged spleen, or esophageal varices, a condition marked by dilated, tortuous veins in the lower esophagus, which may start bleeding and lead to serious consequences.

Causes above the liver
- Incompetence of the heart's tricuspid valve
- Hepatic vein clot
- Constrictive pericarditis (inflammation of the sac surrounding the heart)

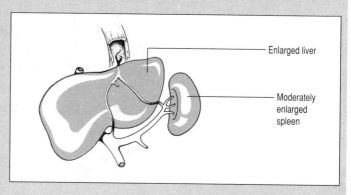

Enlarged liver

Moderately enlarged spleen

Causes within the liver
Cirrhosis

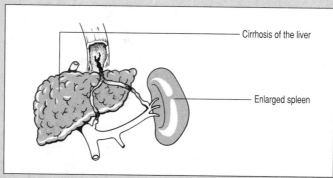

Cirrhosis of the liver

Enlarged spleen

Causes below the liver
Portal vein clot

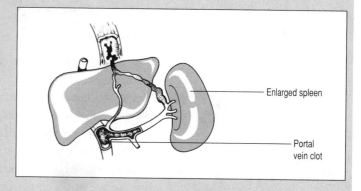

Enlarged spleen

Portal vein clot

Does the test have risks?

■ This test shouldn't be performed on a person with ascites, uncorrectable blood clotting problems, an enlarged spleen caused by infection, markedly impaired liver or kidney function, and an allergy to iodine.

■ This test may cause excessive bleeding that requires transfusion or, occasionally, splenectomy.

What are the normal results?

Spleen pressure normally measures 50 to 180 millimeters of water (3.5 to 13.5 millimeters of mercury). After the dye is injected into the spleen, it outlines splenic tributary veins and drains into the splenic and portal veins. Normal venous flow should be contained within these two vessels, without diversion into collateral veins.

What do abnormal results mean?

In portal hypertension, spleen pressure ranges from 200 to 450 millimeters of water (15 to 34 millimeters of mercury). The presence of collateral veins — often associated with esophageal varices, splenomegaly and, in some cases, an enlarged liver — can also indicate portal hypertension resulting from blocked portal venous flow. Results may also show thrombosis or occlusion in the splenic and portal veins provided venous flow isn't reversed. (See *Understanding portal hypertension: Its causes and complications,* page 45.)

The test may also show cirrhosis and, depending on the specific findings, may help determine its stage.

ANGIOGRAM OF THE ABDOMINAL BLOOD VESSELS

Called *celiac and mesenteric arteriography* by doctors, this X-ray test examines the abdominal blood vessels after the injection of a special dye. Injection of the dye into one or more arteries provides a map of the abdominal vessels. Injection into specific arterial branches, called *superselective angiography,* permits detailed study of a particular area.

This test is performed when endoscopy can't find the source of gastrointestinal bleeding or when barium studies, ultrasound scans, and nuclear medicine or computed tomography (CAT) scans prove inconclusive in evaluating cancer. It's also used to evaluate cirrhosis and portal hypertension, to find blood vessel damage after abdominal injury, and to detect other blood vessel problems.

Why is this test done?

An angiogram of the abdominal blood vessels may be performed for the following reasons:

- To locate the source of gastrointestinal bleeding
- To help distinguish between benign and malignant tumors
- To evaluate cirrhosis and portal hypertension
- To evaluate blood vessel damage after abdominal injury
- To detect other blood vessels abnormalities.

What should you know before the test?

- You'll learn who will perform the test and where and that it takes 30 minutes to 3 hours, depending on the number of vessels studied. You'll receive a local anesthetic and feel a brief, stinging sensation as it's injected. You may also feel pressure when the doctor touches the area (over the femoral artery in the groin area) where the dye will be injected. But the local anesthetic will minimize the pain when the needle is introduced into the artery.
- You'll learn that the injection may cause a brief feeling of warmth or burning, a headache, a salty taste, and nausea and vomiting. Tell the doctor or nurse if you have allergies to anesthetics, iodine, shellfish (such as shrimp or scallops), or the dyes used in any tests.
- You'll need to lie still during the test to avoid blurring the films, and restraints may be used to keep you still. The X-ray equipment makes a loud, clacking sound as the films are taken.
- You'll need to fast for 8 hours before the test.
- Just before the test, put on a hospital gown and remove jewelry and other objects that might obscure anatomic detail on X-ray films. Then go to the bathroom to urinate.
- You'll receive a sedative just before the test, if the doctor prescribed one.
- You'll receive a form that asks your consent to perform the test. Be sure to read this form carefully before signing it. Ask questions if you don't understand any portion of it.

What happens during the test?

- You lie on your back on an X-ray table, and a nurse inserts an intravenous line.
- X-rays are taken of your abdomen, and your pulse rate is checked.

> *You'll need to lie still during the test to avoid blurring the films, and restraints may be used to keep you still. The X-ray equipment makes a loud, clacking sound as the films are taken.*

- The nurse cleans the area around the injection site and shaves it.
- The doctor injects the local anesthetic and locates the femoral artery. Then the doctor inserts the needle and passes a catheter through it to the aorta, the major abdominal blood vessel.
- Next, the doctor injects the dye and takes a series of X-rays. After injecting into one or more major arteries, superselective catheterization may be performed.
- After the X-rays are completed, the doctor removes the catheter and applies a dressing.

What happens after the test?
- The nurse will check on you often to see if your pulses and the temperature and color of your leg are okay.
- You'll rest in bed for 4 to 6 hours. The leg with the puncture site must be kept straight.
- If you don't have an intravenous line, drink lots of fluids to speed the excretion of the dye.
- You may feel some temporary stiffness after the test from lying still on the hard X-ray table.

Does the test have risks?
- The test should be performed cautiously on a person with a blood clotting problem.
- The dye used in the test can cause an allergic reaction, which rarely is severe. Most reactions occur within a half-hour.
- Complications of the test include hemorrhage, thrombosis, an irregular heartbeat, and emboli caused by dislodging atherosclerotic plaques.

After the test, you'll rest in bed for 4 to 6 hours, and you must keep the leg with the puncture site straight.

What are the normal results?
The X-rays show no problems with the abdominal blood vessels.

What do abnormal results mean?
Gastrointestinal bleeding appears on the angiogram as the leakage of the dye from the damaged vessels. Severe upper gastrointestinal bleeding can be caused by conditions such as Mallory-Weiss syndrome, gastric or peptic ulcer, hemorrhagic gastritis, and an eroded hiatal hernia. Severe lower gastrointestinal bleeding can be caused by conditions such as bleeding diverticula and angiodysplasia.

The test can identify changes in blood vessels caused by abdominal cancer. It may also show the progression of cirrhosis.

Abdominal injury often damages the spleen and, less often, the liver. The test can reveal these injuries.

Various abnormalities affecting the diameter and course of an artery may appear on the angiogram. Atherosclerotic plaques or atheromas — fatty deposits inside the vessel — narrow the blood vessel and may block it.

KIDNEYS & URINARY TRACT

X-RAY OF THE KIDNEYS, URETERS, AND BLADDER

Called *KUB* for short, an X-ray of the kidneys, ureters, and bladder is usually the first step in testing the urinary system. This test determines the position of the kidneys, ureters, and bladder and helps detect major abnormalities.

This test has many limitations and nearly always must be followed by more elaborate tests, such as a computed tomography (CAT) scan.

Why is this test done?
An X-ray of the kidneys, ureters, and bladder may be performed for the following reasons:
- To evaluate the size, structure, and position of the kidneys
- To screen for abnormalities in the region of the kidneys, ureters, and bladder.

What should you know before the test?
- You'll learn who will perform the test and where and that it takes only a few minutes.
- You won't need to fast or limit fluids.

What happens during the test?

- You lie on your back on an X-ray table, with your arms extended overhead.
- A single X-ray is taken.

Does the test have risks?

The test does involve exposure to a small amount of radiation. Men will have their groin area shielded by a lead apron to avoid irradiation of the testicles. Women, unfortunately, can't have their ovaries shielded because they're too close to the kidneys, ureters, and bladder.

An X-ray of the kidneys, ureters, and bladder is usually the first step in testing the urinary system.

What are the normal results?

Both kidneys should be about the same size. The ureters are only visible when an abnormality is present. The bladder may or may not be visible.

What do abnormal results mean?

Enlargement of both kidneys seen on the X-ray may be caused by polycystic disease, multiple myeloma, lymphoma, amyloidosis, or hydronephrosis. Enlargement of one kidney may be caused by a tumor, cyst, or hydronephrosis. Decreased size of one kidney suggests possible congenital hypoplasia, pyelonephritis, or ischemia.

This test may detect problems present at birth, such as abnormal location or absence of a kidney. It may also reveal polycystic disease, pyelonephritis, or kidney stones. In most cases, positive identification of kidney stones requires further testing.

NEPHROTOMOGRAPHY

This test provides images of sections or layers of the kidney and its blood vessels. In the test, special X-rays and other films are taken before and after the kidney is coated with a dye. Injected into the arm, this dye has special properties that cause it to show up on X-rays.

Nephrotomography can be performed as a separate test or as an adjunct to a test called *intravenous pyelography*. It's particularly helpful in identifying problems suggested by such other tests.

Why is this test done?

Nephrotomography may be performed for the following reasons:
- To differentiate a simple kidney cyst from a tumor
- To evaluate lacerations of the kidneys
- To find adrenal gland tumors when other tests indicate their presence but not their location.

What should you know before the test?

- You'll learn who will perform the test and where and that it takes less than 1 hour. During the test, you'll be positioned on an X-ray table and may hear loud, clacking sounds as the films are exposed. When the dye is injected, you may feel a burning or stinging sensation at the injection site, flushing, and a metallic taste.
- Tell the doctor or nurse if you have any allergies to shellfish (such as shrimp or scallops), iodine, or the dyes used in other diagnostic tests.
- You'll fast for 8 hours before the test.
- You'll need to sign a form that gives your consent to perform the test. Be sure to read this form carefully and ask questions if you don't understand any portion of it.

What happens during the test?

- You lie on an X-ray table as preliminary X-rays and tomograms are taken.
- After reviewing the preliminary tomograms, the doctor selects five vertical views of the kidney for filming. Then the doctor administers the test dye and takes additional tomograms.

What happens after the test?

- The nurse will check your condition regularly for 24 hours after the test.
- Tell the nurse if you feel flushed, nauseated, or itch or sneeze a lot. If you have these symptoms, the nurse will give you medication for them.

Does the test have risks?

Nephrotomography is performed with extreme caution on a person who has allergies to iodine or shellfish. Caution is also used when the test is being performed on a person with severe cardiovascular disease or multiple myeloma.

By examining images of sections or layers of the kidney, the doctor can differentiate a simple kidney cyst from a tumor.

What are the normal results?

The size, shape, and position of the kidneys should appear normal. No tumors, stones, or other abnormalities should be present.

What do abnormal results mean?

Among the problems detected by the test are simple cysts and tumors, areas of poor circulation, and kidney lacerations that occur following injury.

EXAMINATION OF THE URETHRA

X-ray examination of the urethra is called *retrograde urethrography.* Performed almost exclusively on men, this X-ray study uses a special dye that's injected or instilled into the urethra, the canal that carries urine from the bladder. The test allows the doctor to examine the full length of this canal.

Why is this test done?

X-ray examination of the urethra may be performed for the following reasons:
- To diagnose narrowing of the urethra, blockages, diverticula, and urethral problems present at birth
- To evaluate tears of the urethra or other injury
- To check the condition of the urethra after surgery.

What should you know before the test?

- You'll learn about the test, including who will perform it, where it will take place, and its expected duration (about 30 minutes). During the test, you may experience some discomfort when the catheter is inserted into the urethral opening and when the dye is instilled through the catheter.
- Tell the doctor or nurse if you have any allergies to shellfish (such as shrimp or scallops), iodine, or the dyes used in other diagnostic tests.
- You'll be told about the loud, clacking sounds as X-ray films are made.
- Just before the test, you may receive a sedative. The nurse will tell you to urinate.

- You'll need to sign a form that gives your consent to perform the test. Be sure to read this form carefully and ask questions if you don't understand any portion of it.

What happens during the test?

- You lie on the examining table as X-rays of the bladder and urethra are made. The doctor studies these X-rays to detect any stones, foreign bodies, or other problems.
- The nurse cleans your penis with an antiseptic solution. The doctor then inserts the catheter into the urethra. The catheter has a small balloon at its end. The doctor inflates the balloon with a little water to prevent the catheter from slipping during the test.
- The doctor injects the dye through the catheter. After three-fourths of the dye has been injected, the first X-ray film is exposed. The doctor injects the remainder of the dye and takes additional X-rays.

After the test, you'll be checked on regularly for 12 to 24 hours. Tell the nurse if you feel hot or have chills.

What happens after the test?

You'll be checked on regularly for 12 to 24 hours. Tell the nurse if you feel hot or have chills.

Does the test have risks?

The test is performed cautiously on a person with a urinary tract infection.

What are the normal results?

The urethra should appear normal in size, shape, and course.

What do abnormal results mean?

This test may reveal different problems, such as urethral diverticula, fistulas, narrowing, false passages, stones, and tears. It can identify problems present from birth, such as urethral valves and perineal hypospadias. It can also detect tumors, which are rare in the urethra.

EXAMINATION OF THE BLADDER

X-ray examination of the bladder is called *retrograde cystography*. During this procedure, a doctor inserts a catheter into the urethra, the slender channel through which urine flows from the bladder. After inserting the catheter, the doctor instills a special dye through the catheter into the bladder. The dye possesses properties that cause it to appear on X-rays.

The test can diagnose bladder rupture. It's also done for recurrent urinary tract infections (especially in children) and suspected fistulas, diverticula, and tumors.

The test should show a bladder with normal contours, capacity, and integrity. The bladder wall should be smooth, not thick.

Why is this test done?

This test is performed to evaluate the structure and integrity of the bladder.

What should you know before the test?

- You'll learn about the test, including who will perform it, where it will take place, and its expected duration (about 30 to 60 minutes). During the test, you may experience some discomfort when the catheter is inserted into the urethral opening and when the dye is instilled through the catheter.
- Tell the doctor or nurse if you have any allergies to shellfish (such as shrimp or scallops), iodine, or the dyes used in other diagnostic tests.
- You'll be told that the X-ray machine makes loud, clacking sounds.
- You'll need to sign a form that gives your consent to perform the test. Be sure to read this form carefully and ask questions if you don't understand any portion of it.

What happens during the test?

- You lie on your back on the examining table, and a preliminary X-ray is taken. The doctor checks this X-ray before proceeding with the test.
- Next, the doctor inserts a catheter through the urethra into the bladder, puts a clamp on the catheter to keep it in place, and gently instills the test dye through it.
- The doctor takes one X-ray while you remain on your back and two more while you lie on each side. Next, the nurse may help you assume a jackknife position while the doctor takes yet another X-ray.

- The doctor unclamps the catheter, which allows urine and the test dye to drain, and takes another X-ray. After this, the doctor removes the catheter.

What happens after the test

- A nurse will check on you several times an hour for the first 2 hours after the test, then roughly every 2 hours for up to 24 hours.
- The nurse will check the color and volume of your urine, which will probably contain some blood for a short time.
- Tell the nurse if you feel hot, have chills, or simply don't feel well.

Does the test have risks?

- This test shouldn't be performed during a severe urinary tract infection.
- It also shouldn't be performed on any person with a blockage in the urinary tract.

What are the normal results?

The test should show a bladder with normal contours, capacity, and integrity. The bladder wall should be smooth, not thick.

What do abnormal results mean?

The test can identify pouches in the bladder wall called *diverticula*. It can also find tumors, stones or gravel, and blood clots.

EXAMINATION OF THE URETERS

This X-ray test, called *retrograde ureteropyelography*, examines the ureters, the two slender tubes that carry urine from the kidneys to the bladder. It's performed during cystoscopy, a procedure in which the doctor examines the bladder using a viewing instrument called an *endoscope*. During cystoscopy, the doctor will insert a catheter through one of the endoscope's channels into the ureters and gently instill a special dye. The dye possesses properties that cause it to appear on X-rays. (See *Spotting stones and other obstructions,* page 56.)

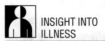

INSIGHT INTO
ILLNESS

Spotting stones and other obstructions

X-ray examination of the ureters may detect blockages of urine flow in the kidneys and ureters. These blockages can be caused by a stricture, a tumor, a blood clot, or stones. Small stones may travel and become lodged in the ureter. A large blockage called a *staghorn stone* may form in the kidney.

Examples of various blockages are shown below.

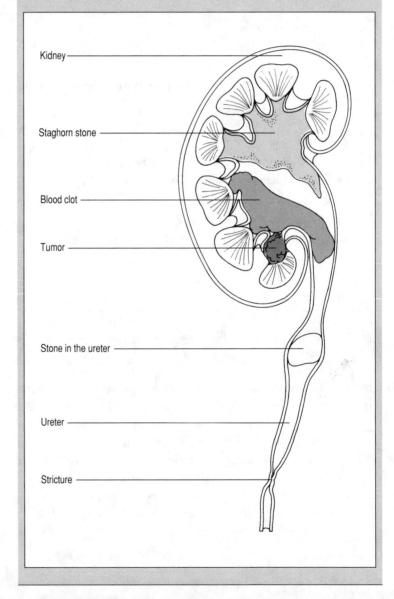

Why is this test done?

This test is performed to check the structure and integrity of the kidneys and the ureters.

What should you know before the test?

- You'll learn who will perform the test and where and that it takes about 1 hour. If a general anesthetic is to be used, you'll need to fast for 8 hours before the test. Generally, you should be well hydrated to ensure adequate urine flow.
- During the test, you'll be positioned on an examining table, with your legs in stirrups. This position may be tiring.
- If you don't receive a general anesthetic, you'll receive a sedative before the test. During the test, you may feel pressure when the endoscope is passed and when the dye is instilled. Also, you may feel an urgency to urinate.
- You'll need to sign a form that gives your consent to perform the test. Be sure to read this form carefully and ask questions if you don't understand any portion of it.

What happens during the test?

- You lie on your back on the examining table, with your legs in the stirrups.
- After you receive an anesthetic, the doctor inserts the endoscope through the urethral opening and advances it into the bladder. Once there, the doctor can look at the bladder and insert a catheter into one or both ureters.
- Next, the doctor instills a tiny amount of the test dye through the catheter and takes a series of X-rays.
- Then the doctor removes the catheter, waits 10 to 15 minutes, and checks for retention of the dye. However, if the doctor finds a blockage in a ureter, the catheter may be kept in place to allow urine to flow.

What happens after the test

- The nurse will check on you often to see how you're feeling. You'll need to drink extra fluids.
- The nurse will check the color and volume of your urine. You'll probably experience pain when you urinate, but the nurse will give you medication for as long as the pain lasts. Your urine will also contain some blood for a short time.
- Tell the nurse if you have any pain or feel hot or have chills.

Does the test have risks?

Examination of the ureters will be done very carefully in a person with an ureteral blockage to prevent further injury.

What are the normal results?

The ureters should fill uniformly and appear normal in size and course.

What do abnormal results mean?

The test can reveal a blockage, most commonly at the junction of a ureter and the kidney. The blockage may be caused by a tumor, a blood clot, narrowing, or a stone.

EXAMINATION OF THE KIDNEYS

This X-ray test, called *antegrade pyelography*, examines the kidneys. It's performed when a blocked ureter makes it impossible to perform cystoscopy.

In this test, the doctor inserts a needle into the kidney, injects a special dye, and takes X-rays. The dye possesses properties that cause it to appear on X-rays.

Why is this test done?

X-ray examination of the kidneys may be performed for the following reasons:
- To evaluate blockages in the kidneys or ureters caused by a stricture, stones, blood clots, or a tumor
- To evaluate hydronephrosis
- To check the condition of the kidneys or ureters before or after surgery.

What should you know before the test?

- You'll learn about the test, including who will perform it and where and that it will take approximately 1 to 2 hours. During the test, the doctor will insert a needle into the kidney after giving you a sedative and a local anesthetic. Urine may be collected from the kidney for testing and, if necessary, a tube will be left in the kidney for drainage.

- You may feel mild discomfort during injection of the local anesthetic and dye and also a brief sensation of burning and warmth from the dye.
- Tell the doctor or the nurse if you have a blood clotting disorder. Also mention if you have any allergies to shellfish (such as shrimp or scallops), iodine, or the dyes used in other diagnostic tests.
- You may need to fast for 6 to 8 hours before the test.
- You may receive antibiotics before and after the test. Just before it, you may get a sedative to help you relax.
- You'll need to sign a form that states your consent to perform the test. Be sure to read this form carefully and ask questions if you don't understand any portion of it.

What happens during the test?

- You lie face down on the X-ray table. The skin over the kidney is cleaned with an antiseptic, and a local anesthetic is injected.
- The doctor inserts a needle into the kidney, attaches tubing to it, and collects a little urine for testing.
- Next, the doctor injects the test dye and takes X-rays.
- If necessary, the doctor will insert a tube into the kidney to allow it to drain. If a tube isn't needed, the doctor removes the needle and tubing and applies a dressing.

What happens after the test?

- The nurse will check on you often to see how you're feeling.
- The nurse will check the color and volume of your urine. You'll probably experience pain when you urinate, but the nurse will give you medication for as long as the pain lasts. Your urine will also contain some blood for a short time.
- Tell the nurse if you have any pain or feel hot or have chills.
- If the doctor leaves a kidney tube in place, the nurse will check that it's draining properly.

Does the test have risks?

This test shouldn't be performed on a person with a bleeding disorder.

As the test begins, you lie face down on the X-ray table. The skin over the kidney is cleaned with an antiseptic, and a local anesthetic is injected.

What are the normal results?

After injection of dye, the kidneys and ureters should fill uniformly and appear normal in size and course. Normal structures should be outlined clearly.

What do abnormal results mean?

The test can show enlarged areas of the kidneys or ureters. This enlargement means a blockage, which can be caused by stricture, stones, blood clots, or a tumor.

The test can detect hydronephrosis. It also shows the results of a recent surgery.

EXAMINATION OF THE URINARY TRACT

The cornerstone of urologic testing, this test, called *intravenous pyelography*, evaluates the structure and function of nearly the entire urinary tract. It's commonly known by the abbreviation IVP. Another name for this test is excretory urography.

In this test, the doctor injects a dye into an arm vein. The dye, which has properties that cause it to appear on X-rays, flows to the kidneys. Once it's there, X-rays are taken. The dye continues to flow through the ureters, the slender tubes that connect the kidneys to the bladder. The doctor takes X-rays of the dye's passage through these structures.

Why is this test done?

Examination of the urinary tract may be performed for the following reasons:
- To evaluate the condition of the kidneys, ureters, and bladder
- To check for suspected kidney or urinary tract disease, such as kidney stones, tumors, urinary problems present at birth, or an injury to the urinary system
- To identify kidney problems as the cause of high blood pressure, a condition called *renovascular hypertension*.

What should you know before the test?

- You'll learn about the test, including who will perform it, where it will take place, and its expected duration.

- You may feel mild discomfort during the injection of the local anesthetic and a brief sensation of burning and warmth and a metallic taste in your mouth from the injection of the dye. During the test, the X-ray machine will make loud, clacking sounds.
- Tell the doctor or the nurse if you have a blood clotting disorder. Also mention if you have any allergies to shellfish (such as shrimp or scallops), iodine, or the dyes used in other diagnostic tests.
- Drink lots of fluids on the day before the test. For 8 hours before the test, you'll need to fast.
- You may receive a laxative on the night before the test to help give clearer X-rays.
- You'll need to sign a form that gives your consent to perform the test. Be sure to read this form carefully and ask questions if you don't understand any portion of it.

What happens during the test?
- You lie on your back on an X-ray table.
- The doctor takes a preliminary X-ray of your kidneys, ureters, and bladder. If this X-ray shows no obvious problems, the doctor goes ahead and injects the dye.
- About a minute later, the dye reaches the kidneys, and the doctor takes an X-ray. Additional X-rays are then taken at regular intervals, usually 5, 10, and 15 or 20 minutes after the injection.
- After the 5-minute X-ray is done, the doctor compresses the ureters. To do this, the doctor inflates two small rubber devices and places them on both sides of your stomach. The inflated devices block the ureters, without causing any discomfort, and keep the dye from flowing farther.
- After the 10-minute X-ray is done, the doctor removes the rubber devices. As the dye flows into the lower urinary tract, the doctor takes another X-ray of the lower halves of both ureters and then, finally, one of the bladder.
- At the end of the test, you'll urinate. The doctor then takes a last X-ray.

What happens after the test?
A nurse will check you for a delayed reaction to the dye.

To prepare for the test, you'll drink lots of fluids the day before, fast for 8 hours and, possibly, take a laxative.

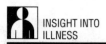

INSIGHT INTO
ILLNESS

Where stones form in the urinary tract

Stones may form in the kidneys or in the ureters, the two slender tubes that connect the kidneys and bladder. Stones can also form in the bladder.

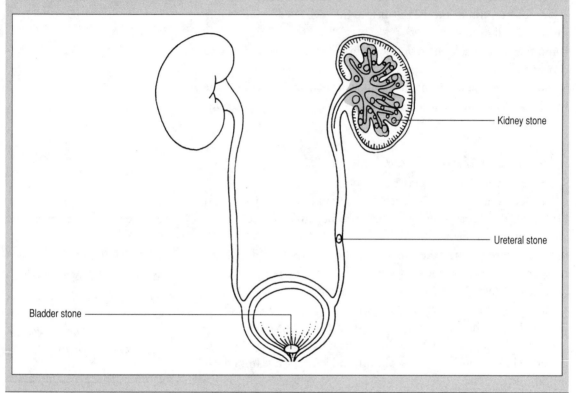

Kidney stone

Ureteral stone

Bladder stone

Does the test have risks?

The test shouldn't be performed on people with severe asthma or an allergy to the dye, unless they receive medication to avoid a serious reaction.

What are the normal results?

The kidneys, ureters, and bladder should show no evidence of tumors or other diseases.

What do abnormal results mean?

This test can demonstrate many abnormalities of the urinary system, including kidney or ureteral stones. (See *Where stones form in the uri-*

nary tract.) It can also show an abnormal size, shape, or structure of the kidneys, ureters, or bladder. It can detect an absent kidney or more than the normal two. Likewise, it can show polycystic kidney disease, tumors, renovascular hypertension, and urinary problems present at birth.

ANGIOGRAM OF THE KIDNEYS

This X-ray test allows examination of the kidneys and their blood vessels. In the test, the doctor injects a special dye into a blood vessel in the groin area. The dye possesses special properties that allow it to be seen on X-rays. When the dye reaches the kidneys, the doctor rapidly takes a series of X-rays.

Why is this test done?
An angiogram of the kidneys may be performed for the following reasons:
- To show the configuration of all the kidneys' blood vessels before surgery
- To determine the cause of renovascular hypertension
- To investigate kidney enlargement and nonfunctioning kidneys
- To evaluate chronic kidney disease or kidney failure
- To investigate kidney masses, blood vessel malformations, pseudo-tumors, and kidney trauma
- To detect complications following a kidney transplant, such as rejection of a new kidney.

What should you know before the test?
- You'll learn about the test, including who will perform it, where it will take place, and its expected duration (about 1 hour).
- You may feel mild discomfort during injection of the local anesthetic and a brief sensation of burning and warmth and a metallic taste in your mouth from the injection of the dye. During the test, the X-ray machine will make loud, clacking sounds.
- Tell the doctor or the nurse if you have a blood clotting disorder. Also mention if you have any allergies to shellfish (such as shrimp or scallops), iodine, or the dyes used in other diagnostic tests.
- For 8 hours before the test, you'll need to fast.

Angiogram of the kidneys may show narrowing of the renal artery by arteriosclerosis. This crucial finding confirms that high blood pressure is caused by a kidney problem.

- You'll put on a hospital gown and be asked to remove all jewelry or other metal objects that may obscure the X-rays.
- Just before the test, you'll receive a sedative and pain medication. The nurse will tell you to urinate.
- You'll need to sign a form that states your consent to undergo the test. Be sure to read this form carefully and ask questions if you don't understand any portion of it.

What happens during the test?

- You lie on the examining table, and a nurse inserts an intravenous line. The skin over the femoral artery, the blood vessel in the groin area where the doctor injects the dye, is cleaned with an antiseptic, and a local anesthetic is injected.
- The doctor then inserts a small tube called a *catheter* into the blood vessel and advances it, using a guide wire, to the aorta, the main blood vessel in the abdomen.
- The doctor injects the dye and takes X-rays.
- Next, to determine the position of the kidneys' arteries, the doctor injects additional dye and rapidly takes a series of X-rays.
- The doctor removes the catheter and applies pressure over the injection site for about 15 minutes to prevent bleeding. Then the doctor applies a dressing.

What happens after the test?

- You'll lie flat in bed for at least 6 hours. A nurse will check on you roughly every 15 minutes for 1 hour, then every 30 minutes for 2 hours.
- The nurse will check the dressing to make sure too much bleeding doesn't occur.

Does the test have risks?

This test shouldn't be done on a pregnant woman or on a person with bleeding tendencies, an allergy to the test dye, or kidney failure.

What are the normal results?

The test should show normal kidneys and blood vessels.

What do abnormal results mean?

An angiogram can show kidney tumors and cysts. The test can also show narrowing of the renal artery by arteriosclerosis. This crucial finding confirms that high blood pressure is caused by a kidney problem.

The test can detect kidney infarction, renal artery aneurysms, and renal arteriovenous fistula. It may show destruction and distortion of parts of the kidney in a person with severe or chronic pyelonephritis. The test may also indicate kidney abscesses or inflammation.

When angiography is used to evaluate kidney injury, it may detect blood clots, lacerations, shattered kidneys, and areas of infarction.

Venogram of the Kidneys

This relatively simple X-ray test examines the main kidney veins and their tributaries. In this test, the doctor injects a special dye through a catheter placed in a blood vessel in the groin area. The dye possesses properties that cause it to appear on X-rays, which are taken when the dye reaches the kidney veins.

Why is this test done?
A venogram of the kidneys may be performed for the following reasons:
- To permit X-ray examination of the renal veins
- To detect renal vein thrombosis
- To evaluate kidney vein compression from tumors or retroperitoneal fibrosis
- To distinguish kidney disease and aneurysms from pressure exerted by an adjacent mass
- To evaluate kidney tumors and detect invasion of the kidney vein or inferior vena cava
- To detect kidney vein anomalies and defects
- To differentiate renal agenesis (absence of a kidney) from an undersized kidney
- To collect blood samples from the kidney to check for renovascular hypertension.

In preparation for these relatively simple X-rays, you'll need to fast for 4 hours and, possibly, follow a low-salt diet.

What should you know before the test?
- You'll learn about the test, including who will perform it, where it will take place, and its expected duration (about 1 hour). During the

test, a catheter will be inserted into a vein in the groin area after you receive a sedative and a local anesthetic.

- You may feel mild discomfort during injection of the local anesthetic and a brief sensation of burning and warmth and a metallic taste in your mouth from the injection of the dye. During the test, the X-ray machine will make loud, clacking sounds.

- Tell the doctor or the nurse if you have a blood clotting disorder. Also mention if you have any allergies to shellfish (such as shrimp or scallops), iodine, or the dyes used in other diagnostic tests.

- For 4 hours before the test, you'll need to fast. However, if a blood sample will be taken as part of the test, you may need to follow a low-salt diet. You may also be instructed to temporarily stop taking any drugs for high blood pressure or, for women, oral contraceptives.

- You may receive a sedative before the test.

- You'll need to sign a form that gives your consent to perform the test. Be sure to read this form carefully and ask questions if you don't understand any portion of it.

What happens during the test?

- You lie on your back on the X-ray table. The skin over the right femoral vein near the groin is cleaned with antiseptic solution and draped.

- After injecting the local anesthetic, the doctor inserts a catheter into the femoral vein. Next, the doctor advances the catheter to the right kidney vein and injects the test dye. X-rays are taken.

- When studies of the right-side veins are completed, the doctor moves the catheter to the left kidney vein. More X-rays are taken.

- Next, the doctor may collect a blood sample from the kidney for testing. Then, the doctor removes the catheter, applies pressure to the site for 15 minutes, and applies a dressing.

What happens after the test?

- A nurse will check on you roughly every 15 minutes for 1 hour, then every 30 minutes for 2 hours. The nurse will also check the dressing to make sure too much bleeding doesn't occur. You'll be given pain medication and antibiotics.

- Tell the nurse if you don't feel well, especially if you have chills, feel hot, have trouble breathing, or feel pain.

Does the test have risks?

The test shouldn't be performed on a person with severe thrombosis of the kidney vein.

> *When studies of the right-side veins are completed, the doctor moves the catheter to the left kidney vein. More X-rays are taken.*

What are the normal results?

After injection of the dye, the kidney vein and tributaries should appear coated and have no abnormalities.

What do abnormal results mean?

The test can detect blockage of the kidney vein, tumors, and various venous anomalies, such as a missing kidney vein.

Lab tests of the kidney blood sample may indicate renovascular hypertension.

VOIDING CYSTOURETHROGRAPHY

This X-ray test examines the bladder and urethra after injection of a special dye through a catheter into the bladder. The dye contains special properties that allow it to be seen on X-rays, which are taken with the person in various positions. X-rays are also taken at the end of the test, during urination.

Why is this test done?

Voiding cystourethrography may be performed for the following reasons:
- To detect certain abnormalities of the bladder and urethra, such as vesicoureteral reflux, neurogenic bladder, an enlarged prostate, or diverticula
- To investigate recurrent urinary tract infection
- To investigate a suspected congenital anomaly of the lower urinary tract, abnormal bladder emptying, and loss of control over urination
- To evaluate an enlarged prostate, a narrowed urethra, and the degree of urinary impairment in men from a narrowed urethra.

What should you know before the test?

- You'll learn about the test, including who will perform it, where it will take place, and its expected duration (about 30 to 45 minutes).
- Tell the doctor or the nurse if you have a blood clotting disorder. Also mention if you have any allergies to shellfish (such as shrimp or scallops), iodine, or the dyes used in other diagnostic tests.
- You won't need to fast before the test.

- You'll need to sign a form that gives your consent to perform the test. Be sure to read this form carefully and ask questions if you don't understand any portion of it.

What happens during the test?

- You lie on your back on the examining table, and a catheter is inserted into the bladder.
- The doctor instills the dye through the catheter until the bladder is full. You may experience a feeling of fullness and an urge to urinate. Next, the doctor clamps the catheter and takes X-rays as you change positions.
- After the doctor removes the catheter, you change position again and urinate. During urination, the doctor takes four high-speed X-rays of the bladder and urethra.

What happens after the test?

- Drink lots of fluids to reduce burning on urination and to flush out any residual dye. The nurse will check the time, color, and volume of your urination.
- Tell the nurse if you feel hot or have chills.

Does the test have risks?

- Voiding cystourethrography shouldn't be performed if the person has a severe urethral or bladder infection, or a severe urethral injury.
- Men should wear a lead shield over their testicles to prevent radiation exposure during the test. Unfortunately, a woman's ovaries can't be shielded without blocking the bladder.

What are the normal results?

The structure and function of the bladder and urethra should be normal. There should be no regurgitation of dye into the ureters.

What do abnormal results mean?

The test may show urethral stricture, vesical or urethral diverticula, ureterocele, an enlarged prostate, vesicoureteral reflux, or neurogenic bladder. The severity and location of these conditions are then evaluated to determine whether surgery is necessary.

WHITAKER TEST OF KIDNEY FUNCTION

Also called a *pressure study* or *flow study,* this test evaluates kidney function. It combines X-rays with measurements of pressure and flow in the kidneys and ureters. (See *How the Whitaker test helps detect kidney blockage,* page 70.)

Why is this test done?

The Whitaker test may be performed for the following reasons:
- To detect a kidney blockage and to help determine if surgery is needed
- To further evaluate a blockage after other tests are done.

What should you know before the test?

- You'll learn about the test, including who will perform it, where it will take place, and its expected duration (about 1 hour).
- You may feel may feel some discomfort during insertion of the urethral catheter and injection of the local anesthetic and a brief sensation of warmth and burning after injection of the dye. During the test, the X-ray machine will make loud, clacking sounds.
- Tell the doctor or the nurse if you have a blood clotting disorder. Also mention if you have any allergies to shellfish (such as shrimp or scallops), iodine, or the dyes used in other diagnostic tests.
- For at least 4 hours before the test, you'll need to fast.
- You'll put on a hospital gown and be asked to remove all jewelry or other metal objects that may obscure the X-rays.
- Just before the test, you'll receive a sedative and antibiotics. The nurse will tell you to urinate.
- You'll be asked to sign a consent form.

What happens during the test?

- You lie on your back on an X-ray table.
- To prepare for measurement of bladder pressure, the doctor inserts a catheter through the urethra into the bladder.
- The doctor takes an X-ray of the urinary tract and then connects the catheter to a pressure-measuring device called a *manometer.*
- The doctor injects the dye into a vein. After a brief wait, the doctor injects a local anesthetic and makes a small incision to insert a cannula into the kidney.

How the Whitaker test helps detect kidney blockage

In the Whitaker test, many X-rays are taken of the upper urinary tract. X-ray results are compared with measurements of kidney and bladder pressures to detect evidence of blockages.

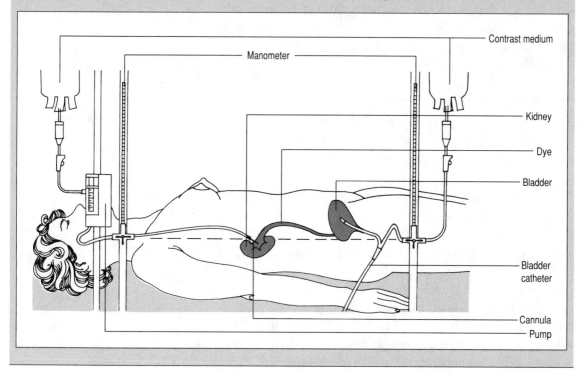

- You'll be asked to hold your breath as the doctor inserts the cannula into the kidney. Next, the doctor connects the tubing to the manometer.
- Now the doctor delivers the dye through the tubing as serial X-rays are taken and kidney pressure is measured. Bladder pressure is then measured.
- After the pressures are measured, the doctor removes the cannula and applies a dressing.

What happens after the test?
- You'll lie in bed on your back for 12 hours after the test.
- The nurse will check on you often, watching the color, frequency, and amount of urination. Some blood in the urine will appear for a brief time.
- Tell the nurse if you have chills, feel hot, or are breathing more rapidly than usual.

- Tell the nurse if you feel any pain. If you do, the nurse will give you pain medication. You'll also take antibiotics for several days to prevent infection.

Does the test have risks?

The test shouldn't be done if a person has a bleeding disorder or severe infection.

What are the normal results?

The test should show normal outlines of the kidneys. The ureters should fill uniformly and appear normal in size and course.

The normal kidney pressure is 15 centimeters of water. The normal bladder pressure ranges from 5 to 10 centimeters of water.

What do abnormal results mean?

Enlargement of the renal pelvis, calyces, or ureteropelvic junction may indicate obstruction. Subtraction of bladder pressure from kidney pressure aids diagnosis. A difference in pressure of 12 to 15 centimeters of water indicates obstruction. A difference of less than 10 centimeters of water indicates a bladder problem, such as hypertonia or neurogenic bladder.

REPRODUCTIVE SYSTEM

MAMMOGRAPHY

This commonly performed X-ray helps to detect breast cysts or cancer. Mammography can detect 90% to 95% of breast cancers. However, a biopsy of suspicious areas may be required to confirm cancer. (See *How to examine your breasts,* pages 72 and 73, and *Using light and sound to detect breast cancer,* page 74.)

If a significant breast lump is present, a mammogram may be done even during pregnancy. A lead shield placed over the mother's abdomen protects the fetus.

(Text continues on page 74.)

How to examine your breasts

Women themselves discover about 90% of breast cancers by using breast self-examination techniques. It's best to examine your breasts once a month. If you haven't reached menopause, the best examination time is immediately after your menstrual period. If you're past menopause, choose any convenient, easy-to-remember day each month — the first of the month, for example. Here's how to proceed.

1 Undress to the waist, and stand or sit in front of a mirror with your arms at your sides. Observe your breasts for any change in their shape or size. Look for any puckering or dimpling of the skin.

2 Raise your arms and press your hands together behind your head. Observe your breasts as before.

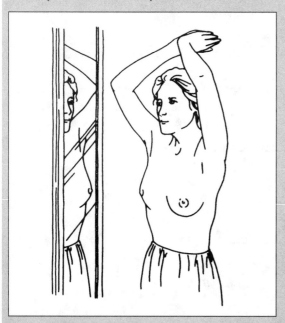

3 Press your palms firmly on your hips and observe your breasts again.

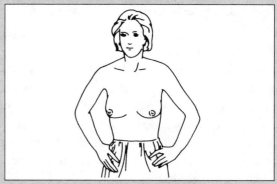

4 Now lie flat on your back. This position flattens and spreads your breasts more evenly over the chest wall. Place a small pillow under your left shoulder, and put your left hand behind your head.

5 Examine your left breast with your right hand, using a circular motion and progressing clockwise. You'll notice a ridge of firm tissue in the lower curve of your breast; this is normal. Now, repeat steps five and six on your right breast.

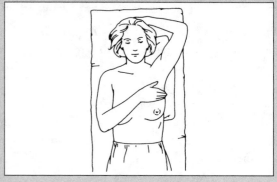

6 Check the area under your arm with your elbow slightly bent. If you feel a small lump that moves freely under your armpit, don't be alarmed. This area contains your lymph glands, which may become swollen when you're sick. Check the lump daily. Call the doctor if it doesn't go away in a few days or if it gets larger.

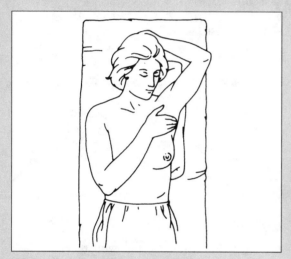

7 Gently squeeze your nipple between your thumb and forefinger, and note any discharge. Repeat this examination on your right breast, using your left hand.

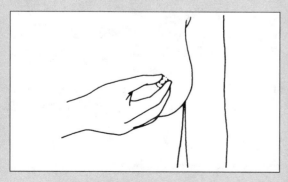

8 Finally, examine your breasts while you're in the shower or bath, lubricating your breasts with soap and water. Using the same circular, clockwise motion, gently inspect both breasts with your fingertips. After you've toweled dry, squeeze each nipple gently, and note any discharge.

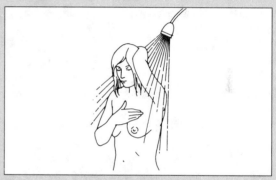

9 If you feel a lump, don't panic — most lumps aren't cancerous. First, note whether you can easily lift the skin covering it and whether the lump moves when you do so.

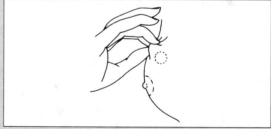

Next, notify your doctor. Be prepared to describe how the lump feels (hard or soft) and whether it moves easily under the skin.

Chances are, your doctor will want to examine the lump. Then he or she can advise you about what treatment (if any) you need.

Although self-examination is important, it's not a substitute for examination by your doctor. Be sure to see him or her annually or semiannually (if you're considered at risk.)

Using light and sound to detect breast cancer

Two noninvasive tests that don't require X-rays allow safe, early detection of cancer and other breast diseases. In most cases, their diagnostic accuracy isn't as high as that of conventional mammography, but they can be repeated as often as needed without risk.

Diaphanography: The light approach

Also known as *transillumination of the breast,* diaphanography directs infrared light through the breast with a fiber-optic device, and the transmitted light is photographed with infrared film. The denser the tissue, the darker it appears on the film, which allows a trained examiner to make the following observations:

- Healthy breast tissue appears reddish yellow and translucent.
- Fluid-filled cysts and fatty tissue appear as bright spots.
- Blood vessels are dark red to black.
- Benign tumors are red.
- Malignant tumors are dark brown or black.
  Diaphanography is a useful tool when used with mammography and a physical exam.

Ultrasonography: A sound technique

This test can detect breast tumors that are less than a quarter-inch in diameter. It can also help distinguish cysts from solid tumors. A transducer focuses a beam of high-frequency sound waves through the skin and into the breast. These waves then bounce back to the transducer as an echo that varies in strength with the density of the underlying tissues. A computer processes these echoes and displays a screen image of them.

Ultrasound can show all areas of a breast, including the difficult area close to the chest wall, which is hard to study with X-rays. When used with mammography, the technique increases diagnostic accuracy. When used alone, it's more accurate than mammography in examining the denser breast tissue of young women.

Why is this test done?

Mammography may be performed for the following reasons:

- To check for breast cancer
- To investigate breast masses, breast pain, or nipple discharge
- To help differentiate between benign breast disease and breast cancer.

What should you know before the test?

- You'll learn who will perform the test and where. The test takes only about 15 minutes to perform, but you may be asked to wait while the films are checked to make sure they're readable.
- Just before the test, you'll put on a hospital gown that opens in the front and be asked to remove all jewelry and clothing above the waist.

What happens during the test?

- You stand up and are asked to rest one breast on a table above an X-ray cassette.

▪ The compression plate is placed on the breast, and you're asked to hold your breath. After one X-ray is taken, the machine is rotated, the breast is compressed again, and another X-ray is taken.
▪ The procedure is repeated on the other breast.
▪ After the X-ray films are developed, they're checked to make sure they're readable.

What are the normal results?

A mammogram should reveal normal ducts, glandular tissue, and fat architecture. No abnormal masses should be seen.

What do abnormal results mean?

Well-outlined, regular, and clear spots on a mammogram suggest benign cysts. Irregular, poorly outlined, and opaque areas suggest cancer. However, before the doctor can make a diagnosis, additional mammograms may be necessary. A biopsy may also be needed.

X-RAYS OF THE UTERUS AND FALLOPIAN TUBES

This type of X-ray is called a *hysterosalpingography*. It assists with examination of the uterus, the fallopian tubes, and the surrounding structures. In this test, X-rays are taken after the doctor injects a special dye that flows through the uterus and the fallopian tubes. The dye possesses properties that allow it to appear on X-rays.

X-rays of the uterus and fallopian tubes are generally taken as part of an infertility study. Although ultrasound tests have virtually replaced this test in detecting foreign bodies, such as a dislodged intrauterine device, they can't evaluate tubal patency, which is the main purpose of this test.

Why is this test done?

This test may be performed for the following reasons:
▪ To confirm tubal abnormalities, such as adhesions and occlusion
▪ To confirm uterine abnormalities, such as the presence of foreign bodies, congenital malformations, and traumatic injuries
▪ To confirm the presence of fistulas or peritubal adhesions
▪ To help evaluate repeated fetal loss

- To check the outcome of surgery, especially uterine repair procedures and tubal reconstruction.

What should you know before the test?

- You'll learn about the test, including who will perform it and where, and that it takes about 15 minutes.
- Tell the doctor or the nurse if you have a blood clotting disorder. Also mention if you have any allergies to shellfish (such as shrimp or scallops), iodine, or the dyes used in other diagnostic tests.
- Be prepared to feel moderate cramping from the procedure. You can receive a mild sedative.
- You'll need to sign a form that gives your consent to perform the test. Be sure to read this form carefully and ask questions if you don't understand any portion of it.

What happens during the test?

- You lie on the examination table with your feet in stirrups. The doctor inserts a speculum into the vagina and cleans the cervix.
- Next, the doctor inserts a catheter into the cervix and injects dye through it. X-rays are then taken.

What happens after the test?

- Tell the nurse if you feel hot or have any pain.
- Any cramps, nausea, and dizziness should go away.

Normally, X-rays reveal a symmetrical uterine cavity, and the dye courses through fallopian tubes of normal caliber.

Does the test have risks?

- This test shouldn't be performed on menstruating women or on women with undiagnosed vaginal bleeding or pelvic inflammatory disease.
- The test can cause uterine perforation and exposure to potentially harmful radiation.

What are the normal results?

Normally, X-rays reveal a symmetrical uterine cavity. The dye courses through fallopian tubes of normal caliber, spills freely into the peritoneal cavity, and doesn't leak from the uterus.

What do abnormal results mean?

An asymmetrical uterus on the X-rays suggests intrauterine adhesions or masses, such as fibroids or foreign bodies. Impaired flow of the dye through the fallopian tubes suggests partial or complete blockage. Leakage of the dye through the uterine wall suggests fistulas. Laparoscopy (insertion of a small fiber-optic telescope) with instillation of contrast dye may help confirm findings.

SKELETAL SYSTEM

X-RAYS OF THE VERTEBRAE

The test permits examination of all or part of the spinal column. A commonly performed test, it's used to evaluate the vertebrae for deformities, fractures, dislocations, tumors, and other abnormalities. Bone X-rays determine bone density, texture, erosion, and changes in bone relationships. Joint X-rays can reveal the presence of fluid, spur formation, narrowing, and changes in the joint structure.

Why is this test done?
X-rays of the vertebrae may be performed for the following reasons:
- To detect fractures, dislocations, subluxations, and deformities
- To detect degeneration, infection, and congenital disorders
- To detect disorders of the intervertebral disks
- To determine the effects of arthritis and other conditions on the vertebrae.

What should you know before the test?
- You'll learn about the test, including who will perform the test and where and that it usually takes 15 to 30 minutes. During the test, you'll be placed in various positions for the X-ray films. Although some positions may be slightly uncomfortable, try to stay still. If you can't, the test may not be accurate.
- You won't need to fast before the test.

What happens during the test?
- Initially, you lie on your back on the table for an X-ray taken from front to back.
- You may be repositioned on your side for additional X-rays, depending on the vertebrae being tested.

What happens after the test?

You'll receive pain medications and a heating pad to relieve any discomfort.

Does the test have risks?

X-rays of the vertebrae shouldn't be performed for a woman in the first 3 months of pregnancy, unless the benefits outweigh the risks of exposing the fetus to X-rays.

What are the normal results?

Normal vertebrae show no fractures, dislocations, curvatures, or other abnormalities. Specific positions and spacing of the vertebrae vary with the person's age.

What do abnormal results mean?

The X-rays readily show vertebral displacements, fractures, dislocations, wedging, and such deformities as kyphosis, scoliosis, and lordosis. Information from the test may be used to help confirm diagnosis of a variety of disorders. These disorders include congenital abnormalities, such as torticollis (wryneck), absence of sacral or lumbar vertebrae, hemivertebrae, and Klippel-Feil syndrome; degenerative processes, such as osteoarthritis and narrowed disk spaces; benign or malignant spinal tumors; ruptured disk and cervical disk syndrome; and rheumatoid arthritis, ankylosing spondylitis, osteoporosis, and Paget's disease.

Depending on X-ray results, a definite diagnosis may require additional tests, such as a computed tomography (CAT) scan.

X-RAYS OF THE JOINTS

This X-ray test, called *arthrography*, examines a joint after the injection of a special dye, air, or both to outline soft-tissue structures and the contour of the joint. The joint is put through its range of motion while a series of X-rays are taken. (See *Major movements of the knee joint.*)

This test is usually done if a person complains of lasting, unexplained joint discomfort or pain.

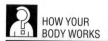

HOW YOUR
BODY WORKS

Major movements of the knee joint

The synovial knee joint moves in three chief directions: It can extend, flex, or rotate to the side.

During extension, both the collateral ligaments and the cruciate ligaments are tensed. During flexion, the collateral ligaments are relaxed while the cruciate ligaments are tensed. During medial rotation, the collateral and cruciate ligaments are twisted.

EXTENSION   **FLEXION**   **MEDIAL ROTATION**

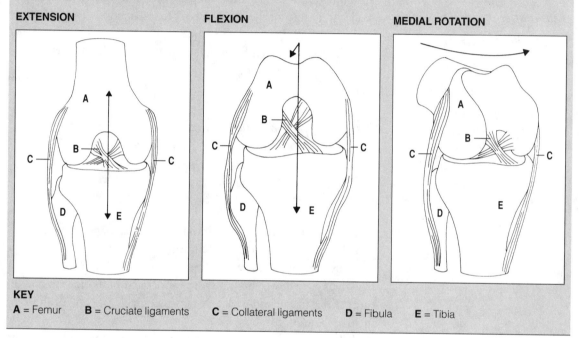

KEY
A = Femur   **B** = Cruciate ligaments   **C** = Collateral ligaments   **D** = Fibula   **E** = Tibia

Why is this test done?

X-rays of the joints may be taken for the following reasons:
- To identify acute or chronic tears or other abnormalities of the joint capsule or supporting ligaments of the knee, shoulder, ankle, hips, or wrist
- To detect internal joint derangements
- To locate synovial cysts.

What should you know before the test?

- You'll learn about the test, including who will perform it, where it will take place, and its expected duration.
- You may feel mild discomfort during injection of the local anesthetic and a brief sensation of burning and warmth and a metallic

The doctor examines a joint after the injection of a special dye, air, or both to outline soft-tissue structures and the contour of the joint.

taste in your mouth from the injection of the dye. During the test, the doctor will track the test dye as it fills the joint space and will take X-rays.

▪ You'll need to remain as still as possible during the procedure, except when following instructions to change position. Your cooperation in assuming various positions is critical because X-rays must be taken quickly to ensure good quality.

▪ Tell the doctor or the nurse if you have a blood clotting disorder. Also mention if you have any allergies to shellfish (such as shrimp or scallops), iodine, or the dyes used in other diagnostic tests.

▪ You won't need to fast before the test.

▪ You'll need to sign a form that gives your consent to perform the test. Be sure to read this form carefully and ask questions if you don't understand any portion of it.

What happens during the test?

The test may be performed on the knee or the shoulder.

Knee arthrography

▪ The knee is cleaned with an antiseptic solution, and the area around the puncture site is anesthetized.

▪ The doctor inserts a needle into the joint space and removes fluid, which is usually sent to a lab for testing.

▪ Next, the doctor injects dye into the joint. You're asked to walk a few steps or to move your knee through a range of motions to distribute the dye in the joint space. X-rays are quickly taken with the knee held in various positions.

▪ If the X-rays show no problems, the knee is bandaged. Keep the bandage in place for several days.

Shoulder arthrography

▪ The skin is prepared, and a local anesthetic is injected. The doctor inserts a needle into the joint and injects dye.

▪ X-rays are taken quickly to achieve maximum contrast.

What happens after the test?

▪ You'll need to rest the joint for at least 12 hours.

▪ You may experience some swelling or discomfort or may hear noises in the joint after the test, but these symptoms usually disappear after 1 or 2 days. Report persistent symptoms.

▪ Apply ice to the joint if swelling occurs and take aspirin or Tylenol (or another brand of acetaminophen) for pain.

Does the test have risks?

- This test shouldn't be performed on a pregnant woman.
- It also shouldn't be performed on a person with arthritis, joint infection, or allergies to the test dye.

What are the normal results?

A normal knee arthrogram shows a characteristic wedge-shaped shadow, pointed toward the interior of the joint, that indicates a normal medial meniscus (cartilage). A normal shoulder arthrogram shows that the bicipital tendon sheath, redundant inferior joint capsule, and subscapular bursa (lubricating sac) are intact.

What do abnormal results mean?

X-rays of the joints almost always accurately detect medial meniscal tears and lacerations. They may also help identify extrameniscal lesions, such as osteochondritis dissecans, chondromalacia patellae, osteochondral fractures, cartilaginous abnormalities, synovial abnormalities, tears of the cruciate ligaments, and disruption of the joint capsule and collateral ligaments.

This test can reveal shoulder abnormalities, such as adhesive capsulitis, bicipital tenosynovitis or rupture, and rotator cuff tears, and can evaluate damage from recurrent dislocations.

LYMPH NODES

ANGIOGRAM OF THE LYMPH NODES

This test examines the lymphatic system (see *The lymphatic system: Its structure and function,* page 82). It involves a series of X-rays taken after the doctor injects a special dye into a lymphatic vessel in each foot or, less commonly, in each hand. Another name for this test is *lymphangiography*.

Dye injected into the foot lets the doctor examine the lymphatics of the leg, inguinal and iliac regions, and the retroperitoneum up to the thoracic duct. Injection into the hand allows examination of the axillary and supraclavicular nodes.

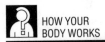

HOW YOUR
BODY WORKS

The lymphatic system: Its structure and function

The lymphatic system does many important jobs:
- It transports fluids and proteins to the veins.
- It produces some of the white blood cells that fight infection and provide other immune defenses.
- It reabsorbs fats from the small intestine.

Structure of the lymphatic system

The system includes the lymphatic vessels, lymph nodes, lymphoid tissue, blood cells called lymphocytes, and reticuloendothelial cells.

Lymphatic vessels, which are like veins, eventually converge into one of two main ducts — the thoracic or right lymphatic. The thoracic duct drains the legs, the pelvis, the abdomen, and the left arm (the white area of the diagram below) as well as the left side of the head, neck, and chest. The right lymphatic duct drains the right side of the head, neck, and chest and the right arm (the shaded area of the diagram). The two ducts then empty into the veins.

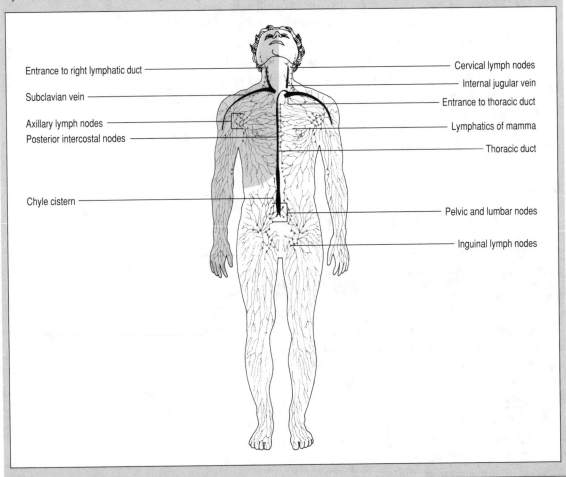

Entrance to right lymphatic duct

Subclavian vein

Axillary lymph nodes
Posterior intercostal nodes

Chyle cistern

Cervical lymph nodes
Internal jugular vein
Entrance to thoracic duct
Lymphatics of mamma
Thoracic duct

Pelvic and lumbar nodes

Inguinal lymph nodes

X-rays are taken immediately after injection to show the filling of the lymphatic system and then again 24 hours later to examine the lymph nodes. Because the dye remains in the nodes for up to 2 years, subsequent X-rays can also be taken.

Why is this test done?

An angiogram of the lymph nodes may be performed for the following reasons:

- To detect and stage lymphomas and to identify the spread of cancer to the lymph nodes
- To suggest surgical treatment or evaluate the effectiveness of chemotherapy and radiation therapy in controlling cancer
- To investigate enlarged lymph nodes that have been detected by a computed tomography (CAT) scan or ultrasound.

What should you know before the test?

- You'll learn about the test, including who will perform this procedure and where and that it takes about 3 hours. Additional X-rays are also taken the following day, but these take less than 30 minutes.
- You'll learn about the blue dye that will be injected into each foot to outline the lymphatic vessels. The injection causes brief discomfort, but the dye discolors urine and stools for 48 hours and may give your skin and vision a bluish tinge for 48 hours.
- A local anesthetic will be injected before a small incision is made in each foot. The dye is then injected for the next 1½ hours using a cannula inserted into a lymphatic vessel. You must remain as still as possible during injection of the dye.
- Tell the doctor or the nurse if you have allergies to shellfish (such as shrimp or scallops), iodine, or the dyes used in other diagnostic tests.
- If this test is performed on an outpatient basis, have a friend or relative accompany you.
- Just before the test, you should urinate. You may receive a sedative and other medication.
- You'll need to sign a form that gives your consent to perform the test. Be sure to read this form carefully and ask questions if you don't understand any portion of it.

What happens during the test?

- A preliminary X-ray of the chest is taken, and the skin on each foot is cleaned with an antiseptic.

- The doctor injects a blue dye into the area between the toes, usually the first and fourth toe webs.
- The dye infiltrates the lymphatic system and, within 15 to 30 minutes, the lymphatic vessels appear as small blue lines on the upper surface of the instep of each foot.
- The doctor injects a local anesthetic into each foot and makes a small incision to expose the lymphatic vessel. Next, the doctor inserts a cannula into the vessel and slowly delivers the dye. Fluoroscopy may be used to monitor filling of the lymphatic system.
- The needles are removed, the incisions stitched, and sterile dressings applied.
- X-rays are taken of the legs, pelvis, abdomen, and chest.
- You are then taken to your room but must return 24 hours later for additional X-rays.

What happens after the test?

- You'll be checked on often. Tell the nurse if you feel short of breath, have chest pains, or feel warm.
- You'll stay in bed for 24 hours with your feet elevated to help reduce swelling. The nurse will apply ice packs to the incision sites to help reduce swelling and will give you pain medication.
- The incision site may be sore for several days after the test. The dressings usually remain in place for 2 days, making sure the wounds stay dry.
- You'll be given a follow-up X-ray, as needed.

Does the test have risks?

This test shouldn't be performed on a person with an allergy to the test dye, breathing problems, heart disease, or severe kidney or liver disease.

What are the normal results?

The lymphatic system normally fills fully and evenly with dye on the initial X-rays. On the 24-hour X-rays, the lymph nodes are fully opacified and well circumscribed.

What do abnormal results mean?

Enlarged, foamy-looking nodes indicate lymphoma, a type of cancer that originates in the lymphatic system. Other tests are needed to stage the cancer.

2

CAT & MRI SCANS:
Diagnosing with
High-Tech Help

BRAIN & SPINE

CAT SCAN OF THE BRAIN

Doctors use a CAT scan (short for a computed tomography scan) to study an area of the body, such as the brain, in much greater detail than they could by using conventional X-rays. In a CAT scan, a narrow X-ray beam is directed at the brain; at the same time, a scintillation counter, located exactly opposite the X-ray source, measures the amount of radiation that's unabsorbed as it passes through the skull and brain tissues. As the X-ray source and the scintillation counter revolve around the person's head, data from the counter is processed by a computer to create images of various sections of the brain, which are then displayed on a computer monitor.

Tumors and other brain lesions, or tissue damage, show up as areas of altered density. A CAT scan of the brain may eliminate the need for other procedures that can be painful and hazardous.

Another emerging test for obtaining detailed images of the brain is positron emission tomography. (See *Positron emission tomography: New insights into brain function.*)

Why is this test done?
A CAT scan of the brain may be performed for the following reasons:
- To check the brain's function
- To find tumors and abnormalities within the brain
- To monitor the effects of surgery, radiotherapy, or chemotherapy on brain tumors
- To detect possible blood clots after a head injury.

What should you know before the test?
- There are usually no dietary restrictions before the test. However, if a contrast dye will be used during the test, you'll be asked to fast for 4 hours before the test.
- A contrast dye — a special substance that enhances the images of the brain — may be used. You may feel flushed and warm and may experience a brief headache, a salty taste, or nausea and vomiting after this dye is injected.

Positron emission tomography: New insights into brain function

Positron emission tomography (also known by the acronym PET) is a technique for viewing the brain without surgery. Positron emission tomography produces sophisticated computer-generated images showing the details of brain function as well as brain structures.

How it works
Positron emission tomography involves the use of the radioactive forms of certain elements — oxygen, nitrogen, carbon, and fluorine — which emit tiny particles called *positrons*.

During the test, a device called a *positron emission tomography scanner* detects radiation and relays the information to a computer. The computer translates the information into an image. Positron-emitters can be used as chemical "tags" to trace the fate of various metabolites in the brain. For example, chemically tagged glucose — a form of sugar that penetrates the brain rapidly — allows the study of brain function because positron emission tomography can pinpoint glucose in the brain under various conditions.

Uses and limitations
Researchers expect this test to be useful in diagnosing many problems, such as psychiatric disorders, Parkinson's disease, MS, seizure disorders, and Alzheimer's disease.

Positron emission tomography is a costly test that has limited use, except as a research tool. However, it has already provided valuable information about the brain and may someday be widely used.

- This test involves taking a series of X-ray films of your brain. The test causes very little discomfort and lasts 15 to 30 minutes.
- A nurse or technician will explain the procedure to you.
- Your medical history will be checked for past allergic reactions to shellfish, iodine, or certain dyes.
- You may be asked to wear a hospital gown or any comfortable clothing and to remove all metal objects from the CAT scan field.
- You'll be asked to sign a consent form before the test takes place.

What happens during the test?
- You're asked to lie still on a special table; your head is held gently in place by straps and your face is left uncovered.
- The head of the table is moved into the scanner. The scanner rotates around your head, taking X-rays. It makes clacking sounds.
- If contrast dye is used, another series of scans is taken after the dye is injected and is taken up by the appropriate area of the brain.
- Information from the scans is fed into a computer and converted into images on a monitor. Photographs of selected views are taken for further study.

What happens after the test?

- If contrast dye was used, you're watched for side effects such as headache, nausea, and vomiting. You'll also be monitored for reactions such as hives, rash, or difficulty breathing. Reactions usually develop within 30 minutes.
- You may resume your usual diet.

Does the test have risks?

A pregnant woman should not undergo a CAT scan of the brain with contrast dye, especially during the first 3 months. People who are allergic to iodine or the contrast dye should also avoid the procedure.

What are the normal results?

The density of brain tissue affects its appearance on the scan. Brain tissue may appear as white, black, or shades of gray. The doctor evaluates structures according to their density, size, shape, and position.

What do abnormal results mean?

Displaced tissues or areas of altered density may indicate a tumor, blood clot, cerebral damage, infarction, swelling, or hydrocephalus.

CAT SCAN OF THE SPINE

This test provides detailed, high-resolution images of the spine. During the procedure, multiple X-ray beams are directed at the spine from different angles. X-rays pass through the body and are intercepted by radiation detectors, which produce electrical impulses that are converted by a computer into three-dimensional images. These images are displayed on a video monitor.

Why is this test done?

A CAT scan of the spine may be performed for the following reasons:
- To allow visualization of the spine
- To diagnose spinal lesions, tissue damage, and other abnormalities
- To monitor the effects of spinal surgery or therapy.

What should you know before the test?

- If contrast dye isn't ordered, you don't need to restrict food or fluids. If contrast dye is ordered, you'll be asked to fast for 4 hours before the test.
- A nurse or technician will describe the procedure, which takes 30 to 60 minutes.
- The procedure is painless, but having to remain still for a prolonged period may be slightly uncomfortable.
- If contrast dye is used, you may feel flushed and warm and may experience a brief headache, a salty taste, and nausea or vomiting after injection of the contrast dye. These reactions are normal.
- During the test, you'll be asked to wear an examining gown and to remove all metal objects and jewelry.
- Your history will be checked for past allergic reactions to iodine, shellfish, or contrast dye. If such reactions have occurred, you may receive alternative medications or the test may be performed without contrast dye.
- If you seem restless or apprehensive about the procedure, the doctor may prescribe a mild sedative.
- You'll be asked to sign a consent form before the test takes place.

You're positioned on an X-ray table inside a body scanning unit. The table slides into an opening and the scanner revolves around you, taking images at preselected intervals.

What happens during the test?

- You're positioned on an X-ray table inside a body CAT scanning unit and asked to lie very still.
- The table slides into the circular opening of the CAT scanner and the scanner revolves around you, taking images at preselected intervals.
- After the first set of scans is taken, you're removed from the scanner. Contrast dye may be administered.
- You're observed for signs and symptoms of a hypersensitivity reaction — including hives, rash, and respiratory difficulty — for 30 minutes after the contrast dye has been injected.
- After the dye is injected, you're moved back into the scanner, and another series of scans is taken. The images obtained from the scan are displayed on a video monitor during the procedure and stored on magnetic tape.

What happens after the test?

- After a scan with contrast dye, you'll be observed for side effects of the dye, such as headache, nausea, and vomiting.
- You may resume your usual diet.

Does the test have risks?

- CAT scanning with contrast dye is not recommended for a person who is hypersensitive to iodine, shellfish, or contrast dye used in radiographic studies.
- Some people experience strong feelings of claustrophobia or anxiety when they're inside the CAT scanner. A mild sedative may be given to help reduce the person's anxiety.
- For people with significant back pain, painkillers are prescribed before the scan.

What are the normal results?

In the computed tomography image, spinal tissue appears white, black, or gray, depending on its density.

What do abnormal results mean?

By highlighting areas of altered density and depicting structural malformations, a CAT scan can reveal different types of spinal tissue damage and abnormalities. It's particularly useful in detecting and identifying tumors. CAT scans also reveal degenerative processes and structural changes, such as spinal cord compression. Other types of disorders show as soft-tissue changes, bony overgrowth, and spurring of the vertebrae, which result in nerve root compression. Blood vessel malformations, evident after contrast dye, show as masses or clusters. Congenital spinal malformations, such as spina bifida, show as abnormally large, dark gaps between the vertebrae.

MRI SCAN OF THE BRAIN AND SPINE

MRI (which is the abbreviation for *magnetic resonance imaging*) produces computerized images of various sections of the brain and spine. These images are highly detailed. Unlike a CAT scan, which uses X-rays, an MRI scan uses magnetic fields and radio waves to produce images of the brain and spine. The magnetic fields and radio waves aren't noticed by the person undergoing the test, and no harmful effects have been reported.

The doctor uses an MRI scan to diagnose brain tumors, abscesses, swelling, bleeding, nerve damage, and other disorders that increase the fluid content of tissues. The test can also show irregularities of the spinal cord.

Why is this test done?

An MRI scan of the brain and spinal cord may be performed to diagnose brain and spinal tumors, tissue damage, or soft-tissue abnormalities.

What should you know before the test?

- This test takes up to 90 minutes to complete.
- Although MRI is painless and involves no exposure to radiation from the scanner, a radioactive contrast dye may be used. The contrast dye is injected, usually near the organ or tissue that is being observed.
- The opening for your head and body in most MRI scanners is small and deep. If you've ever experienced claustrophobia, you may need a sedative to help you relax before the test. Some of the newer MRI scanners, though, are transparent.
- During the test, you'll hear the scanner clicking, whirring, and thumping as it moves inside its housing.
- You'll be able to talk with the technician at all times during the test.
- You'll be asked to remove all metallic objects, including jewelry, hair pins, and watches. You'll also asked if you have any surgically implanted joints, pins, clips, valves, pumps, or pacemakers containing metal that could be attracted to the strong MRI magnet. If you do, you won't be able to undergo the test.
- You'll be asked to sign a consent form before the test takes place.

What happens during the test?

- You're asked to lie on a narrow bed, which then slides into the desired position inside the scanner. (See *Undergoing MRI.*)
- During the procedure you're asked to remain very still.
- The images that are generated are displayed on a monitor and recorded on film or magnetic tape for permanent storage; the radiologist may use the computer to manipulate and enhance the images.

What happens after the test?

- You may resume normal activity.
- If the test took a long time, you'll be watched for signs of lightheadedness or fainting when you sit or stand up.

Undergoing MRI

The illustration below shows a person being moved into an MRI, or magnetic resonance imaging, scanner. MRI is an imaging technique based on the response of various elements to a generated magnetic field and radio signal.

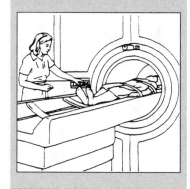

Does the test have risks?

▪ Because MRI works through the use of powerful magnets, it can't be performed on people with pacemakers, intracranial aneurysm clips, or other iron implants or on a person with gunshot wounds to the head.
▪ Because of the strong magnetic field, metallic or computer-based equipment — for example, ventilators — can't be used in the MRI area.

What are the normal results?

An MRI scan can distinctly show the brain and spine. Tissue color and shading vary, depending in part on the magnetic strength used and the amount of computer enhancement. MRI can detect nerve-related disorders, for example, MS.

What do abnormal results mean?

MRI clearly shows changes that result when water accumulates in an organ or tissue. Examples include certain brain tumors and disorders such as cerebral edema, in which fluid accumulates in the brain.

DIGESTIVE SYSTEM

CAT SCAN OF THE LIVER AND BILIARY TRACT

This test checks for problems in the biliary tract and liver. In a CAT scan (called *computed tomography* by doctors), a series of X-rays pass through the body and show differences in tissue densities. Images of the tissues appear on a computer screen. A special dye — called a *contrast medium* — may be given intravenously or by mouth to accentuate the images.

Why is this test done?

A CAT scan of the liver and biliary tract may be performed for the following reasons:
▪ To detect biliary tract and liver disease
▪ To distinguish between two types of jaundice
▪ To clarify previously detected defects
▪ To detect suspected blood clots after abdominal injury.

What should you know before the test?

- If you'll be receiving a contrast dye by mouth, you'll be asked to fast after midnight before the test. If a dye won't be used, fasting won't be necessary.
- If an intravenous contrast dye is used, you may experience slight discomfort from the needle puncture and a feeling of warmth on injection. Immediately report nausea, vomiting, dizziness, headache, and itching or hives.
- You'll be asked about any past allergies to iodine, shellfish, or the contrast dye used in other diagnostic tests.
- The test is painless and takes approximately 90 minutes to complete.
- A nurse or technician will explain the procedure before the test.
- You'll be told to remain very still during the test and to hold your breath at certain intervals.
- You'll be asked to sign a consent form before the test takes place.

What happens during the test?

- You're positioned on an adjustable table, which is moved into a scanning chamber.
- A series of X-ray films is taken and recorded. The information is reconstructed by a computer and appears as images on a monitor.
- These images are studied, and selected ones are photographed.
- The test may be repeated with contrast dye to enhance results. After the contrast dye is injected, a second series of films is taken.

What happens after the test?

- You'll be carefully observed for allergic reactions if contrast dye was used.
- You may resume your usual diet.

Does the test have risks?

- A CAT scan of the biliary tract and liver is usually not recommended during pregnancy.
- Use of an intravenous contrast dye is not recommended for people with allergies to iodine or with severe kidney or liver disease.

What are the normal results?

Normally, the liver has a uniform density that's slightly denser than the pancreas, kidneys, and spleen. Like the biliary ducts, the gallbladder is visible as a round or elliptical low-density structure. A contracted gallbladder may be impossible to visualize.

What do abnormal results mean?

Most liver defects appear as areas that are less dense than normal, and CAT scans can detect small defects. Some lesions have the same density as the liver and may be undetectable. Other defects may distort the liver or change the character of the biliary duct. Use of an intravenous contrast dye helps detect even slight biliary duct dilation.

Usually, a CAT scan can identify the cause of biliary obstructions. However, if an obstruction must be located before surgery, other tests may be performed as well.

CAT SCAN OF THE PANCREAS

During this test, a series of X-rays penetrate the upper abdomen and enable the doctor to distinguish different tissue thicknesses. Computerized images of the findings are then displayed on a monitor. A series of these cross-sectional images can provide a detailed look at the pancreas.

A CAT (computed tomography) scan may be used to distinguish the pancreas and surrounding organs and vessels if enough fat is present between the structures. A type of dye, called a *contrast medium,* may be given intravenously or orally to further accentuate differences in tissue density and clarify the images.

Why is this test done?

A CAT scan of the pancreas may be performed for the following reasons:
- To detect disorders of the pancreas, such as cancer or abnormal structures called *pseudocysts*
- To detect or evaluate pancreatitis.

What should you know before the test?

- You'll be asked to fast after midnight before the test.
- A nurse or technician will explain the procedure, which is painless.
- You'll be asked to remain still during the test and to periodically hold your breath.
- You may be given an intravenous or oral contrast dye, or both, to enhance images of the pancreas. Report side effects of the dye, such as nausea, flushing, dizziness, and sweating, to the doctor or nurse.

- Your medication history will be checked for recent barium studies and for past allergic reactions to iodine, shellfish, or contrast dye used in prior tests.
- If an oral contrast dye is used, it's given before the test.

What happens during the test?

- You're positioned on an adjustable table that is placed inside a scanning booth.
- A series of X-rays is taken and recorded. The information is reconstructed as images on a monitor. These images are studied, and selected ones are photographed.
- After the first series of X-rays is completed, the images are reviewed. Then contrast dye may be administered, followed by another series of X-rays. You're observed for allergic reactions, such as itching, blood pressure changes, sweating, or dizziness.

Changes in pancreatic size and shape help the doctor diagnose certain types of cancer.

What happens after the test?

After a CAT scan of the pancreas, you may resume your usual diet.

Does the test have risks?

A CAT scan of the pancreas should not be performed during pregnancy or, if a contrast dye is needed, on people with a history of allergic reactions to iodine or severe kidney or liver disease.

What are the normal results?

Usually, the pancreas has a uniform density, especially when an intravenous contrast dye is used. The gland normally thickens from its tail to its head and has a smooth surface.

Use of a contrast dye administered by mouth helps distinguish the stomach and duodenum and outlines the pancreas, particularly in people with little fat, such as children and thin adults.

What do abnormal results mean?

Because the tissue density of pancreatic cancer resembles normal tissue, changes in pancreatic size and shape help the doctor diagnose certain cancers and pseudocysts (abnormal or dilated cavities).

This test may also help the doctor to diagnose pancreatitis. Acute pancreatitis produces widespread enlargement of the pancreas. In chronic pancreatitis, the pancreas may appear normal, enlarged, or shrunken, depending on the severity of the disease.

SKELETON

CAT SCAN OF THE SKELETON

This test takes a series of X-ray images of the bones of the skeleton. A computer constructs these images into cross-sectional views, which are displayed on a monitor. (See *Understanding your bones and joints*.)

Special techniques — such as using dyes called *contrast media* — improve the resolution and accuracy of the images. Hundreds of thousands of readings may be combined to provide three-dimensional views of the bones.

Why is this test done?

A CAT scan of the skeleton may be performed for the following reasons:
- To allow the doctor to view the bones and joints
- To check for bone tumors, the spread of cancer through the skeleton, and soft-tissue tumors
- To diagnose joint abnormalities that are difficult to detect by other methods.

What should you know before the test?

- If a contrast dye isn't ordered, you don't need to restrict food or fluids before this test. If contrast dye is ordered, you'll be asked to fast for 4 hours before the test.
- The test takes 30 to 60 minutes and is painless.
- A nurse or technician will explain the procedure to you. You'll be asked to lie as still as possible during the test because movement may cause distorted images.
- If contrast dye is used, you may feel flushed and warm and may experience a brief headache, a salty taste, and nausea or vomiting after the injection. These reactions are normal.
- You'll be given a gown to wear and asked to remove all metal objects and jewelry that may appear in the X-ray field.
- You'll be asked to sign a consent form before the test.
- Your medical history will be checked for past allergic reactions to iodine, shellfish, or the contrast dye in previous tests. If you've had such reactions, your doctor may prescribe medications before the test or choose not to use a contrast dye.

If contrast dye is injected, you may feel flushed and warm and may have a brief headache, a salty taste, and nausea or vomiting. These reactions are normal.

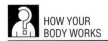

HOW YOUR
BODY WORKS

Understanding your bones and joints

There are 206 bones in the normal human body. They form an underlying supporting structure called the *skeleton*. Most bones are classified by shape.

- *Long bones* consist of a shaft and two bulbous ends. The parts of the shaft that flare to join the ends contain the bone's growth zones. Long bones are composed primarily of compact bone, which is strong and dense. Examples of long bones in the arms and legs are the humerus, radius, ulna, femur, tibia, fibula, phalanges, and metatarsals.
- *Short bones* consist mainly of cancellous — or spongy — bone with a thin, compact bone shell, and include the tarsal and carpal bones of the feet and hands.
- *Flat bones* have a large surface area and provide protection for soft body parts. They're made up of an inner layer of cancellous bone surrounded by compact bone. Examples are the bones of the skull over the brain area and the ribs, sternum, scapulae, ilium, and pubis, which form the torso.
- *Irregular bones* are of various shapes and composition and include bones of the spine and certain skull bones, such as those that make up the jaw.

Joints

Joints consist of two bones joined in various ways. Like bones, joints have several forms:
- Fibrous joints can move only slightly. This type of joint provides stability when a tight juncture is necessary. Examples of fibrous joints are the irregular "seams" between the bones of the skull.
- *Cartilaginous joints* allow limited movement. Examples of cartilaginous joints are those between the vertebrae, or bones of the spine.
- *Synovial joints* are the most common type. These joints allow angular and circular movement. To allow

freedom of movement, synovial joints have special characteristics: They're covered with a material called *cartilage* that resists pressure; where the bones meet, they glide smoothly on each other; and a fibrous capsule holds the joint together.

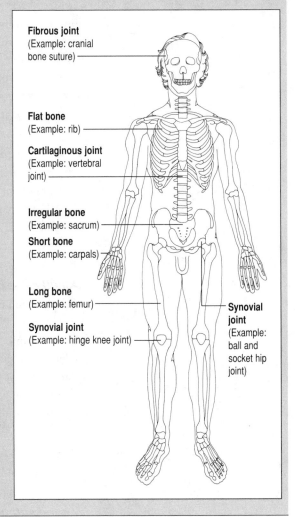

Fibrous joint
(Example: cranial bone suture)

Flat bone
(Example: rib)

Cartilaginous joint
(Example: vertebral joint)

Irregular bone
(Example: sacrum)

Short bone
(Example: carpals)

Long bone
(Example: femur)

Synovial joint
(Example: hinge knee joint)

Synovial joint
(Example: ball and socket hip joint)

- If you're restless or apprehensive about the procedure, a mild sedative may be prescribed.

What happens during the test?

- You're positioned on an X-ray table and asked to lie still.
- The table slides into the circular opening of the CAT scanner. The computer-controlled scanner revolves around you, taking multiple scans.
- After the first set of scans is taken, you're removed from the scanner and contrast dye is administered if necessary.
- You're observed for signs and symptoms of a hypersensitivity reaction — including itching, rash, and respiratory difficulty — for 30 minutes after the contrast dye is injected.
- After the dye is injected, you're moved back into the scanner, and another series of scans is taken. The images obtained from the scan are displayed on a video monitor during the procedure and stored on magnetic tape to create a permanent record for further study.

What happens after the test?

- If contrast dye was used, you'll be observed for a possible delayed allergic reaction and will be given appropriate treatment if necessary.
- You'll be encouraged to drink fluids to help eliminate the dye from your system.
- You may resume your usual activity level and diet following the test.

Does the test have risks?

- People who are allergic to iodine, shellfish, or contrast dye should not undergo a CAT scan with contrast enhancement.
- Some people may experience strong feelings of claustrophobia or anxiety when inside the CAT scan machine. For such people, a mild sedative may be ordered to help reduce anxiety.
- For a person with significant bone or joint pain, painkillers are given so the person can lie still comfortably during the scan.

What are the normal results?

The scan should reveal no problem in the bones or joints.

What do abnormal results mean?

Because it's able to display cross-sectional views of the body, CAT scanning is useful for assessing the shoulder, spine, hip, and pelvis. The scan can reveal some bone tumors and soft-tissue tumors as well as cancer that has spread from one part of the skeletal system to another. It can also reveal joint disorders that are difficult to detect by other tests.

MRI SCAN OF THE SKELETON

MRI stands for *magnetic resonance imaging*. This is a noninvasive diagnostic technique (a test in which nothing enters your body) that produces clear images of bone and soft tissue. MRI scans of the skeleton allow three-dimensional imaging of areas that can't be easily viewed with X-rays or CAT scans. It eliminates any risks associated with exposure to X-ray beams and causes no known harm to cells.

During an MRI, a powerful magnetic field is used to generate images of a person's bones on a monitor.

Why is this test done?
MRI of the skeleton may be performed for the following reasons:
- To check the bones and soft tissue
- To evaluate bone and soft-tissue tumors
- To identify changes in bone marrow composition
- To identify spinal disorders.

What should you know before the test?
- This test takes up to 90 minutes. Although MRI is painless and involves no exposure to radiation, a radioactive contrast dye may be used, depending on the type of tissue being studied.
- A nurse or technician will explain the procedure. You'll learn that the opening for your head and body in the MRI scanner is small and deep. If claustrophobia has ever been a problem for you, a sedative may help you to tolerate the scan.
- While being tested, you'll hear the scanner clicking, whirring, and thumping as it moves inside its housing. You'll be able to communicate with the technician at all times, though.
- You'll be asked to remove all metallic objects, including jewelry, hair pins, or watches before the test.

- Inform the technician if you have any surgically implanted joints, pins, clips, valves, pumps, or pacemakers containing metal. If you do, you won't be able to undergo this test.
- You'll be asked to sign a consent form before the test.

What happens during the test?

- At the scanner room door, you're checked one last time for metal objects.
- You're positioned on a narrow, padded table that moves into the scanner tunnel. Fans continuously circulate air in the tunnel, and a call bell or intercom is used to maintain verbal contact.
- You must remain still throughout the procedure.

What happens after the test?

- If the test has been prolonged, you're watched for signs of light-headedness or fainting when you stand or sit up.
- You may resume normal activity after the test.

Does the test have risks?

- MRI can't be performed on people with pacemakers, intracranial aneurysm clips, or other iron-based metal implants. Ventilators, intravenous infusion pumps, and other metallic or computer-based equipment must be kept out of the MRI area.
- If necessary, the level of oxygen in the blood, heart rhythm, and respiratory status are monitored during the test. An anesthesiologist may monitor a heavily sedated person.

What are the normal results?

Normally, MRI reveals no disorders in bones, muscles, and joints.

What do abnormal results mean?

MRI is excellent for visualizing diseases of the spinal canal and spinal cord and for identifying bone tumors. It helps delineate muscles, ligaments, and bones. The images sharply define healthy, benign, and malignant tissues.

MRI can't be performed on people with pacemakers, intracranial aneurysm clips, or other iron-based metal implants. Devices such as ventilators and intravenous infusion pumps are also kept out of the MRI area.

CHEST & HEART

CAT SCAN OF THE CHEST

This test provides cross-sectional views of the chest by passing an X-ray beam from a computerized scanner through the body at different angles. Another name for this test is *thoracic computed tomography.*

CAT scanning may be done with or without an injected contrast dye. Contrast dyes are special dyes that highlight blood vessels and produce clearer images.

This test provides a three-dimensional image and is especially useful in detecting small differences in tissue density. It may provide information for diagnosing masses in the chest and Hodgkin's disease. It's also valuable for evaluating lung disorders. (See *Looking at the respiratory system,* page 102.)

Why is this test done?
A CAT scan of the chest may be performed for the following reasons:
- To provide cross-sectional views of the chest that distinguish small differences in tissue density
- To locate suspected tumors, such as those in Hodgkin's disease
- To differentiate tumors from other soft-tissue changes, such as those that indicate tuberculosis
- To distinguish tumors near the aorta from aortic aneurysms
- To detect the movement of a neck mass into the thorax
- To evaluate cancer that may move to the lungs
- To evaluate the lymph nodes in the chest area.

What should you know before the test?
- If a dye isn't used, you won't need to restrict food or fluids before the test. If the test is performed with a dye, you'll be asked to fast for 4 hours before the test.
- A nurse or technician will describe the procedure to you. The test usually takes 90 minutes and will not cause you any discomfort. Radiation exposure is minimal.
- A dye may be injected into a vein in your arm. If so, you may experience nausea, warmth, flushing of the face, or a salty taste.
- You'll be asked to keep still during the test and to breathe normally.

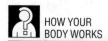

HOW YOUR
BODY WORKS

Looking at the respiratory system

Several organs are involved in the act of breathing — the exchange of gases between the atmosphere and the blood. These are the nose, pharynx, larynx, trachea, bronchi, and lungs. The trachea is branched, like a tree, into smaller and smaller "tubes" that carry air into the lungs. These are the primary bronchi, secondary and tertiary bronchi, bronchioles, terminal bronchioles and, finally, the alveolar sacs.

The alveolar sacs are composed of *alveoli,* which make up the main tissue of the lungs. The exchange of gases between inhaled air and the blood takes place in the alveoli. The alveoli are covered by a network of the smallest blood-carrying vessels, called *capillaries.*

In the lungs, the capillaries are further divided into *arterioles* — which carry the oxygen-rich blood away from the lungs — and *venules* — which bring oxygen-depleted blood that needs "recharging" to the lungs.

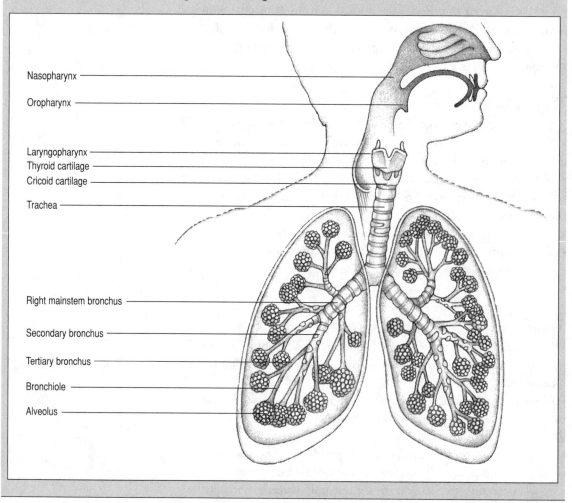

- You'll be asked to remove all jewelry and metal in the X-ray field.
- You'll be asked to sign a consent form before the test takes place.
- Your history will be checked for past allergic reactions to iodine, shellfish, or contrast dyes.

What happens during the test?

- You're positioned on an X-ray table and the dye is injected. The table then moves into the center of a large ring-shaped piece of X-ray equipment. The equipment may be noisy as it scans you from different angles.
- The computer detects small differences in the densities of various tissues, water, fat, bone, and air. This information is displayed as a printout of numbers and as an image on a screen. Images may be recorded for further study.

What happens after the test?

- You'll be monitored for signs of a delayed allergic reaction to the dye, such as itching, blood pressure changes, or respiratory distress.
- You may resume your usual diet.
- You'll drink fluids to help eliminate the dye from your system.

Does the test have risks?

A CAT scan of the chest is not recommended for pregnant women or — if a dye is used — in people with a history of allergies to iodine, shellfish, or the dyes used in X-ray tests.

What are the normal results?

Black and white areas on a CAT scan of the chest help the radiologist to distinguish the density of air and bone. Shades of gray correspond to water, fat, and soft-tissue densities.

What do abnormal results mean?

A CAT scan may reveal tumors, nodules, cysts, aortic aneurysms, enlarged lymph nodes, pleural effusion, and accumulations of blood, fluid, or fat.

MRI SCAN OF THE HEART

This test helps the doctor diagnose certain heart disorders. MRI, or *magnetic resonance imaging,* uses a powerful but harmless magnetic field to "see through" bone and to show fluid-filled soft tissue in great detail, as well as produce images of organs and vessels in motion.

In this noninvasive procedure, cross-sectional images of your heart are displayed on a monitor and recorded. No X-rays are used.

Why is this test done?

An MRI scan of the heart may be performed for the following reasons:
- To check the heart's function and structure
- To identify signs of a heart attack
- To detect and evaluate cardiomyopathies (heart muscle disorders)
- To detect and evaluate diseases of the pericardium, the fluid-filled sac that surrounds the heart
- To identify masses in or around the heart
- To detect heart disease that's present at birth
- To check major blood vessels and identify vascular disorders.

What should you know before the test?

- A nurse or technician will describe this procedure to you. The test takes up to 90 minutes.
- Although MRI is painless, you may feel uncomfortable because you must remain still inside a small space throughout the test.
- If you suffer from claustrophobia, discuss this with your doctor or a nurse. You may need a sedative to tolerate the test.
- You'll be able to talk with the technician who performs the test at all times, and the procedure will be stopped if you experience problems.
- Immediately before the test, you must remove all metal objects. If you have a pacemaker or any surgically implanted joints, pins, clips, valves, or pumps containing metal that could be attracted to the strong magnetic field, you won't be able to undergo the test.
- You'll be asked to sign a consent form before the test takes place.

What happens during the test?

- You're positioned on a narrow bed, which slides into a large cylinder that houses the MRI magnets.
- You must remember to hold still throughout the procedure.
- The scanner makes clicking, whirring, and thumping noises as it moves inside its housing.
- The resulting images are displayed on a monitor and recorded on film or magnetic tape for permanent storage.
- The technician may use the computer to manipulate and enhance the images.

What happens after the test?

If you were sedated, your status is monitored until the effects of the sedative wear off.

Does the test have risks?

- Claustrophobic people may experience anxiety.
- People with heart conditions are watched for signs of distress, such as chest pressure, shortness of breath, or changes in blood movement.
- MRI can't be performed on people with pacemakers, intracranial aneurysm clips, or other iron-based metal implants.

What are the normal results?

An MRI scan should reveal a healthy heart.

What do abnormal results mean?

MRI can be used to detect and evaluate the extent of various heart diseases and defects. For example, the doctor may use information from this test in the diagnosis of cardiomyopathy, pericardial disease, and congenital heart defects. In addition, information from this test may help determine the extent of heart or blood vessel disorders.

Although MRI is painless, you may feel uncomfortable because you must remain still inside a small space throughout the test. If you suffer from claustrophobia, you may need a sedative to tolerate the test.

OTHER CAT SCANS

CAT SCAN OF STRUCTURES AROUND THE EYES

This test provides three-dimensional images of structures around the eye, especially the ocular muscles and the optic nerve. It helps the doctor identify abnormalities earlier and more accurately than other techniques, such as standard X-ray.

This test may also be called an *orbital computed tomography scan.* The orbit is the bony structure that contains the eyeball.

A computer generates a series of cross-sectional images depicting the size and position of structures around the eye and their relationship to each other. In some cases, a special dye called a *contrast dye* is injected near the area that is being observed to clarify the images that are produced.

In evaluating fractures around the eye, CAT scans allow a complete three-dimensional view of the affected structures...even the circulation of blood through abnormal tissues.

Why is this test done?
A CAT scan of the structures around the eye may be performed for the following reasons:
- To view the anatomy of the eye and its surrounding structures
- To evaluate disorders of the orbit and eye — especially expanding tissue damage and bone destruction
- To evaluate fractures of the orbit and adjoining structures
- To determine the cause of a condition called unilateral exophthalmos, which is an abnormal protrusion of the eyeball
- To help diagnose brain-related disorders that affect vision
- To evaluate conditions such as suspected circulatory disorders.

What should you know before the test?
- If contrast dye won't be used, you don't need to restrict food or fluids before this test. If the dye will be used, food and fluids are withheld for 4 hours before the test.
- A nurse or technician will describe how a series of X-ray films will be taken of your eye. During the test, a scanner rotates around your head and makes loud, clacking sounds.
- The test causes no discomfort and takes 15 to 30 minutes to perform.

- If a dye is used, you'll be warned that you may feel flushed and warm and experience a brief headache, a salty taste, and nausea or vomiting after the dye is injected. These reactions to the contrast dye are typical.
- You'll be asked to sign a consent form before the test takes place.
- Your history will be checked for reactions to iodine, shellfish, or contrast dyes.
- Before the test, you'll be asked to remove jewelry, hairpins, or other metal objects in the X-ray field to allow for precise imaging of the structures around the eye.

What happens during the test?
- You're positioned on a special table, with your head held gently in place by straps. During the test you're asked to lie as still as possible.
- The head of the table is moved into the scanner, which rotates around your head taking X-rays.
- The information is stored on magnetic tapes, and the images are displayed on a screen. Photographs may be made if a permanent record is desired.
- After this series of images is taken, a contrast dye is injected and a second series of scans is recorded.

What happens after the test?
- If a contrast dye was used, you'll be monitored for side effects of the dye, including headache, nausea, or vomiting.
- You may resume your usual diet.

Does the test have risks?
Use of contrast dyes is not recommended in people with known allergy to iodine, shellfish, or dyes used in other tests.

What are the normal results?
Structures around the eye are evaluated for size, shape, and position by the radiologist.

What do abnormal results mean?

A CAT scan can help the doctor identify tissue damage that obscures the normal eye structures or causes orbital enlargement, indentation of the orbital walls, or bone destruction. This test can also help determine the type of lesion, including some tumors and enlargement of the optic canal.

In evaluating fractures around the eye, CAT scans allow a complete three-dimensional view of the affected structures.

Enhancement with a contrast dye may provide information about the circulation of the blood through abnormal eye structures.

CAT SCAN OF THE KIDNEYS

In this test, a series of cross-sectional X-ray views of the kidneys are displayed on a monitor. The images of the kidneys make it possible to identify masses, such as tumors, and other lesions, or tissue damage.

An intravenous contrast medium, or dye, may be injected into your body to infiltrate the kidneys and accentuate the images that are generated. This highly accurate test is usually performed to investigate diseases found by other diagnostic procedures.

Why is this test done?

A CAT scan of the kidneys may be performed for the following reasons:
- To permit examination of the kidneys
- To detect and evaluate kidney disorders, such as tumors, obstructions, kidney stones, and fluid accumulation around the kidneys
- To guide needle placement before a biopsy
- To determine the kidney's size and location in relation to the bladder after a kidney transplant
- To locate abscesses for drainage.

What should you know before the test?

- If use of a contrast dye isn't scheduled, you won't need to restrict your diet before this test. If use of a contrast dye is scheduled, you'll be asked to fast for 4 hours before the test.
- A nurse or technician will describe the procedure to you. Expect the procedure to take about an hour, depending on the purpose of the scan.

- You may experience brief side effects from the dye, such as flushing, metallic taste, and headache, after it's injected.
- You'll be asked to sign a consent form before the test takes place.
- Your medical history will be checked for past allergic reactions to shellfish, iodine, or dyes.
- Just before the procedure, you'll be asked to put on a hospital gown and to remove any metallic objects that could interfere with the scan.
- The doctor may prescribe sedatives to reduce your anxiety about the test. They'll be given to you at the appropriate time before the test.

What happens during the test?

- You're positioned on an X-ray table and held gently in place with straps.
- The table is moved into the scanner.
- You're asked to lie still while the scanner rotates around your body.
- The scanner takes multiple images — called *tomograms* — from different angles. The equipment may make loud, clacking sounds as it rotates.
- When one series of tomograms is complete, a dye may be injected, usually through a vein. Another series of tomograms is then taken.
- After the intravenous dye is injected, you're monitored for allergic reactions, such as respiratory difficulty, hives, or rashes.
- Information from the scan is stored on a disk or on magnetic tape, fed into a computer, and converted into an image for display on a viewing screen. Photographs are taken of selected views for future reference.

The scanner takes multiple images — called tomograms — from different angles. The equipment may make loud, clacking sounds as it rotates.

What happens after the test?

- If a dye was used, you'll be monitored for signs of a possible allergic reaction.
- You may resume your usual diet.

What are the normal results?

The radiologist evaluates the position of the kidneys in relation to the surrounding structures. Normally, the density of the kidneys is slightly greater than that of the liver but less than that of bone. The size and shape of the kidneys are also determined.

What do abnormal results mean?

Kidney masses, such as tumors, appear as areas of different density than normal tissue. Such masses may alter the kidneys' shape or size.

A CAT scan may also identify other abnormalities, including obstructions, kidney stones, polycystic kidney disease, congenital anomalies, and abnormal accumulations of fluid around the kidneys. After surgical removal of a kidney, a CAT scan can detect abnormal masses, such as recurrent tumors, in a space that should be empty.

3

NUCLEAR MEDICINE SCANS:
Picturing Internal Organs

SCANNING THE THYROID

IODINE TEST OF THE THYROID GLAND

This test — which doctors call the *radioactive iodine uptake test* — is used to evaluate the thyroid gland. This important gland, located in the neck, releases two major hormones that regulate the body's metabolism. (See *Learning about the thyroid.*)

As the test begins, you receive a capsule or liquid that contains a tiny amount of radioactive iodine. After you swallow the iodine, a percentage of it accumulates in the thyroid gland, indicating the thyroid's ability to trap and retain iodine.

The test is used to accurately diagnose hyperthyroidism, a condition in which the thyroid is overactive and releases too much of its hormones. However, the test is less accurate for diagnosing hypothyroidism, a condition in which the thyroid is underactive and releases too little of its hormones.

Why is this test done?
The radioactive iodine uptake test may be performed for the following reasons:
- To check the function of the thyroid gland
- To help diagnose hyperthyroidism or hypothyroidism
- To help differentiate Graves' disease from a tumor that releases thyroid hormones.

What should you know before the test?
- You must fast after midnight on the night before the test. At the start of the test, you'll receive radioactive iodine in a capsule or liquid form. Six hours later, your thyroid will be scanned. Then, 18 hours after the first scan, your thyroid will be scanned again.
- The test is painless and exposes you to only a small, harmless amount of radiation. Its results will be available within 24 hours.
- The nurse will ask if you've ever been exposed to iodine. For instance, you may have been exposed to iodine if you had an X-ray test in which the doctor injected a special dye. Similarly, you may have

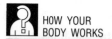

HOW YOUR
BODY WORKS

Learning about the thyroid

The thyroid gland is located in the neck. It has two portions called *lobes* that straddle the trachea (windpipe). The right lobe is a bit larger and higher in the neck than the left.

About 50% of normal persons have a third lobe, which has the shape of a pyramid and is called the *pyramidal lobe.*

The four small parathyroid glands, two upper and two lower, sit behind the thyroid. They're closely connected to the thyroid.

Powerful hormones released by the thyroid
The thyroid controls the body's metabolism by releasing two powerful hormones: thyroxine and triiodothyronine. Besides controlling the body's metabolism, thyroxine helps control physical and mental development, resistance to infection, and vitamin requirements. Triiodothyronine, though, is an even more potent form of thyroxine.

FRONT VIEW

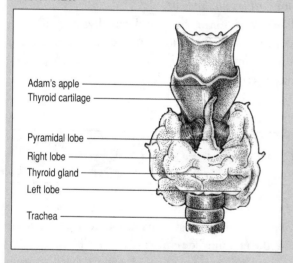

Adam's apple
Thyroid cartilage

Pyramidal lobe
Right lobe
Thyroid gland
Left lobe

Trachea

BACK VIEW

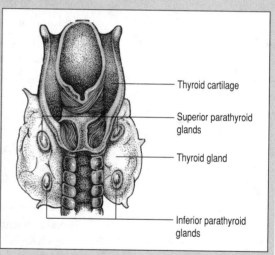

Thyroid cartilage

Superior parathyroid glands

Thyroid gland

Inferior parathyroid glands

been exposed if you had a previous scan, used iodine preparations, or took medication for a thyroid problem.

What happens during the test?

- After you take the dose of radioactive iodine, your thyroid gland is scanned after 6 hours and then after 24 hours.
- During each scan, the front of your neck is placed in front of a device that detects and measures the radioactivity in your thyroid gland.

What happens after the test?

You'll be able to resume a light diet 2 hours after swallowing the iodine. When the study is complete, you'll resume a normal diet.

Does the test have risks?

The test shouldn't be performed during pregnancy and breast-feeding because the radiation could cause developmental defects in the fetus or baby.

What are the normal results?

After 6 hours, 3% to 16% of the radioactive iodine should accumulate in the thyroid. After 24 hours, the accumulation should be 8% to 29%. The rest of the iodine is excreted in the urine.

What do abnormal results mean?

Below-normal levels of iodine may indicate hypothyroidism, subacute thyroiditis, or iodine overload. Above-normal levels may indicate hyperthyroidism, early Hashimoto's thyroiditis, hypoalbuminemia, lithium ingestion, or iodine-deficient goiter.

THYROID SCAN

This test is used to examine the thyroid gland after a person ingests a small amount of a radionuclide that contains iodine or technetium. For a brief period, the radionuclide emits radiation. This radioactivity in the thyroid gland is detected by a special camera (called a *gamma camera*).

The doctor may order this scan after the discovery of a lump in the thyroid area, an enlarged thyroid gland, or an asymmetrical goiter. It's performed at the same time as the radioactive thyroid uptake test and blood tests of thyroid hormones.

Why is this test done?

The thyroid scan may be performed for the following reasons:

- To check the size, structure, and position of the thyroid gland
- To evaluate thyroid function along with other tests.

What should you know before the test?

▪ You'll learn about the test, including who will perform it and where. The test itself takes about 30 minutes, but you'll need to ingest the radionuclide 20 to 30 minutes earlier (if technetium is used) or 24 hours earlier (if iodine is used). You'll need to fast after midnight on the night before the test if iodine is used, but not if technetium is used.

▪ The nurse will ask about your diet and any medications that you take. Medications such as thyroid hormones and iodine preparations (Lugol's solution, some multivitamins, and cough syrups) will be discontinued 2 to 3 weeks before the test. Aspirin, blood-thinning drugs, steroids, and antihistamines will be discontinued 1 week before the test.

▪ Don't use iodized salt or iodine-containing salt substitutes for 1 week before the test, and don't eat seafood during this period.

▪ Just before the test, remove any jewelry, dentures, or other materials that may interfere with the scan.

After the discovery of a lump in the thyroid area, the doctor may order a thyroid scan.

What happens during the test?

▪ You lie on your back with your neck extended.

▪ The doctor or technician positions the gamma camera above your neck. The camera projects images of the gland on a monitor and records them on X-ray film. The doctor takes three views of the thyroid: a straight-on, frontal view and two side views.

What happens after the test?

You may resume any medications suspended for the test. And you may resume your normal diet.

Does the test have risks?

The test shouldn't be performed during pregnancy and breast-feeding because the radioactivity could cause developmental defects in the fetus or baby.

What are the normal results?

Normally, the scan shows a thyroid gland that is about 2 inches (5 centimeters) long and 1 inch (2.5 centimeters) wide. The gland should have two portions, which are called *lobes,* and should have a butterfly shape. Occasionally, a third lobe may be present; this is normal, too.

What do abnormal results mean?

The test can show areas of the thyroid that retain too much iodine. These areas are called *hot spots*. Their discovery requires follow-up testing.

The test can also show areas of the thyroid that retain little or no iodine. These areas, in contrast, are called *cold spots*. Their discovery requires an ultrasound scan to rule out cysts. In addition, a biopsy (removal and analysis of tissue) of the cold spot may be done to rule out cancer.

SCANNING THE LUNGS & HEART

BLOOD FLOW TO THE LUNGS

This test — which doctors call the *lung perfusion scan* — is used to evaluate lung perfusion, the movement of blood through the arteries that supply blood to the lungs.

The lung perfusion scan produces an image of this blood flow after the doctor injects a slightly radioactive drug into an arm vein. The drug emits tiny amounts of radiation, which is recorded by a special camera.

Why is this test done?

A lung perfusion scan may be performed for the following reasons:
- To check lung perfusion
- To detect a pulmonary embolism
- To check lung function before surgery on a person with marginal lung reserves.

What should you know before the test?

- You'll learn about the test, including who will perform it, where it will take place, and its expected duration (15 to 30 minutes). During the test, the doctor will inject a slightly radioactive drug into a vein in your arm and you'll sit in front of a camera or lie under it. Neither the camera nor the probe is radioactive.
- You won't need to fast before the test.

What happens during the test?

- The doctor injects the drug and takes a series of single stationary images with the gamma camera.
- The images, which are projected on a screen, show the distribution of radioactive particles.

What happens after the test?

If swelling occurs at the needle puncture site, warm soaks may be applied to the area.

Does the test have risks?

A lung perfusion scan shouldn't be performed in a person with allergies to the test drug.

What are the normal results?

"Hot spots" — areas with normal blood perfusion — show a high uptake of the test drug. A normal lung shows a uniform uptake pattern.

What do abnormal results mean?

"Cold spots" — areas with poor perfusion — suggest a blood clot. However, a lung ventilation scan must be done to confirm the diagnosis.

Areas of decreased blood flow without vessel blockage may indicate pneumonitis.

LUNG VENTILATION SCAN

This test is used to evaluate lung ventilation, one of the three processes that occur during breathing. (The other two processes are called *diffusion* and *perfusion*.) Ventilation refers to the movement of air from outside the body into the alveoli, the grapelike clusters in the farthest reaches of the lungs that exchange oxygen for carbon dioxide. (See *The lungs in action*, page 118.)

This scan is performed after a person inhales a mixture of air and a mildly radioactive gas that outlines areas of the lung ventilated during breathing. The scan records the distribution of the gas during three phases: the buildup of gas (wash-in phase), the time after

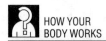

HOW YOUR
BODY WORKS

The lungs in action

The lungs provide your body with a continuous supply of oxygen. The lungs also remove carbon dioxide from your body quickly and efficiently. This switching of the two gases takes place in grapelike clusters at the end of your breathing passages.

Alveoli do the work

These clusters, called *alveoli,* contain a network of capillaries, the body's tiniest blood vessels. The cap-

illaries bring blood containing carbon dioxide to the alveoli. At the same time, the breathing passages transport oxygen to the alveoli. When blood passes through the alveoli, it releases its carbon dioxide and takes on the oxygen. The now-fresh blood travels to the heart and, from there, circulates throughout the rest of body, releasing oxygen. Carbon dioxide, the other gas, passes into the breathing passages and leaves your body when you exhale.

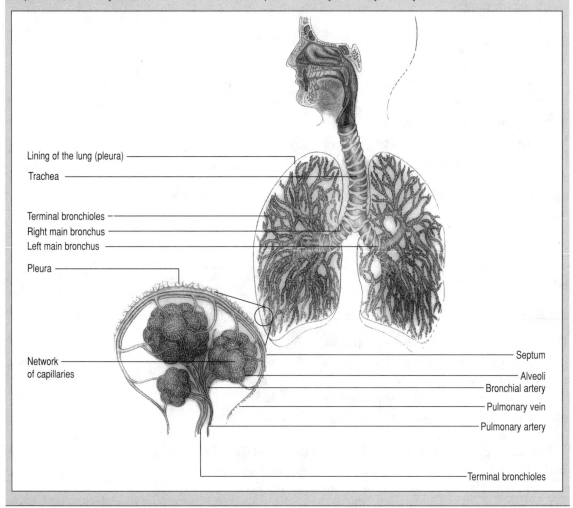

Lining of the lung (pleura)

Trachea

Terminal bronchioles

Right main bronchus

Left main bronchus

Pleura

Network
of capillaries

Septum

Alveoli

Bronchial artery

Pulmonary vein

Pulmonary artery

Terminal bronchioles

rebreathing when radioactivity reaches a steady level (equilibrium phase), and after removal of the gas from the lungs (wash-out phase).

Why is this test done?

A lung ventilation scan may be performed for the following reasons:
- To help diagnose pulmonary emboli, identify areas of the lung capable of ventilation, and help evaluate breathing in a lung region
- To locate a lung region marked by poor ventilation (usually caused by smoking, chronic asthma, or emphysema)
- To distinguish between parenchymal disease, such as emphysema, sarcoidosis, lung cancer, and tuberculosis, and conditions caused by blood vessel problems such as pulmonary emboli.

What should you know before the test?

- You'll learn who will perform the test, where it will take place, and that it takes 15 to 30 minutes. During the test, you'll be asked to hold your breath for a short time after inhaling a gas and to remain still while a machine scans your chest. The test uses only a small amount of radioactive gas.
- You won't need to fast before the test.
- Before the test, remove all jewelry or metal from your neck and chest.

What happens during the test?

- You inhale the air-gas mixture through a mask. As you hold your breath, the doctor checks the distribution of the gas in your lungs on a monitor.
- When you exhale, the doctor again views your lungs on the monitor.

What are the normal results?

Normal findings include an equal distribution of gas in both lungs and normal wash-in and wash-out phases.

What do abnormal results mean?

Unequal gas distribution in both lungs indicates poor ventilation or a blocked airway.

Test results may be compared to those from a lung perfusion scan. In a pulmonary embolism, perfusion is decreased but ventilation is maintained. In pneumonia or other parenchymal lung diseases, ventilation is abnormal.

During a lung ventilation scan, you must inhale a mixture of air and a mildly radioactive gas.

TECHNETIUM SCAN OF THE HEART

Also called *hot-spot myocardial imaging* or *infarct avid imaging*, a technetium scan is used to detect a recent heart attack and determine its extent. In this test, the doctor injects a mildly radioactive element called *technetium* into a person's arm vein. The technetium accumulates in damaged heart tissue, where it shows up as "hot spots" on a scan done with a special camera.

Why is this test done?
The technetium scan may be performed for the following reasons:
- To confirm a recent heart attack in a person suffering from puzzling cardiac pain or when an electrocardiograph and blood tests don't give enough information
- To identify the size and location of a heart attack
- To determine a prognosis after a heart attack.

A technetium scan of the heart may enable the doctor to detect a recent heart attack.

What should you know before the test?
- You'll learn about the test, including who will perform the 30- to 60-minute procedure and where. Two to three hours before the test, the doctor will inject the technetium into a vein in your forearm. The injection causes only brief discomfort, and the scan itself is painless. The test involves less exposure to radiation than a chest X-ray.
- You'll need to remain quiet and motionless during the test.
- You won't need to fast before the test.
- You'll be asked to sign a form that gives your consent to do the test. Carefully read the form and ask questions if any portion of it isn't clear.

What happens during the test?
- The doctor injects the technetium into an arm vein. After 2 or 3 hours, you lie on your back on the test table and electrocardiogram electrodes are attached to your skin for continuous monitoring during the test.
- Generally, the scans are taken with you in several positions. Each scan takes 10 minutes.

What are the normal results?
A normal scan shows no technetium in the heart.

What do abnormal results mean?

The scan can reveal hot spots in a damaged heart, particularly 2 to 3 days after the start of a heart attack. However, hot spots become apparent as early as 12 hours after a heart attack. In most people who've had a heart attack, these areas disappear after 1 week. In some, they last for several months.

THALLIUM SCAN OF THE HEART

Also called *cold spot myocardial imaging,* this test helps determine if any areas of the heart aren't receiving enough blood. In the test, the doctor injects a mildly radioactive solution called *thallium* into a person's arm vein. Because thallium accumulates in healthy heart tissue but not in damaged tissue, areas of the heart with a normal blood supply and intact cells rapidly absorb it. Areas of the heart with poor blood flow and injured cells don't absorb thallium and appear as "cold spots" on a scan.

This test can be performed at rest or during exercise on a treadmill.

Persistent "cold spots" indicate a heart attack.

Why is this test done?

A thallium scan during rest may be performed for the following reasons:
- To evaluate blood flow in the heart and check for damaged areas
- To demonstrate the location and extent of a heart attack.

A thallium scan during exercise, a type of stress test, may be performed for the following reasons:
- To diagnose coronary artery disease
- To check the condition of vein grafts after bypass surgery
- To evaluate the effectiveness of drugs for chest pain
- To evaluate the effectiveness of balloon angioplasty, a procedure in which a catheter with a balloon at the tip is used to open blocked coronary arteries.

What should you know before the test?

- You'll learn about the test, including who will perform it and where it will take place. The test usually takes 45 to 90 minutes. Sometimes it's done in two stages. When that happens, additional scans are taken 3 to 6 hours after the first stage.

Treadmill stress test

The illustration below shows a stress test being performed on a treadmill. Here, the doctor is preparing to perform a special test called a *thallium scan*. The doctor injects thallium into a vein while the person continues exercising. Next the doctor will take pictures of the person's heart with a special scanner. These pictures show how well the coronary arteries supply blood to the heart during exercise.

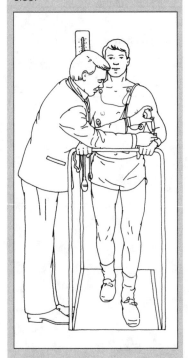

- During the test, the doctor will inject thallium into an arm vein and take scans of the heart. You may experience discomfort from the injection. During the treadmill test, you may feel some discomfort from the abrasion of your skin when electrodes are applied to your body.
- If you'll be having a treadmill test, don't drink alcohol, smoke, or take any unprescribed medications for 24 hours before the test. Don't eat or drink anything for 3 hours before the test. Before this fasting period, you should eat a light meal.
- Wear sneakers and lightweight clothing for the treadmill test. During the test, tell the doctor or nurse right away if you feel tired, are short of breath, or have chest pains.
- You'll be asked to sign a form that gives your consent to do the test. Carefully read the form and ask questions if any portion of it isn't clear.

What happens during a resting scan?

- The doctor injects thallium into a vein in your arm. After about 5 minutes, the scans are taken.
- If the doctor decides that additional scans are required, you rest and fast for several hours before they are done.

What happens during an exercise scan?

- The nurse attaches electrocardiograph electrodes to different parts of your body. These electrodes record your heart's response to different levels of exercise.
- You walk on the treadmill. (See *Treadmill stress test.*) As you reach your peak exercise level, the doctor injects thallium into a vein in your forearm. Tell the doctor or the nurse at once if you feel confused or faint, are short of breath, or have chest pains. The test is stopped for these symptoms.
- You exercise for another minute and then lie on your back under a special camera. After about 5 minutes, the scans are taken as you assume different positions on the table.
- Additional scans may be taken after you rest for 3 to 6 hours.

Does the test have risks?

- The test shouldn't be performed on a pregnant woman. It also shouldn't be done if a person has a neuromuscular impairment, an acute heart attack, an inflammation of the heart called myocarditis, narrowing of a heart valve, or a severe infection.
- The test can cause fainting, chest pain, an irregular heartbeat, and even a heart attack.

What are the normal results?

The test should show no cold spots.

What do abnormal results mean?

Persistent cold spots indicate a heart attack. Cold spots that disappear after a 3- to 6-hour rest indicate coronary artery disease, a condition that can eventually cause a heart attack.

The test can show the results of bypass surgery. For instance, if blood flow to an area of the heart improves after bypass surgery, then the new blood vessel inserted during surgery is working well.

The test can also judge how well drugs for chest pain are working and how well an alternative to bypass surgery, called *angioplasty,* improves blood flow in a previously blocked artery in the heart.

PERSANTINE-THALLIUM SCAN OF THE HEART

This test provides a way of examining the heart's blood vessels for people who can't tolerate exercise or a stress test. It involves the injection of two substances: the drug Persantine, then mildly radioactive thallium.

Persantine causes the body to respond as if it were actually exercising. Thallium is then used to evaluate how well the heart's blood vessels respond. Diseased vessels can't deliver thallium to the heart, and thallium lingers in diseased areas of the heart. Diseased areas appear as "cold spots" on the scan.

Why is this test done?

The Persantine-thallium scan may be performed for the following reasons:
- To identify irregular heartbeats caused by exercise or stress
- To check for damage to the heart.

What should you know before the test?

- You'll learn about the test, including who will perform it and where it will take place. The test may be done in two stages, with scans taken several hours apart.

- The nurse will tell you about the drug Persantine, which the doctor injects at the start of the test. After you get this drug, you may feel dizzy, flushed, and a little nauseated, or have a headache. These symptoms only last a brief time.
- You'll need to fast before the test. Avoid coffee and other caffeinated drinks because they may cause irregular heartbeats.
- Continue to take all your regular medications.

What happens during the test?
- At the start of the test, you lie on a table or sit. A nurse attaches electrodes to your body and performs a routine electrocardiograph, which takes 5 or 10 minutes.
- You receive Persantine and are asked to get up and walk. After Persantine takes effect, the doctor injects the thallium.
- Next, you lie on a table for about 40 minutes while the scan is performed. Then the scan is reviewed. If necessary, a second scan is performed.
- If you must return for further scanning, you should rest and not eat or drink anything in the interim.

Does the test have risks?
- The most serious risks are irregular heartbeats, chest pain, and difficulty breathing. If any of these problems occurs, the doctor will immediately treat it.
- The test can also cause nausea, headache, flushing, dizziness, and stomach pain.

What are the normal results?
The test should show no heart problems.

What do abnormal results mean?
The presence of "cold spots" usually points to coronary artery disease. However, this result could be caused by other conditions, such as sarcoidosis, myocardial fibrosis, cardiac contusion, or a spasm of one of the heart's arteries.

CARDIAC BLOOD POOL SCAN

This test is used to check the function of the ventricles, the heart's two lower chambers. (The two upper chambers are called the *atria*.) To perform this test, the doctor first gives an injection of red blood cells or a protein (albumin) that's tagged with a mildly radioactive substance called *technetium*. A scintillation camera records radioactivity as the technetium passes through the left ventricle.

Gated cardiac blood pool imaging, performed after a first-pass scan or as a separate test, has several forms. The basic principle is that multiple images are taken to show the heart in motion. This helps the doctor find problem areas in the ventricle.

Another variant of the cardiac blood pool scan, called a *MUGA scan*, may be done. (See *What is a MUGA scan?*)

Why is this test done?

A cardiac blood pool scan may be performed for the following reasons:
- To check the function of the left ventricle, the chief pumping chamber of the heart
- To detect aneurysms of the left ventricle and other motion abnormalities of the heart wall.

What should you know before the test?

- You'll learn about the test, including who will perform it, where it will take place, and its expected duration. During the test, the doctor will inject the test solution into a vein in your forearm. Then a detector positioned above your chest will record the circulation of this solution through the heart. The solution, although slightly radioactive, poses no radiation hazard and rarely produces side effects.
- You'll be directed to remain silent and motionless during the test, unless otherwise instructed.
- You'll be asked to sign a consent form. Carefully read the form and ask questions if any portion of it isn't clear.

What happens during the test?

- At the start of the test, a nurse attaches electrodes to your body so that an electrocardiogram can be performed during the test.
- You lie beneath the detector of a scintillation camera, and the doctor injects the solution.

What is a MUGA scan?

MUGA stands for a multiple-gated acquisition scan. In this test, a special camera records sequential images of the heart wall that can be studied like motion picture films. These images capture events in the heart's pumping cycle: the contraction of the heart, followed by its relaxation.

MUGA under stress
The MUGA test can be performed in two stages: at rest and after exercise. The stress MUGA test is done to detect changes in the heart's pumping performance.

Nitro MUGA
Nitro is an abbreviation for the powerful drug nitroglycerin, which is widely prescribed by doctors for chest pain. In the nitro MUGA test, a special camera records different points in the cardiac cycle after a person takes nitroglycerin. The test tells the effect nitroglycerin has on heart function.

The camera records the movement of a radioactive element called technetium *as it circulates through the heart.*

- For the next minute, the camera records the first pass of the solution through the heart so that heart valves can be located.
- Then the camera records the end of the contraction and relaxation stages of the heartbeat. In all, it records 500 to 1,000 cardiac cycles on X-ray or Polaroid film. An electrocardiograph is used to help time the taking of pictures.
- You may be asked to change your position during the test. You may also be asked to take the drug nitroglycerin or to exercise briefly.

Does the test have risks?
The test shouldn't be performed on a pregnant woman.

What are the normal results?
Normally, the left ventricle contracts symmetrically, and the technetium appears evenly distributed in the scans. Higher counts of radioactivity occur during the heart's contraction because there's more blood in the ventricle. Lower counts occur during its relaxation as the blood is ejected.

What do abnormal results mean?
The test can be used to detect coronary artery disease, which causes asymmetrical distribution of blood to the heart. The test also can detect cardiomyopathies and shunting of blood within the heart.

MISCELLANEOUS TESTS

BONE SCAN

A bone scan is used to examine the skeleton and helps doctors detect cancer and other problems long before X-ray detection is possible. In this procedure, a doctor injects a slightly radioactive solution into an arm vein. The solution accumulates in bone tissue where an abnormality is present. A special camera passes over the entire body during the test and can pinpoint these abnormal sites, which are called "hot spots."

Why is this test done?

A bone scan may be done for the following reasons:
- To detect or rule out malignant bone tumors when X-rays are normal but cancer is confirmed or suspected
- To detect difficult-to-find bone fractures
- To monitor degenerative bone disorders
- To detect bone infection
- To evaluate unexplained bone pain.

What should you know before the test?

- You'll learn about the scan, including who will perform the test and where. During the test, you may have to assume various positions on a scanner table. You must keep still for the scan.
- You'll be told that the scan, which takes about 1 hour, is painless and that the radioactive solution emits less radiation than a standard X-ray machine.
- The nurse will tell you to urinate just before the test and will give you a painkiller.
- You'll be asked to sign a form that gives your consent to do the test. Carefully read the form and ask questions if any portions of it aren't clear.

What happens during the test?

- The doctor injects the solution into a vein in your forearm. During the next 1 to 3 hours, you need to drink four to six 8-ounce glasses (about 2 liters) of water or tea.
- After this period, you lie on the scanning table. The scanner moves back and forth over your body. As it does, it detects low-level radiation emitted by the skeleton and translates this onto a film or paper chart, or both.
- The scanner takes as many views as needed to cover the specified area. You may change positions several times during the test to obtain adequate views.

What happens after the test?

You may have redness or swelling where the doctor injected the solution.

A bone scan examines the skeleton and enables the doctor to detect cancer and other problems long before they can be detected by X-rays.

Does the test have risks?

The test shouldn't be performed on a pregnant or breast-feeding woman.

What are the normal results?

The solution concentrates in bone tissue at sites of new bone formation or increased metabolism.

What do abnormal results mean?

Although a bone scan shows hot spots that identify sites of bone formation, it doesn't distinguish between normal and abnormal bone formation. But scan results can identify all types of bone cancer, infection, fracture, and other disorders if viewed in light of a person's medical and surgical history, X-rays, and other tests.

LIVER AND SPLEEN SCAN

In this test, a special camera shows images of the liver and spleen. These images show the distribution of radioactivity within the liver and spleen after a doctor injects a mildly radioactive solution of technetium into a person's arm. Roughly 80% to 90% of the solution is absorbed by the liver, 5% to 10% by the spleen, and 3% to 5% by bone marrow.

Although a person's symptoms may aid a diagnosis, results from a liver and spleen scan frequently require confirmation by an ultrasound test, a computed tomography scan (commonly called a CAT scan), a gallium scan, or a biopsy (removal and analysis of tissue).

Why is this test done?

A liver and spleen scan may be performed for the following reasons:
- To screen for liver cancer and liver diseases, such as cirrhosis and hepatitis
- To detect tumors, cysts, and abscesses in the liver and spleen
- To demonstrate enlargement of the liver or spleen
- To assess the condition of the liver and spleen after abdominal injury.

What should you know before the test?

▪ You'll learn about the test, including who will perform it and where it will take place. The test takes about 1 hour. You don't need to fast beforehand.

▪ You'll find out that the injection isn't dangerous because the test solution contains only tiny amounts of radioactivity.

▪ During the test, you must lie still and breathe quietly to ensure images of good quality; you may also be asked to briefly hold your breath. The detector head of the camera may touch your abdomen but isn't dangerous.

▪ You'll be asked to sign a form that gives your consent to do the test. Carefully read the form and ask questions if any portion of it isn't clear.

What happens during the test?

The doctor injects the technetium into a vein in your arm. After 10 to 15 minutes, your abdomen is scanned. You change positions on the table several times to get the best views of the liver and spleen.

What happens after the test?

The doctor reviews the images for clarity. If they're clear, you're allowed to leave.

Does the test have risks?

▪ The test shouldn't be performed on children or on pregnant or breast-feeding women.

▪ Rarely, severe reactions result from a stabilizer, such as dextran or gelatin, that's added to the technetium.

What are the normal results?

Both the liver and spleen normally appear equally bright on the image. However, distribution of the technetium is generally more uniform in the spleen than in the liver.

What do abnormal results mean?

Although the scan may fail to detect early liver disease, it shows characteristic, distinct patterns as the disease progresses. The test can also show the effects of hepatitis and cirrhosis. The spread of cancer to the liver or spleen may appear on the scan, but a biopsy must be performed to confirm the diagnosis.

Results of a liver and spleen scan frequently require confirmation by an ultrasound or other tests.

The scan can identify cysts, abscesses, and tumors because they fail to absorb the technetium. Cysts appear on the scan as single or multiple defects, but an ultrasound test is required to confirm the diagnosis. Abscesses can appear in the liver or spleen, but both require a gallium scan or ultrasound test to confirm the diagnosis. Tumors require a confirming biopsy or flow studies.

The scan can demonstrate an enlarged liver or spleen, a large dependent gallbladder, and infarction of the spleen. It can evaluate liver and spleen damage after an abdominal injury.

KIDNEY SCAN

This test is used to evaluate the structure, blood flow, and function of the kidneys. It involves injection of a mildly radioactive solution into an arm vein, followed by scans of the kidneys.

Why is this test done?
A kidney scan may be performed for the following reasons:
- To detect functional and structural kidney problems (such as lesions)
- To detect renovascular hypertension and acute and chronic kidney disease, such as pyelonephritis and glomerulonephritis
- To check on the condition of a kidney transplant
- To evaluate kidney injury from trauma and blockage of the urinary tract.

What should you know before the test?
- You'll learn about the test, including who will perform it and where, and that it takes about 90 minutes. However, if certain scans are ordered, there will be a delay of 4 or more hours before the images are taken.
- You'll find out that the doctor will give you an injection that contains a tiny amount of radioactive solution. During the injection, you may feel a brief sensation of warmth and nausea.
- If you're taking any drugs for high blood pressure, the doctor may tell you to discontinue them before the test.
- You'll be asked to sign a form that gives your consent to do the test. Carefully read the form and ask questions if any portion of it isn't clear.

What happens during the test?

- You lie facedown on the examination table.
- The doctor performs a test to study blood flow through the kidneys and takes rapid-sequence photographs (one per second) for 1 minute.
- Next, the doctor does a test to measure the transit time of the radioactive solution through the kidneys.
- After the doctor injects the solution into an arm vein, images are taken for 20 minutes.
- Additional images may be obtained 4 or more hours later.

What happens after the test?

After you urinate, flush the toilet immediately as a radiation precaution. You should do this every time you urinate for the next 24 hours.

What are the normal results?

The test should reveal no problems in the structure, blood flow, and function of the kidneys.

What do abnormal results mean?

The kidney scan can show poor circulation of blood through the kidneys. This circulatory problem can be caused by a kidney injury, the narrowing of the main artery in the kidneys, or a kidney infarction.

Because malignant kidney tumors usually have blood vessels within them, the test can help differentiate tumors from cysts. It can also identify the site of an obstruction in a ureter and point out congenital abnormalities, abscesses, polycystic kidney disease, acute tubular necrosis, severe infection, or rejection of a transplanted kidney.

In the first stage, the doctor takes rapid-sequence photographs of blood flow through your kidneys.

GALLIUM SCAN OF THE BODY

This test, a total body scan, is used to check for certain tumors and inflammations that attract a mildly radioactive solution of gallium. The test is usually performed 24 to 48 hours after the doctor injects gallium into an arm vein.

Because gallium has an affinity for both benign and malignant tumors and inflammatory lesions, an exact diagnosis requires additional tests, such as ultrasound and a computed tomography scan (commonly called a CAT scan).

Why is this test done?

A gallium scan may be performed for the following reasons:
- To detect cancer and its spread and inflammation when the site of the disease hasn't been clearly defined
- To evaluate malignant lymphoma and identify recurrent tumors after chemotherapy or radiation therapy
- To clarify defects in the liver when liver and spleen scanning and ultrasound tests prove inconclusive
- To evaluate lung cancer when the results of other tests conflict.

What should you know before the test?

- You'll learn about the test, including who will perform it and where, and that the scan takes 30 to 60 minutes. The scan is usually performed 24 to 48 hours after the injection of gallium.
- During the test, you may experience discomfort from the injection of gallium. However, the dosage is only slightly radioactive and isn't harmful.
- You'll receive a laxative before the test.
- You'll be asked to sign a form that gives your consent to do the test. Carefully read the form and ask questions if any portion of it isn't clear.

What happens during the test?

- The doctor injects the gallium solution into a vein in your forearm. After 24 to 48 hours, scans are taken.
- If the initial scan suggests bowel disease and additional scans are necessary, you receive a cleansing enema before continuing the test.

Does the test have risks?

A gallium scan shouldn't usually be done on children or pregnant or breast-feeding women. However, it may be performed if its potential diagnostic benefit outweighs the risks of exposure to radiation.

What are the normal results?

Gallium normally appears in the liver, spleen, bones, and large bowel.

The total body scan is usually performed 24 to 48 hours after the doctor injects gallium into an arm vein.

What do abnormal results mean?

A gallium scan may reveal inflammatory diseases. Abnormally high gallium accumulation is characteristic in inflammatory bowel diseases, such as ulcerative colitis and Crohn's disease, and in a number of cancers.

Abnormal gallium activity may be present in various sarcomas, Wilms' tumor, and neuroblastomas; cancer of the kidney, uterus, vagina, or stomach; and testicular tumors. In Hodgkin's disease and malignant lymphoma, a gallium scan may reveal abnormal activity in one or more lymph nodes.

After chemotherapy or radiation therapy, a gallium scan may be used to detect new or recurrent tumors. In a person with liver disease, the results of a gallium scan may help the doctor pinpoint the diagnosis.

In suspected lung cancer, abnormal gallium activity confirms the presence of a tumor. However, a chest X-ray should be performed to distinguish a tumor from an inflammatory lesion.

RED BLOOD CELL SURVIVAL TIME

Red blood cells, one of the main components of blood, normally die from old age. In hemolytic diseases, however, red blood cells of all ages randomly die, resulting in anemia. This test helps identify the cause of this anemia.

The test measures the lifespan of red blood cells that are removed from the body, tagged with a slightly radioactive solution of chromium, and injected back into the body. Then, over the next 3 to 4 weeks, blood samples are collected to measure the percentage of tagged cells until half of the cells disappear.

During the test period, a special camera scans the body for sites of abnormally high radioactivity, which indicates excessive red blood cell storage and destruction. Other tests may be performed with this one.

Why is this test done?

The test for red blood cell survival time may be performed for the following reasons:
- To help evaluate unexplained anemia, particularly hemolytic anemia
- To identify sites of abnormal red blood cell storage and destruction.

What should you know before the test?

- You'll learn that the test requires regular blood samples at 3-day intervals for 3 to 4 weeks. Collecting each sample takes less than 3 minutes, and the small amount of radioactive solution used is harmless.
- You don't need to fast before the blood tests.
- You'll be asked to sign a form that gives your consent to do the test. Carefully read the form and ask questions if any portion of it isn't clear.

What happens during the test?

- A blood sample is drawn from you and mixed with radioactive chromium. The mixture is injected into your arm.
- A blood sample is drawn 30 minutes after this injection to determine blood and red blood cell volumes.
- Additional blood samples are usually collected a day later and then at 3-day intervals for 3 to 4 weeks. (The intervals between samples may vary.) Radioactivity is calculated in each blood sample and the values are plotted to determine how long red blood cells last. Simultaneous scans are done of the chest, sacrum, liver, and spleen to detect radioactivity at sites of excessive red blood cell storage.

Does the test have risks?

This test shouldn't be done during pregnancy because it exposes a developing fetus to radiation, which may cause birth defects.

What are the normal results?

Normally, red blood cells have a half-life of 25 to 35 days.

What do abnormal results mean?

Shorter lifespans for the red blood cells indicate a blood disease. It could be leukemia, hemolytic anemia, hemoglobin C disease, spherocytosis, paroxysmal nocturnal hemoglobinuria, elliptocytosis, pernicious anemia, sickle cell anemia, or hemolytic-uremic syndrome.

HEART & BLOOD VESSELS

HEART SCAN

Called an *echocardiogram* by doctors, this test evaluates the size, shape, and motion of various structures within the heart. (See *The pump that keeps you going.*) It's a noninvasive test, which means that nothing enters your body during the procedure.

In an echocardiogram, a microphone-like transducer directs extremely high-pitched sound waves (which can't be heard by the human ear) toward the heart, which reflects these waves, producing echoes. The echoes are converted to images that are displayed on a monitor and recorded on a strip chart or videotape.

The doctor may use an echocardiogram when evaluating people with chest pain, enlarged heart silhouettes on X-rays, suspicious changes on electrocardiograms, and abnormal heart sounds.

Why is this test done?
An echocardiogram may be performed for the following reasons:
- To help the doctor diagnose and evaluate abnormalities of the heart's valves
- To measure the size of the heart's chambers
- To evaluate chambers and valves in congenital heart disorders
- To help diagnose hypertrophic and related cardiomyopathies
- To detect tumors in the atria
- To evaluate cardiac function or wall motion after a heart attack
- To detect pericardial effusion, a disorder marked by excessive fluid in the sac surrounding the heart.

What should you know before the test?
- You won't need to change your diet before the test.
- The test usually takes 15 to 30 minutes, and it's safe and painless.

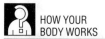

HOW YOUR
BODY WORKS

The pump that keeps you going

Your heart is the mechanism and the arteries, veins, and capillaries are the pathway by which blood circulates in your body. Together, they deliver oxygen and nutrients to the body's cells and remove waste.

The heart is a hollow, muscular organ located between the lungs. It's enclosed by a membranous sac called the *pericardium*, which consists of two layers, one inside the other. Pericardial fluid lubricates the layers as they glide over each other during heart movements.

The chambers
The heart pump system is made up of four chambers and an intricate set of valves:
- The atria — the two smaller upper chambers — receive blood from the systemic circulation and the pulmonary circulation.
- The two larger, thicker lower chambers — the ventricles — receive blood from the atria.

The valves
The interventricular septum divides the heart into right and left halves, and two valves separate the atria from the ventricles:
- The tricuspid valve separates the top chamber from the bottom in the right side.
- The mitral valve separates the top from bottom chambers in the left side of the heart.

The mitral valve has two movable leaflets; the tricuspid valve has three. Two crescent-shaped valves (the aortic and pulmonic) guard the entrances to the aortic and pulmonary arteries.

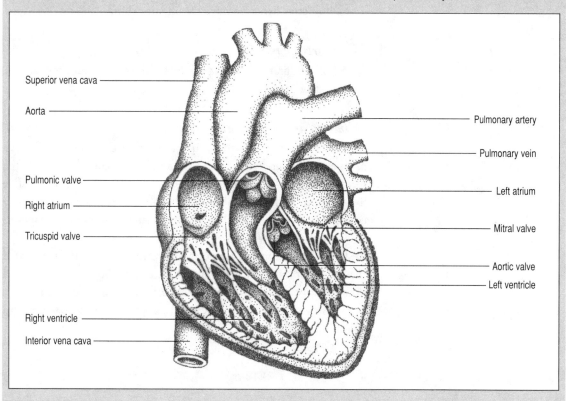

Superior vena cava

Aorta

Pulmonic valve

Right atrium

Tricuspid valve

Right ventricle

Interior vena cava

Pulmonary artery

Pulmonary vein

Left atrium

Mitral valve

Aortic valve

Left ventricle

What happens during the test?

- The room may be darkened slightly to help the examiner see the oscilloscope screen. Other procedures, such as electrocardiography, may be performed at the same time.
- You lie on an examining table for the test.
- Conductive jelly is applied to your chest and a transducer is placed on it.
- The transducer is systematically angled to direct ultrasonic waves at specific parts of your heart.
- Significant findings are recorded on a strip chart recorder or on a videotape recorder.
- To record heart function under various conditions, you may be asked to inhale and exhale slowly or to hold your breath.
- You may be asked to inhale a gas with a slightly sweet odor (amyl nitrite) while changes in your heart function are recorded. The gas can cause dizziness, flushing, and an abnormally rapid heartbeat, but these symptoms quickly subside.

What happens after the test?

The conductive jelly is removed from your skin.

What are the normal results?

An echocardiogram can show the doctor the normal motion patterns and the structures of the four heart valves.

What do abnormal results mean?

Abnormalities in heart valves, such as mitral stenosis, readily appear on the echocardiogram. The test may also indicate that one of the heart's chambers is especially large, possibly indicating congestive heart failure. Other chamber or valve abnormalities may indicate a congenital heart disorder. The doctor can use these and other signs to chose more definitive tests.

   The echocardiogram is especially sensitive in detecting pericardial effusion. Normally, the heart linings are continuous membranes, and thus produce a single or near-single echo. When fluid accumulates between these membranes, it causes an abnormal echo-free space to appear.

HEART SCAN WITH ENDOSCOPY

This test allows the doctor to see the heart's structure and function without opening the body. It combines ultrasound with endoscopy to provide a better view of your heart's structures. The medical name for this test is *transesophageal echocardiography.*

During the test, a small, microphone-like transducer is attached to the end of an endoscope and inserted into your esophagus, allowing images to be taken from the back of the heart. This causes less interference from bones and other structures near the heart and produces high-quality images of the thoracic aorta.

Why is this test done?

The test may be performed to evaluate the following conditions:
- thoracic and aortic disorders, such as dissection and aneurysm
- conditions that affect the heart's valves, especially in the mitral valve and in people with prosthetic devices
- endocarditis
- congenital heart disease
- intracardiac clots
- cardiac tumors
- valve repairs.

Heart scan with endoscopy combines two diagnostic techniques — ultrasound and endoscopy — to give the doctor a better view of your heart's structures.

What should you know before the test?

- You'll need to fast for 6 hours before the test.
- The doctor or nurse will ask if you have any conditions that might interfere with the test, such as esophageal obstruction, gastrointestinal bleeding, previous radiation therapy, severe cervical arthritis, or allergies.
- If you're having the procedure as an outpatient, arrange to have someone take you home.

What happens during the test?

- Your throat is sprayed with a topical anesthetic. You may gag when the endoscope is inserted.
- An intravenous line is inserted to sedate you before the procedure; you may feel some discomfort from the needle puncture and the pressure of the tourniquet.

- You're made as comfortable as possible during the procedure and your blood pressure and heart rate are monitored continuously.
- After the endoscope is put down your throat, ultrasound images are recorded. These images are reviewed by the doctor after the procedure.

What happens after the test?

- You'll remain in bed until the sedative wears off.
- The nurse will encourage you to cough after the procedure, either while lying on your side or sitting upright.
- You can have food or water after your gag response returns.

What are the normal results?

The test should reveal no cardiac problems.

What do abnormal results mean?

The test can reveal thoracic and aortic disorders, endocarditis, congenital heart disease, intracardiac clots, or tumors, or it can be used to evaluate valvular disease or repairs. Findings may indicate aortic dissection or an aneurysm, mitral valve disease, or congenital defects such as patent ductus arteriosus.

BLOOD VESSEL SCAN

This test — which doctors call *Doppler ultrasonography* — evaluates blood flow in your arms and legs or neck. It's a noninvasive procedure, which means nothing enters your body. It's safer, less costly, and faster than invasive tests, such as arteriography and venography. The test can accurately detect artery and vein disease that reduces blood flow by at least 50%.

In a blood vessel scan, a microphonelike transducer directs extremely high-pitch sound waves to the artery or vein being tested. The sound waves strike moving red blood cells and are reflected back to the transducer. The doctor can actually listen to the blood flow. (See *How the Doppler probe works*.)

How the Doppler probe works

If the doctor has suggested that you have this non-intrusive test, here's how it works:
- The Doppler ultrasonic probe directs high-frequency sound waves through layers of tissue.
- When these waves strike red blood cells moving through the bloodstream, their frequency changes in proportion to the rate of blood flow.
- Recording echoing waves helps the doctor detect arterial and venous obstruction, but doesn't measure the quantity of blood flowing by.

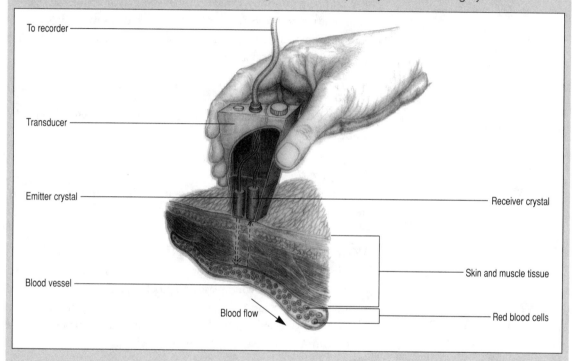

To recorder

Transducer

Emitter crystal

Blood vessel

Blood flow

Receiver crystal

Skin and muscle tissue

Red blood cells

Why is this test done?

A blood vessel scan may be performed for any of the following reasons:
- To help the doctor diagnose chronic venous insufficiency and superficial and deep vein blood clots
- To help diagnose artery disease and arterial blockage
- To monitor people who've had arterial reconstruction and bypass grafts
- To detect abnormalities of carotid artery blood flow linked to conditions such as aortic stenosis
- To evaluate possible injury to the arteries.

What should you know before the test?

The test takes about 20 minutes and doesn't involve any risk or discomfort.

What happens during the test?

- You're asked to move your arms to different positions and to perform breathing exercises as measurements are taken. A small ultrasonic probe resembling a microphone is placed at various sites along veins or arteries, and blood pressure is checked at several sites.
- You're asked to remove clothing from the area to be tested, you're draped, and you lie on an examining table or bed.

What happens after the test?

The nurse will remove all the conductive jelly left on your skin by the probe.

What are the normal results?

The examiner can hear and see that blood flow and blood pressure are within normal limits.

What do abnormal results mean?

The doctor can use the sounds of blocked arteries and veins revealed by the test to track down disease and blockages. For example, arterial narrowing or blockage reduces the blood flow velocity signal. At the lesion, the signal is high-pitched and, occasionally, turbulent. The doctor can use the test to tell how badly circulation is blocked and where.

Abdominal aorta scan

This test uses extremely high-pitched sound waves to examine your abdominal aorta, one of the main vessels for carrying blood away from your heart. It's safe and noninvasive, which means that nothing enters your body.

During the test, a microphone-like transducer directs the sound waves, which can't be heard by human ears, into your abdomen over a wide area from your breastbone to your navel. The echoing sound waves are displayed on a monitor to indicate internal organs, the spinal column, and the size and course of the abdominal aorta and other major vessels.

Why is this test done?

The scan may be performed for the following reasons:
- To detect and measure a suspected abdominal aortic aneurysm
- To detect and measure expansion of a known abdominal aortic aneurysm and so assess the risk of rupture.

What should you know before the test?

- You'll be asked to fast for 12 hours before the test to minimize bowel gas and movement.
- The lights in the examining room may be lowered; you'll feel only slight pressure as the transducer is moved across your abdomen. The test will take 30 to 45 minutes.
- Be assured that, if you've been diagnosed with an aneurysm, the sound waves will not cause rupture.

What happens during the test?

- You're asked to remain still during scanning and to hold your breath when requested.
- You lie on your back, and acoustic coupling gel or mineral oil is applied to your abdomen.
- After several scans of your abdomen, you may be placed on your right side and then on your left for more scans.

What happens after the test?

- The nurse will remove the acoustic coupling gel.
- You may resume your usual diet.

What are the normal results?

The examiner can see a normally sized and shaped abdominal aorta and four of its major branches.

What do abnormal results mean?

If the diameter of the abdominal aorta is too great, it suggests an aneurysm and the risk of rupture.

In a person with an abdominal aortic aneurysm, ultrasound of the abdominal aorta can help to determine the risk of rupture.

DIGESTIVE SYSTEM

GALLBLADDER AND BILE DUCT SCAN

This procedure uses extremely high-pitched sound waves to examine your gallbladder and your bile ducts. In this test, a focused beam of sound waves that can't be heard by human ears passes into the right upper quarter of your abdomen, creating echoes that vary with changes in tissue density. These echoes are converted to images on a monitor, indicating the size, shape, and position of the gallbladder and bile ducts.

Why is this test done?

A scan of the gallbladder and bile ducts may be performed for the following reasons:

- To help the doctor confirm a diagnosis of gallstones
- To diagnose acute inflammation of the gallbladder
- To distinguish between obstructive and nonobstructive jaundice.

What should you know before the test?

- You'll be asked to eat a fat-free meal in the evening and then to fast for 8 to 12 hours before the procedure. This diet change promotes accumulation of bile in your gallbladder and enhances the ultrasonic images.
- The test takes 15 to 30 minutes.
- The room may be darkened slightly to help the examiner read the screen.

What happens during the test?

- You feel only mild pressure as the transducer passes over your skin.
- You're asked to remain as still as possible during the procedure and to hold your breath at times to ensure that the gallbladder is in the same position for each scan.
- You lie on your back and the water-soluble lubricant on the face of the transducer will feel slick and cool on your skin.
- You may be asked to lie on your sides and to sit up for some of the scans.

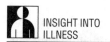
INSIGHT INTO
ILLNESS

Sites of gallstone formation

The illustration below shows potential sites of gallstone formation within the bile ducts.

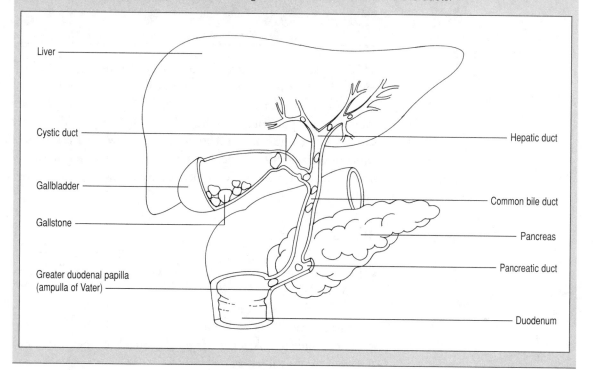

Liver

Cystic duct

Gallbladder

Gallstone

Greater duodenal papilla
(ampulla of Vater)

Hepatic duct

Common bile duct

Pancreas

Pancreatic duct

Duodenum

What happens after the test?

- The nurse will remove the lubricating jelly from your skin.
- You may resume your usual diet.

What are the normal results?

The radiologist can see that the gallbladder is of a normal shape and size, and the cystic duct and common bile ducts are properly visible.

What do abnormal results mean?

Gallstones within the gallbladder's tubes or the bile ducts typically appear as moving shadows. (See *Sites of gallstone formation*.) The doctor can also see stones in the bile ducts. The size, shape, density, and movement of shadows in the gallbladder and ducts can lead the doctor to a long list of disorders, such as cancer, inflammation, and sludge-filled bile ducts that can lead to gallstones.

LIVER SCAN

This procedure uses extremely high-pitched sound waves, which can't be heard by human ears, to examine your liver. Images are produced on a monitor by directing these high-pitched sound waves into the right upper quarter of the abdomen. Different shades of gray show various tissue densities. Ultrasound can show the liver's internal structures and its size, shape, and position. (See *Learning about the liver.*) This test is noninvasive, which means that nothing enters your body.

Why is this test done?
A liver scan may be performed for any of the following reasons:
- To help the doctor distinguish between obstructive and non-obstructive jaundice
- To screen for liver disease
- To detect liver cancer and injury
- To determine if "cold spots" detected during liver-spleen scanning represent tumors, abscesses, or cysts.

What should you know before the test?
- You'll be asked to fast for 8 to 12 hours before the test to reduce bowel gas, which hinders the transmission of ultrasound.
- The test takes 15 to 30 minutes. It's not harmful or painful, although you may feel mild pressure as the microphone-like transducer is pressed against your skin.
- You'll be asked to remain as still as possible during the procedure and to hold your breath at times.

What happens during the test?
You lie on your back, while a water-soluble lubricant is applied to the face of the transducer and the probe is moved across your skin.

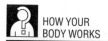

HOW YOUR
BODY WORKS

Learning about the liver

The liver is your body's largest organ. It performs more than 300 functions. The liver can function even if 90% damaged. However, removal or total destruction of the liver leads to death within about 10 hours.

Locating the liver
The liver lies on your right side, just under your ribs. An adult's liver weighs about 3 pounds (1.4 kilograms) and is divided into two lobes. The right lobe has three sections and the left lobe has two. Lobules (the liver's working units) subdivide each lobe section.

You can feel the edge of your own liver, following these directions: Lie down, take a deep breath, and wrap your fingers over the lower edge of your rib cage. In a normal liver, the edge is smooth and firm.

Liver fluids: Where they go
The portal vein and the hepatic artery supply blood to the liver (about one-third of the heart's output). About 3 pints (1.4 liters) of blood flow through your liver each minute. The portal vein delivers nutrient-rich blood from the digestive tract, while the hepatic artery carries oxygen-rich blood to liver cells. The blood flows through lobular channels called *sinusoids,* which drain into the liver's central vein.

The liver also makes bile, a fluid that helps us digest fats. Bile flows through small bile ducts between liver cell plates, and then drains into large bile ducts.

Liver cells: What they do
Special cells called *hepatocytes* do the liver's work. They work as the following:
- a factory — making chemical compounds, such as blood proteins, bile, and enzymes
- a warehouse — storing glycogen, iron, and vitamins
- a waste disposal plant — breaking down and excreting old red blood cells and urea and detoxifying drugs, poisons, and alcohol
- a power plant — burning carbohydrates, proteins, and fats
- a regulatory agency — maintaining blood sugar levels and regulating several hormones.

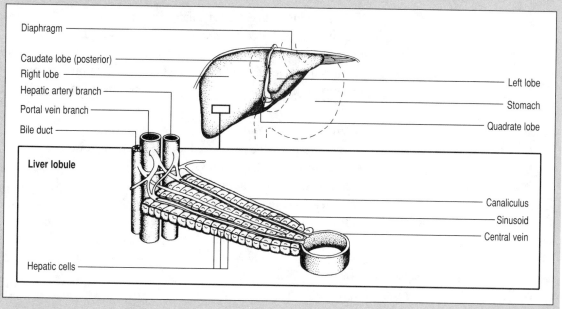

Diaphragm

Caudate lobe (posterior)
Right lobe
Hepatic artery branch
Portal vein branch
Bile duct

Left lobe
Stomach
Quadrate lobe

Liver lobule

Canaliculus
Sinusoid
Central vein

Hepatic cells

What happens after the test?

- The nurse will remove the lubricating jelly from your skin.
- You may resume your usual diet.

What are the normal results?

The liver normally appears as a homogeneous, low-level echo pattern, interrupted only by the different echo patterns of its portal and hepatic veins, the aorta, and the inferior vena cava.

What do abnormal results mean?

The doctor will look for images that indicate a long list of disorders. Dilated bile ducts point to obstructive jaundice. In cirrhosis, the scan may show variable liver size and dilated, tortuous portal branches linked to portal high hypertension. Signs of cancer in the liver vary widely — they may appear as strong or weak echoes, poorly defined or well defined. Tumors also present a varied appearance and may mimic cancers. Abscesses, cysts, and bleeding injuries all have their own characteristic look.

Spleen scan

This procedure uses extremely high-pitched sound waves to examine your spleen. A focused beam of these sound waves passes into the left upper quarter of your abdomen, creating echoes that vary with changes in tissue density. The echoes are displayed on a monitor as images that indicate the size, shape, and position of the spleen.

Why is this test done?

A spleen scan may be performed for the following reasons:

- To confirm an enlarged spleen
- To help the doctor monitor the progression of disease of the spleen and to evaluate the effectiveness of therapy
- To evaluate the spleen after abdominal injury
- To help detect cysts and an abscess of the spleen.

What should you know before the test?

- You'll be asked to fast for 8 to 12 hours before the procedure. Fasting reduces the amount of gas in the bowel, which hinders transmission of ultrasound.
- The procedure takes about 15 to 30 minutes.

What happens during the test?

- You lie on an examining table with your chest uncovered.
- The technician applies a water-soluble lubricant to the face of the microphone-like transducer and moves the ultrasound probe across your body.
- You're asked to remain as still as possible during the procedure. You're also asked to hold your breath periodically to help the examiner get a sharp image on the screen.
- The examining room may be darkened slightly to help the examiner see the screen.
- Because the procedure varies depending on the size of the spleen or your physique, you may be repositioned several times. The transducer scanning angle or path is also changed.

Because the procedure for ultrasound varies depending on the size of the spleen or your physique, you may be repositioned on the examining table several times.

What happens after the test?

- A nurse or technician will remove the lubricating jelly from your skin.
- You may resume your usual diet.

What are the normal results?

The spleen usually shows a homogeneous, low-level echo pattern, with few of its veins apparent. Its shape is usually indented by surrounding organs.

What do abnormal results mean?

The scan can show an enlarged spleen, but it usually doesn't indicate the cause. A computed tomography scan (commonly called a CAT scan) can provide more specific information. The doctor may find evidence of many disorders, including an abdominal injury that's ruptured the spleen and an abscess. Used with liver-spleen scanning, ultrasound can tell cysts from solid lesions. However, ultrasound usually fails to identify tumors associated with lymphoma and chronic leukemia.

PANCREAS SCAN

In this test, extremely high-pitched sound waves are used to examine the pancreas, the organ that secretes insulin into the bloodstream. These sound waves can't be heard by the human ear.

During the test, the doctor looks at images of the pancreas that are produced by directing the high-pitched sound waves toward the organ. When the sound waves strike the pancreas, they produce echoes, which a computer converts to visual images and displays on a monitor. The pattern varies with tissue density and indicates the size, shape, and position of the pancreas and surrounding structures. This test is noninvasive, which means that nothing enters your body.

For the ultrasound, you lie on a bed or examining table in a room that's darkened slightly to help the examiner see the screen.

Why is this test done?
A pancreas scan may be performed for any of the following reasons:
- To help the doctor detect anatomic abnormalities and diagnose pancreatitis, pseudocysts, and pancreatic cancer
- To guide the insertion of biopsy needles.

What should you know before the test?
- You'll be asked to fast for 8 to 12 hours before the procedure to reduce bowel gas.
- If you smoke, you'll be asked not to before the test.
- The test takes 30 minutes.
- The procedure isn't harmful or painful, but you may feel mild pressure from the scanner.
- You'll be asked to inhale deeply during scanning and to remain still during the procedure.

What happens during the test?
- You lie on a bed or examining table.
- The room is darkened slightly to help the examiner see the screen.
- The technician applies a water-soluble lubricant or mineral oil to your abdomen and then moves the scanner, which looks like a microphone, across your body.

What happens after the test?
- The nurse will remove the lubricating jelly from your skin.
- You may resume your usual diet.

What are the normal results?

The pancreas normally shows up as a coarse, uniform echo pattern.

What do abnormal results mean?

Changes in the size, contour, and texture of the pancreas characterize pancreatic disease. An enlarged pancreas with decreased echo strength and distinct borders suggests pancreatitis. A well-defined mass with an essentially echo-free interior indicates a pseudocyst. An ill-defined mass with scattered internal echoes or a mass in the head of the pancreas (obstructing the common bile duct) and a large gallbladder that doesn't contract suggest pancreatic cancer. A computed tomography scan (commonly called a CAT scan) and a biopsy (removal and analysis) of pancreatic tissue may be necessary to confirm a diagnosis.

MISCELLANEOUS SCANS

THYROID SCAN

This test helps the doctor define the size and shape of your thyroid gland. Ultrasonic pulses emitted from a microphone-like transducer are directed at the thyroid gland and reflected back to produce images of the organ's structure on a monitor. The test is noninvasive, which means that nothing enters your body.

After the doctor locates a lump in your neck, an ultrasound scan can help tell the difference between a cyst and a tumor. This test is also used to evaluate thyroid nodules during pregnancy because it doesn't require the use of radioactive iodine.

Why is this test done?

An ultrasound scan of the thyroid may be performed for the following reasons:

- To help the doctor evaluate thyroid structure
- To differentiate between a cyst and a tumor
- To check the size of the thyroid gland during therapy.

What should you know before the test?
- You won't need to change your diet before the test.
- The test takes approximately 30 minutes, it's painless and safe, and results are usually available within 24 hours.

What happens during the test?
- You lie on the examining table with a pillow under your shoulder blades to extend your neck.
- Your neck is coated with water-soluble gel. The technician passes the scanner across the area above your thyroid.
- The image on the monitor is photographed for later, thorough examination by the doctor.

What happens after the test?
A nurse will remove the gel from your neck.

What are the normal results?
Normally, thyroid ultrasound shows a uniform echo pattern throughout the gland.

What do abnormal results mean?
Cysts appear as smooth-bordered, echo-free areas with enhanced sound transmission. Adenomas and cancers appear either solid and well marked or, less frequently, solid with cystic areas. Identification of a tumor is generally followed up by fine needle aspiration or surgical removal and a biopsy (removal and analysis of tissue) to determine if it's cancerous.

After the doctor locates a lump in your neck, an ultrasound scan of the thyroid can help tell the difference between a cyst and a tumor.

PELVIC SCAN

This test enables the doctor to examine the pelvic organs, such as the reproductive organs and the bladder. If you're pregnant, it helps with examination of the fetus.

In pelvic ultrasound, extremely high-pitched sound waves are reflected via a microphone-like transducer to provide images of the interior pelvic area on a monitor. This test is noninvasive, which means that nothing enters your body. Selected views may be photo-

Seeing inside the womb

Imagine seeing what you can't normally see using sounds that you can't hear. Well, that's exactly what happens when an ultrasound scan of a developing fetus is performed. When very high-pitched sound waves from a microphone-like transducer are directed at the fetus's skull, echoes return and appear as spikes on a monitor. The distance between spikes is equivalent to the distance between the top and bottom cranial walls and indicates head size. The doctor uses that measurement to determine the fetus's age.

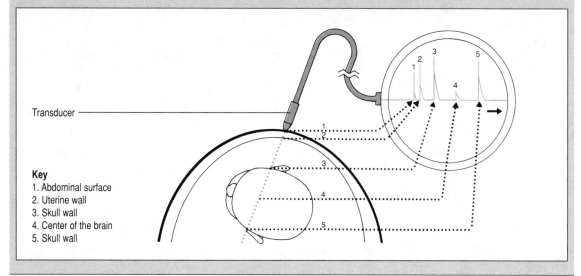

Transducer

Key
1. Abdominal surface
2. Uterine wall
3. Skull wall
4. Center of the brain
5. Skull wall

graphed for later examination by the doctor and as a permanent record of the test.

Why is this test done?

A pelvic ultrasound scan may be performed for the following reasons:
- To help the doctor evaluate symptoms that suggest pelvic disease and to confirm a tentative diagnosis
- To detect foreign bodies and distinguish between cysts and tumors
- To measure organ size
- To evaluate fetal strength, position, gestational age, and growth rate (See *Seeing inside the womb,* above, and *How a fetus grows and develops,* pages 154 and 155.)
- To detect multiple pregnancy
- To confirm fetal abnormalities and maternal abnormalities
- To guide amniocentesis by determining placental location and fetal position.

How a fetus grows and develops

The first month

At the end of 1 month, the embryo has a definite form. The head and trunk are apparent, and the tiny buds that will become the arms and legs are discernible. The heart and blood vessels have begun to work, and the umbilical cord is visible in its most primitive form.

10 TIMES ACTUAL SIZE

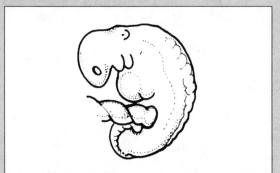

The second month

In the next month, the embryo — called a *fetus* from the seventh week on — grows to 1 inch (2.5 centimeters) in length and weighs $\frac{1}{30}$ of an ounce. The head and facial features develop as the eyes, ears, nose, lips, tongue, and tooth buds form. The arms and legs also take shape, with the fingers and toes becoming visible. Although the gender of the fetus is not yet visible, all external genitalia are present. Heart and blood vessel function is complete, and the umbilical cord has a definite form. At the end of 2 months, the fetus resembles a full-term baby except for its size.

ACTUAL SIZE

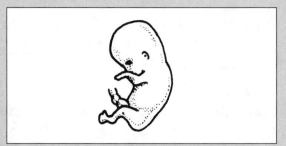

What should you know before the test?

- Because this test requires a full bladder as a reference point to help the examiner define pelvic organs, you'll be asked to drink liquids and not to empty your bladder before the test.
- The test can vary in length from a few minutes to several hours.
- A water enema may be necessary to produce a better outline of the large intestine.
- Be assured that the test will not harm a fetus.

The third month

During the third month, the fetus grows to 3 inches (7.6 centimeters) in length and weighs 1 ounce (28.4 grams). Teeth and bones begin to appear, and the kidneys start to work. Although the mother can't yet feel its activity, the fetus is moving. It opens its mouth to swallow, grasps with its tiny, but fully developed, hands, and — even though its lungs don't yet function — it prepares for breathing by inhaling and exhaling. At the end of the first trimester (3 months), its gender is apparent.

ACTUAL SIZE

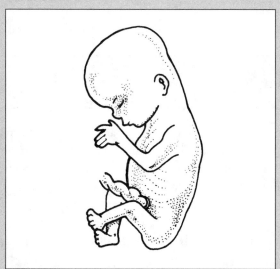

The remaining 6 months

In the remaining 6 months, fetal growth continues as internal and external structures develop at a rapid rate. In the third trimester, the fetus stores fats and minerals it will need to live outside the womb. At birth, the average full-term fetus measures 20 inches (50.8 centimeters) and weighs 7 to 7½ pounds (3.2 to 3.4 kilograms).

ONE-THIRD ACTUAL SIZE

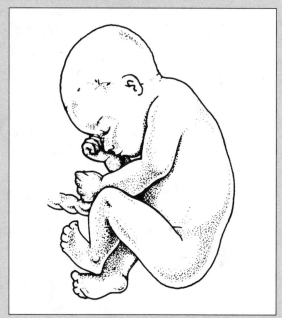

What happens during the test?

▪ You lie on an examining table, and your pelvic area is coated with mineral oil or water-soluble jelly to increase sound wave conduction.

▪ The technician guides the microphone-like transducer over the pelvic area. Images are observed on the oscilloscope screen.

What happens after the test?

You'll be allowed to empty your bladder immediately after the test.

Because this test requires a full bladder to help the examiner define pelvic organs, you'll drink a lot of liquids. You'll be allowed to empty your bladder immediately after the test.

What are the normal results?

The uterus is normal in size and shape. The ovaries' size, shape, and density are normal. No other masses are visible. If you're pregnant, the examiner can see that the gestational sac and fetus are of normal size in relation to gestational age.

What do abnormal results mean?

Both cystic and solid masses have homogeneous densities, but solid masses (such as fibroids) appear more dense. Inappropriate fetal size may indicate miscalculated conception or delivery date or a dead fetus. Abnormal echo patterns may indicate foreign bodies (such as an intrauterine device), multiple pregnancy, maternal abnormalities, fetal abnormalities, and fetal malpresentation (such as a breech or shoulder presentation).

KIDNEY SCAN

In this test, extremely high-pitch sound waves are transmitted from a microphone-like transducer to the kidneys and surrounding structures. The resulting echoes are converted into anatomic images and displayed on a monitor.

The doctor may use an ultrasound scan of the kidneys to detect abnormalities or to clarify those detected by other tests. Ultrasound of the ureter, bladder, and gonads also may be used to evaluate urologic disorders.

Why is this test done?

A kidney scan may be performed for any of the following reasons:
- To help the doctor determine the size, shape, and position of the kidneys, their internal structures, and surrounding tissues (See *Learning about the kidneys.*)
- To evaluate and localize urinary obstruction and abnormal fluid accumulation
- To assess and diagnose complications after kidney transplantation.

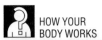

HOW YOUR
BODY WORKS

Learning about the kidneys

The kidneys are reddish brown, bean-shaped organs situated in the back of the abdomen. Each kidney is about the size of a closed hand and weighs 4 to 6 ounces (113 to 170 grams). In the kidneys, the body's waste products are filtered out of the blood and excreted in the urine in combination with water.

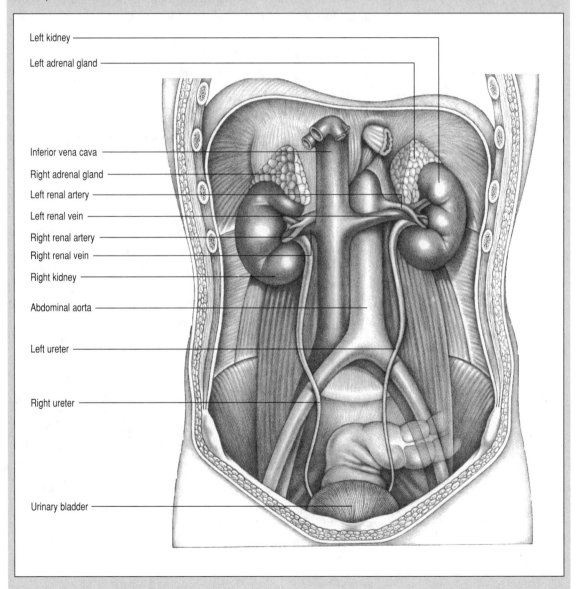

Left kidney

Left adrenal gland

Inferior vena cava

Right adrenal gland

Left renal artery

Left renal vein

Right renal artery

Right renal vein

Right kidney

Abdominal aorta

Left ureter

Right ureter

Urinary bladder

What should you know before the test?

- You won't need to change your diet before the test.
- The test takes about 30 minutes, and it's safe and painless.

What happens during the test?

- You lie on the examining table and ultrasound jelly is applied to the area to be scanned.
- You may be asked to breathe deeply to show the kidneys' movement during respiration.

What happens after the test?

The nurse will remove the ultrasound jelly from your skin.

What are the normal results?

The radiologist can see that the kidneys are of normal size and in the normal location.

What do abnormal results mean?

Cysts are usually fluid-filled, circular structures that don't reflect sound waves. Tumors produce multiple echoes and appear as irregular shapes. Abscesses found within or around the kidneys usually echo sound waves poorly. A perirenal abscess may be discovered because it displaces the kidneys.

Generally, acute kidney diseases are not detectable by ultrasound unless the kidneys are significantly scarred and decreased in size.

This test can also be used to detect inherited defects and to check the progress of a transplanted kidney.

*B*RAIN CIRCULATION SCAN

This scan provides information about the presence, quality, and changing nature of blood circulation to your brain by measuring the rate of blood flow through cerebral arteries. The medical name for this test is a *transcranial Doppler study.*

Narrowed blood vessels produce high blood flow rates, indicating possible narrowing or a spasm of a blood vessel. High rates may also indicate an arteriovenous malformation.

Why is this test done?

A brain circulation scan may be performed for the following reasons:
- To measure the rate of blood flow through certain vessels in the brain
- To help the doctor detect and monitor the progression of a spasm in one of the brain's blood vessels
- To determine whether a secondary route of blood flow exists before surgery for diseased vessels
- To help determine brain death.

What should you know before the test?

- The test will be done while you lie on a bed or a stretcher or sit in a reclining chair. It can be performed at the bedside if you're too ill to be moved to the lab.
- The procedure usually takes less than 1 hour, depending on the number of vessels to be examined.
- You won't have to change your diet before the test.

What happens during the test?

- While you recline in a chair or on an examining table, a small amount of gel is applied to the transcranial window—an area of your head where the bone is thin enough to allow the Doppler signal to enter and be detected.
- The technician directs the signal toward the artery being studied and records the rates detected. Waveforms may be printed for later analysis.

What happens after the test?

The nurse will clean the conductive gel from your skin.

What are the normal results?

The type of waveforms and blood flow rates should indicate that vessels are functioning adequately and that spasms are absent.

This test provides information about the circulation in your brain. If blood's moving too quickly, it may signal narrowing or spasm of a blood vessel.

What do abnormal results mean?

Although this test often is not definitive, high blood flow rates are typically abnormal and suggest that blood flow is too turbulent or the blood vessel is too narrow.

After the test and before surgery, the person may undergo an angiogram of the brain to further define cerebral blood flow patterns and to locate the exact blood vessel abnormality.

5

HEART & BRAIN MONITORING:
Checking Vital Functions

HEART MONITORING

ELECTROCARDIOGRAPHY

An electrocardiogram, commonly known as an EKG, is the most common test of the heart's condition. It's used to graphically record the electrical current generated by the beating heart. (See *The heart's electrical impulses.*) This current radiates from the heart in all directions and, on reaching the skin, is measured by electrodes. These electrodes are connected to an amplifier and strip chart recorder, which prints tracings. The doctor interprets the tracings to obtain information about the heart's functioning.

Why is this test done?

An electrocardiogram may be performed for the following reasons:
- To help identify irregular heartbeats, an enlarged or inflamed heart, heart damage, and the site and extent of a heart attack
- To check on recovery from a heart attack
- To evaluate the effectiveness of drugs for heart problems
- To check the performance of a cardiac pacemaker.

What should you know before the test?

- You'll learn about the test, including who will perform it, where it will take place, and its expected duration (5 to 10 minutes). During the test, electrodes will be attached to your arms, legs, and chest. The procedure is painless and you should relax, lie still, and breathe normally.
- Don't talk during the test because the sound of your voice may distort the electrocardiogram tracing.
- Tell the doctor or nurse if you're taking any medications.

What happens during the test?

- You lie on your back, and a nurse attaches electrodes to your chest, ankles, and wrists.
- The nurse connects leadwires after all electrodes are in place and may secure the limb electrodes with rubber straps, but won't tighten them too much.

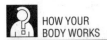

HOW YOUR
BODY WORKS

The heart's electrical impulses

Like a power plant, the heart generates and conducts its own electricity. This electricity travels through the heart to create the heartbeat.

The beat begins
The sinoatrial node, which is located in the right atrium (one of the two upper chambers of the heart), normally controls the heart rate and is called the *pacemaker.* This node has special tissue that allows it to create and send an electrical impulse through the atrium to the atrioventricular node. As an impulse passes through the atrial muscles, the atria contract.

The beat goes on
After a short delay in the atrioventricular node, the impulse travels down the bundle of His, which divides into right and left branches. Finally, the impulse reaches the Purkinje fibers, which send the impulse to the ventricles, causing them to contract.

Momentary relaxation
After contracting, the ventricles relax and begin to fill with blood, in preparation for the next impulse from the sinoatrial node.

Backup systems
The sinoatrial node fires about 60 to 100 impulses every minute. If it fails to generate the expected impulses, the atrioventricular node can take over, but at a slower rate of 40 to 60 impulses each minute. If both nodes fail, the Purkinje fibers can produce 15 to 40 impulses per minute.

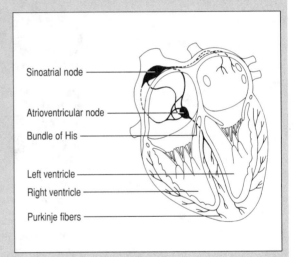

Sinoatrial node

Atrioventricular node

Bundle of His

Left ventricle

Right ventricle

Purkinje fibers

- The nurse presses the START button and the machine records and prints the electrocardiogram. (See *Performing electrocardiography*, page 164.)
- When the machine finishes, the nurse removes the electrodes.

What are the normal results?
An electrocardiogram should show no disturbances in the heart's function.

Performing electrocardiography

The photograph below shows a nurse pressing a button to start an electrocardiograph recording, a graphic recording of the electrical impulses that originate in the heart. Note the electrodes attached to the person's chest.

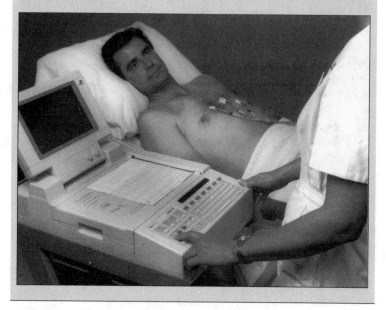

What do abnormal results mean?

An electrocardiogram may show evidence of a heart attack, enlargement of the right or left ventricle, irregular heartbeats, inflammation of the heart, and other problems. Sometimes, an electrocardiogram may only show problems during exercise or an episode of chest pain.

STRESS TEST

Referred to as an *exercise electrocardiogram* or an *exercise EKG* by doctors, this test evaluates the heart's response to physical stress. It provides important information that can't be obtained from a resting electrocardiogram.

In this test, an electrocardiogram and blood pressure readings are taken while a person walks on a treadmill or pedals a stationary bicycle. (See *Comparing two types of stress tests*, page 166.) In the multi-stage treadmill test, the speed and incline of the treadmill increase at predetermined intervals. In the bicycle test, the resistance in pedaling increases gradually as a person tries to maintain a specific speed.

Unless complications develop, the test goes on until a person reaches the target heart rate (set by the doctor) or feels chest pain or fatigue. A person who's had a recent heart attack or bypass surgery may walk the treadmill at a slow pace to determine his or her activity tolerance before being discharged from the hospital.

Why is this test done?

A stress test may be performed for the following reasons:
- To help diagnose the cause of chest pain
- To determine the heart's condition after surgery or a heart attack
- To check for blockages in the heart's arteries, particularly in men over age 35
- To help set limits for an exercise program
- To identify irregular heartbeats that develop during physical exercise
- To evaluate the effectiveness of drugs given for chest pain or irregular heartbeats.

What should you know before the test?

- You'll learn who will perform the test, where it will take place, and its expected duration. Electrodes will be attached to several areas on your chest and, possibly, your back. You won't feel any current from the electrodes; however, they may itch slightly.
- Expect that the test will make you tired, sweaty, and out of breath, but it poses few risks. The doctor may, in fact, stop the test if you feel tired or get chest pains.
- Don't eat, smoke, or drink alcohol or caffeinated beverages for 3 hours before the test. Continue to take any prescribed medications unless your doctor tells you otherwise.
- Wear comfortable socks and sneakers and loose, lightweight shorts or slacks. Men usually don't wear a shirt during the test, and women generally wear a bra and a lightweight short-sleeved blouse or a hospital gown with a front closure.
- Tell the doctor or nurse how you feel during the test.
- You'll be asked to sign a form that gives your permission to do the test. Read the form carefully and ask questions if any portion of it isn't clear.

Unless complications develop, the test goes on until a person reaches the target heart rate or feels chest pain or fatigue.

Comparing two types of stress tests

Treadmill test

Advantages

- Standardized and most reproducible
- Walking is familiar activity
- Constant work rate
- Attains highest maximum oxygen uptake
- Involves muscles commonly used; less chance of fatigue

Disadvantages

- Possibility of person losing balance and falling off
- Workload depends on weight; as weight increases, workload increases
- Noisy, makes communication more difficult

Bicycle test

Advantages

- Workload doesn't depend on weight
- Quieter than treadmill

Disadvantages

- Constant rate of pedaling required to maintain power
- Induces greater stress
- Attains lower maximum oxygen uptake
- Involves muscles less commonly used; greater chance of fatigue

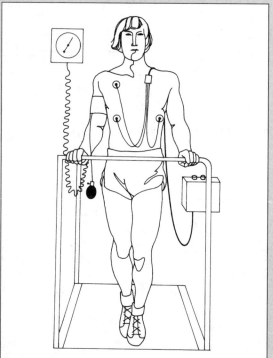

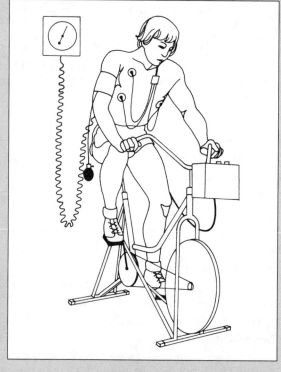

What happens during the test?

- The electrode sites are cleaned with an alcohol swab, and excess skin oils are removed with a gauze pad or fine sandpaper.
- Electrodes are placed on your chest. The leadwire cable is placed over your shoulder and the leadwire box is placed on your chest. The cable is secured by pinning it to your clothing or taping it to your shoulder or back. Then the leadwires are connected to the chest electrodes.
- The monitor is started, and a tracing is obtained. The doctor checks this tracing, takes your blood pressure, and listens to your heart.
- In a treadmill test, the treadmill is turned on to a slow speed, and you're shown how to step onto it and how to use the support railings to maintain your balance. Then the treadmill is turned off. Next, you step onto the treadmill, and it's turned on to slow speed until you get used to walking on it.
- For a bicycle test, sit on the bicycle while the seat and handlebars are adjusted to comfortable positions. Don't grip the handlebars tightly; just use them for maintaining your balance. Pedal until you reach the desired speed, as shown on the speedometer.
- During both tests, the doctor checks the monitor for changes in the heart's rhythm. The doctor also checks blood pressure at the end of each test level. Tell the doctor if you feel dizzy, light-headed, short of breath, or unusually tired. If your symptoms become severe, the doctor will halt the test.
- Usually, testing stops when you reach the target heart rate. As the treadmill speed slows, you may be instructed to continue walking for several minutes to prevent nausea or dizziness. When the treadmill is turned off, you are helped to a chair, and your blood pressure and electrocardiogram are monitored for 10 to 15 minutes.

What happens after the test?

- You may resume your usual diet.
- If any drugs were discontinued before the test, you may resume taking them.

Does the test have risks?

- Because a stress test places considerable demands on the heart, it's not usually performed if a person has an aneurysm, uncontrolled irregular heartbeats, an inflammation of the heart, severe anemia, uncontrolled high blood pressure, unstable angina, or congestive heart failure.

- You may become exhausted from the test, experience chest pain or irregular heartbeats, or have significant changes in your blood pressure. The doctor will stop the test if any of these conditions develops.

What are the normal results?

In a normal exercise electrocardiogram, a person's heart rate rises in direct proportion to the workload and increased need for oxygen. Blood pressure also rises as workload increases. A normal person attains the endurance levels appropriate for his or her age.

What do abnormal results mean?

The test can detect the damage caused by a heart attack. Specific changes in electrocardiogram waveforms may indicate disease in the left coronary artery or in multiple blood vessels in the heart.

The usefulness of the test for predicting coronary artery disease varies. Much depends on the person's medical history. However, inaccurate test results are common. To detect coronary artery disease accurately, a thallium scan and stress test, exercise multiple-gated acquisition scan, or an angiogram may be necessary.

HOLTER MONITORING

This test continuously records the heart's electrical activity as a person goes about a normal routine. In effect, Holter monitoring is an around-the-clock electrocardiogram.

During the test period, which usually lasts for 24 hours but can extend up to 7 days, a person wears a small reel-to-reel or cassette tape recorder that's connected to electrodes placed on the chest. The person also keeps a diary of his or her activities and any associated symptoms. At the end of the recording period, the tape is analyzed by a computer that correlates heart abnormalities, such as irregular beats, with the activities in the diary.

Why is this test done?

Holter monitoring may be performed for the following reasons:
- To detect irregular heartbeats missed by a stress test or resting electrocardiogram
- To evaluate chest pain

- To check the heart's condition after a heart attack or insertion of a pacemaker
- To evaluate the effectiveness of drugs given for irregular heartbeats.

What should you know before the test?

- You'll learn that you'll wear a small tape recorder for 24 hours (or for 5 to 7 days if a self-activated monitor is being used). The nurse will show you how to position the recorder when you lie down.
- The nurse or doctor will demonstrate the proper use of specific equipment, including how to mark the tape (if applicable) at the onset of symptoms.
- If a self-activated monitor is being used, you'll be shown how to press the event button to activate the monitor if you experience any unusual sensations. Don't tamper with the monitor or disconnect the leadwires or electrodes.
- If you won't be returning to the office or hospital right after the test, the nurse or doctor will show you how to remove and store the equipment.

In effect, Holter monitoring is an around-the-clock electrocardiogram.

What happens during the test?

- The nurse or doctor cleans the electrode sites, applies the electrodes to your skin, attaches the leadwires to the electrodes, and shows you how to wear the monitor on a belt or over your shoulder.
- Continue your routine activities during the test period.
- Write in a diary your usual activities (such as walking, climbing stairs, urinating, sleeping, and sexual activity) and their time. Also write down any emotional upsets, physical symptoms (dizziness, palpitations, fatigue, chest pain, and fainting), and use of medication.
- Wear loose-fitting clothing with front-buttoning tops during the test.
- Avoid magnets, metal detectors, high-voltage areas, and electric blankets during the test.
- Check the recorder to make sure it's working properly. If the monitor light flashes, one of the electrodes may be loose and you should depress the center of each one. Notify the nurse if one comes off.

What happens after the test?

The nurse will remove all chest electrodes and clean the area.

What are the normal results?

Electrocardiogram readings are compared with the person's diary. These readings reveal changes in heart rate that normally occur during various activities. The electrocardiogram should show no significant irregular heartbeats.

What do abnormal results mean?

The test can detect many different types of irregular heartbeats. During recovery from a heart attack, this test can help determine the prognosis and the effectiveness of drug therapy.

Although Holter monitoring matches symptoms and electrocardiogram changes, it doesn't always identify the symptoms' causes. If initial monitoring proves inconclusive, the test may be repeated.

IMPEDANCE TEST OF BLOOD FLOW

This test, which doctors call *impedance phlebography* or *plethysmography*, is a painless, safe, and reliable way to measure blood flow in the leg veins. In this widely used test, electrodes are applied to the leg to record changes in electrical resistance (impedance) caused by changes in blood volume variations. These changes occur during breathing and from blocked veins.

Why is this test done?

Impedance plethysmography may be performed for the following reasons:
- To detect blood clots in the deep veins of the leg, a condition called *deep vein thrombosis*
- To check people who have a high risk of thrombophlebitis, a condition in which a vein is inflamed and a blood clot lodges there
- To check for pulmonary emboli, a serious condition in which a blood clot lodges in a blood vessel in the lung. Most blood clots originate in the leg veins and travel to the lungs.

What should you know before the test?

- You'll learn who will perform the test and where and that it takes 30 to 45 minutes. The test examines both legs and requires three to five tracings for each leg.
- Accurate testing requires that leg muscles be relaxed and breathing be normal. If you have any pain that interferes with leg relaxation, you'll receive a mild pain reliever during the test.

- You'll be asked to put on a hospital gown.
- Just before the test, you should urinate.

What happens during the test?

- You lie on your back and raise the leg to be tested 30 degrees. Your calf should be above the level of your heart.
- Flex your knee slightly and rotate your hips by shifting weight to the same side as the leg being tested.
- Your skin will be prepped with electrode gel, and electrodes will be loosely attached to your calf. Then a pressure cuff is wrapped snugly around your thigh.
- The pressure cuff is inflated and maintained for 45 seconds or until the tracing stabilizes.
- A strip chart tracing records the increase in venous volume following cuff inflation and the decrease in venous volume 3 seconds after deflation. The test is repeated for the other leg. If necessary, 3 to 5 tracings for each leg are obtained. The tracing showing the greatest rise and fall in venous volume is reported as the test result.

What happens after the test?

A nurse will remove the gel from your skin.

What are the normal results?

A temporary blockage of a vein normally produces a sharp rise in the vein's blood volume. Release of the blockage produces a rapid flow of blood in the vein.

What do abnormal results mean?

When blood clots in a major deep vein block blood flow, the pressure in the calf veins rises, and these veins become distended. Such veins can't expand further when additional pressure is applied with an occlusive thigh cuff.

Blockage of major deep veins also decreases the rate at which blood flows from the leg. If significant blood clots are present in a major deep vein of the lower leg, both calf vein filling and outflow rate are reduced.

You lie on your back and raise the leg to be tested 30 degrees. Your calf should be above the level of your heart.

HEART CATHETERIZATION

This lengthy test checks the function of the heart and its blood vessels. In particular, it determines blood pressures and blood flow in the chambers of the heart, permits collection of blood samples, and records X-rays of the heart's ventricles or arteries. (See *The heart's blood supply*.)

To start the test, the doctor inserts a plastic catheter into a blood vessel in the arm or groin area and advances it slowly to the left or the right side of the heart. Then, the doctor injects a special dye through the catheter. The dye, which has properties that cause it to appear on X-rays, flows through a ventricle and coronary arteries, during which X-rays are taken.

The test may be done on either side of the heart. Testing the left side of the heart checks the coronary arteries, mitral and aortic valves, and left ventricle. It helps diagnose enlargement of the left ventricle, narrowing of aortic valve, insufficiency of the aortic or mitral valve, an aneurysm, and shunting (diversion) of blood from one side of the heart to the other.

Testing the right side of the heart checks the other heart valves — the tricuspid and pulmonic valves — and measures the pressure in the pulmonary artery.

Why is this test done?

Cardiac catheterization may be performed for the following reasons:
- To check for insufficiency or narrowing of the heart valves
- To identify septal defects and heart problems present at birth
- To evaluate the heart's blood supply, heart wall motion, and overall function.

What should you know before the test?

- You'll learn about the test, including who will perform it, where it will take place, and its duration (2 to 3 hours).
- You may receive a mild sedative but will remain conscious during the test. You'll be strapped to a padded table, and the table may be tilted so your heart can be examined from different angles.
- The doctors and nurses who perform the catheterization will wear gloves, masks, and gowns to protect you from infection.
- The changing X-ray plates and advancing film will make clacking noises.

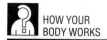

HOW YOUR
BODY WORKS

The heart's blood supply

Most people think of the heart as the pump that supplies the rest of the body with blood. But the heart itself has an intricate web of blood vessels to ensure that it receives its own share of blood (with accompanying oxygen and nutrients). Coronary artery disease results from conditions that slow blood flow and thus interfere with the heart's blood supply.

The illustrations show the network of vessels that supply blood to the heart.

FRONT VIEW

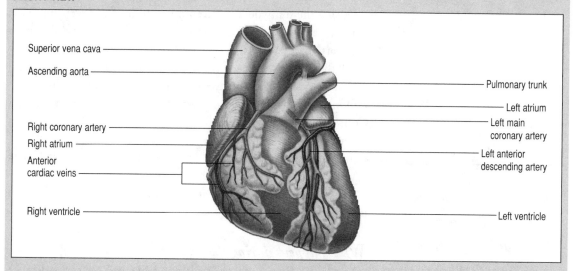

Superior vena cava

Ascending aorta

Pulmonary trunk

Left atrium

Left main coronary artery

Right coronary artery

Right atrium

Left anterior descending artery

Anterior cardiac veins

Right ventricle

Left ventricle

BACK VIEW

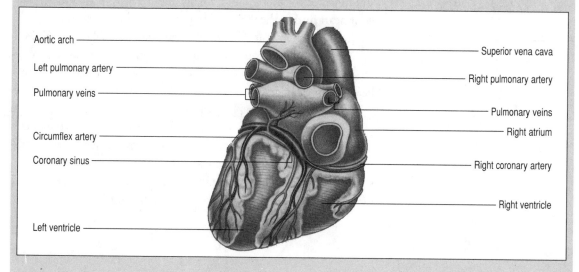

Aortic arch

Superior vena cava

Left pulmonary artery

Right pulmonary artery

Pulmonary veins

Pulmonary veins

Right atrium

Circumflex artery

Coronary sinus

Right coronary artery

Right ventricle

Left ventricle

■ For the test, you'll have an intravenous needle inserted in your arm to allow administration of medication. Electrodes for an electrocardiogram will be attached to your chest but will cause no discomfort.

■ A catheter will be inserted into an artery or vein in your arm or leg. If the skin above the vessel is hairy, it will be shaved and cleaned with an antiseptic. You'll feel a brief stinging sensation when a local anesthetic is injected to numb the incision site for catheter insertion, and you may feel pressure as the catheter moves along the blood vessel.

■ During the injection of the dye, you may feel a hot, flushing sensation or nausea that quickly passes. Follow directions to cough or breathe deeply.

■ During the test, you'll be given medication if you feel chest pain. You may also receive nitroglycerin periodically to expand the size of the heart's blood vessels.

■ Tell the doctor or nurse if you're allergic to shellfish (such as shrimp or scallops), iodine, or the dyes used in other diagnostic tests.

■ Don't eat or drink anything for at least 6 hours before the test. Continue to take any prescribed drugs unless your doctor tells you otherwise.

■ Just before the test, you should urinate and put on a hospital gown.

■ You'll be asked to sign a form that gives your permission to do the test. Read the form carefully and ask questions if any portion of it isn't clear.

What happens during the test?

■ You lie on your back on a tilt-top table and are secured by restraints. Electrocardiograph leads are applied to your skin to monitor your heart during the test and an intravenous line is inserted.

■ After injecting the local anesthetic, the doctor makes a small incision or puncture in an artery or vein. Then the doctor passes a catheter through the needle into the vessel and guides the catheter to a heart chamber or artery.

■ When the catheter is in place, the doctor injects the dye and X-rays are taken. You may be asked to cough or breathe deeply. Coughing helps counteract nausea or light-headedness caused by the dye. Deep breathing moves the diaphragm downward, making the heart easier to see.

■ During the test, you may be given nitroglycerin. After the test, the doctor removes the catheter and applies a dressing.

During the test, you may receive nitroglycerin periodically to expand the size of the heart's blood vessels.

What happens after the test?

- The nurse will check on you regularly.
- You'll rest in bed for 8 hours. If the doctor inserted the catheter into a blood vessel in the groin area, keep your leg extended for 6 to 8 hours. If the doctor inserted the catheter into a blood vessel in the arm, keep your arm extended for at least 3 hours.
- If you feel any pain, tell the nurse, who can give you medication to relieve it.
- Drink plenty of fluids high in potassium, such as orange juice.

Does the test have risks?

- A bleeding disorder, poor kidney function, or debilitation usually rules out performing the test.
- If a person has heart valve disease, antibiotics may be given before the test to guard against endocarditis.
- Complications of the test, such as a heart attack or blood clots, are rare.

Normally, the coronary arteries should have smooth and regular outlines.

What are the normal results?

Cardiac catheterization should reveal no abnormalities of heart chamber size or configuration, wall motion or thickness, direction of blood flow, or valve motion. The coronary arteries should have smooth and regular outlines.

Cardiac catheterization provides information on pressures in the heart's chambers and vessels. Higher pressures than normal are clinically significant. Lower pressures, except in shock, usually aren't significant.

The test also helps determine the ejection fraction — a comparison of the amount of blood ejected from the left ventricle during its contraction phase with the amount of blood remaining in the left ventricle at the end of its relaxation phase. A normal ejection fraction is 60% to 70%.

What do abnormal results mean?

The test can confirm coronary artery disease, poor heart function, disease of the heart valves, and septal defects.

In coronary artery disease, catheterization shows narrowing or blockages in the coronary arteries. Narrowing greater than 70% is especially significant. Narrowing of the left main coronary artery and blockage or narrowing high in the left anterior descending artery is often an indication for surgery.

Impaired wall motion can indicate coronary artery disease, aneurysm, an enlarged heart, or a heart problem present at birth. An ejection fraction under 35% generally increases the risk of complications and decreases the probability of successful surgery.

Heart valve disease is detected by a difference in pressure above and below the heart valve. The higher the difference, the greater the degree of narrowing.

Septal defects can be confirmed by measuring oxygen content in both sides of the heart. Elevated oxygen on the right side indicates a left-to-right atrial or ventricular shunt. Decreased oxygen on the left side indicates a right-to-left shunt.

HIS BUNDLE ELECTROGRAPHY

This test is used to measure the electrical impulses that produce the heartbeat and rhythm. To perform the test, the doctor inserts a small plastic catheter into a vein in the groin area and then advances the catheter into the right ventricle, one of the heart's two lower chambers.

The test measures separate conduction times as the doctor slowly withdraws the catheter from the right ventricle through the bundle of His to the sinoatrial node.

Why is this test done?
His bundle electrography may be performed for the following reasons:
- To detect irregular heartbeats
- To determine the need for a pacemaker and drug therapy and to evaluate their effects on the heart
- To find disturbances in the heart's conduction system
- To locate an abnormal site in the heart that has taken over as the heart's pacemaker
- To evaluate fainting
- To detect and locate abnormal conduction tissue in the heart.

What should you know before the test?
- You'll learn about the test, including who will perform it, where it will take place, and its duration (1 to 3 hours).
- You'll be conscious during the test. If you feel any pain, tell the doctor or nurse right away.

- Don't eat or drink anything for at least 6 hours before the test.
- Your groin area will be shaved, a catheter will be inserted into a vein, and an intravenous line may be started. You'll receive a local anesthetic but may still feel some pressure when the doctor inserts the catheter.
- Just before the test, you should urinate.
- You'll be asked to sign a form that gives your permission to do the test. Read the form carefully and ask questions if any portion of it isn't clear.

What happens during the test?

- You lie on a special X-ray table. Electrodes are applied for an electrocardiogram, which will be done during the test. The insertion site is shaved, scrubbed, and sterilized.
- The doctor injects the local anesthetic, inserts the catheter, and advances it into the right ventricle. Then the doctor slowly withdraws the catheter as recordings of conduction intervals are made. (See *A view of His bundle catheterization*, page 178.)
- After recordings and measurements are completed, the catheter is removed and a dressing is applied to the site.

This test is used to find disturbances in the electrical system that produces your heartbeat.

What happens after the test?

- You'll rest in bed for 4 to 6 hours. A nurse will check on you regularly during this period. Tell the nurse if you feel short of breath or have chest pains.
- You may resume your usual diet.
- You'll be scheduled for a follow-up electrocardiogram to monitor your heart's functioning.

Does the test have risks?

- This test shouldn't be done if a person has a severe bleeding disorder, recent thrombophlebitis, or a pulmonary embolism.
- Possible complications of the test include irregular heartbeats, vein inflammation, bloods clots in the lungs, and severe bleeding.

What are the normal results?

The test should demonstrate normal conduction intervals.

A view of His bundle catheterization

In this view, the doctor has inserted an electrode catheter through the superior vena cava, right atrium, and tricuspid valve. When the doctor slowly withdraws the catheter, the tip moves downward along the ventricle wall. As it passes the bundle of His, a characteristic spike appears on the electrogram.

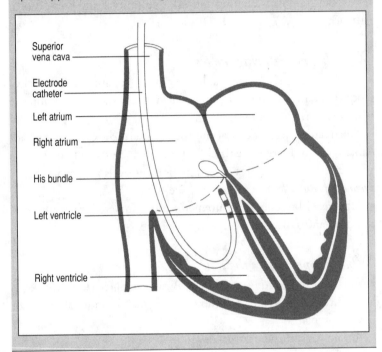

Superior vena cava

Electrode catheter

Left atrium

Right atrium

His bundle

Left ventricle

Right ventricle

What do abnormal results mean?

Longer-than-normal conduction intervals can be caused by acute or chronic heart disease. Shorter-than-normal intervals can be caused by atrial pacing, chronic conduction system disease, carotid sinus pressure, a recent heart attack, diseases of the atria, and use of certain drugs.

PULMONARY ARTERY CATHETERIZATION

Also known as *Swan-Ganz catheterization,* this test evaluates heart function and provides information necessary to determine therapy. It's usually performed at bedside in an intensive care unit.

During the test, the doctor slowly advances a small catheter through an arm or neck vein into the heart. Once the catheter is positioned, the doctor intermittently blocks and releases the flow of blood through the pulmonary artery. The test measures both pulmonary artery pressure and pulmonary artery wedge pressure. The catheter usually stays in place for 2 or 3 days.

Why is this test done?

Pulmonary artery catheterization may be performed for the following reasons:
- To help evaluate heart failure
- To monitor therapy for complications of a heart attack
- To check fluid status in a person with serious burns, kidney disease, or fluid accumulation in the lungs after open heart surgery
- To check the effects of drugs such as nitroglycerin.

What should you know before the test?

- You'll learn about the test, including who will perform it and where. You'll be conscious during catheterization and may feel brief local discomfort from the administration of the local anesthetic.
- The catheter insertion takes about 30 minutes but the catheter will remain in place, causing little or no discomfort, for 48 to 72 hours. You'll need to stay in bed during this period to avoid dislodging the catheter.
- While the catheter is in place, tell the doctor or nurse right away if you feel any pain.
- You'll be asked to sign a form that gives your permission to do the test. Read the form carefully and ask questions if any portion of it isn't clear.

What happens during the test?

- You lie on your back. The doctor inserts the catheter into a vein in your arm or neck.
- The doctor advances the catheter through the heart into the pulmonary artery. At each stage of the journey, the doctor checks the monitor for characteristic waveform changes.
- Next, the doctor inflates a tiny balloon at the end of the catheter and measures arterial pressures.
- When the catheter's correct position and function is established, the doctor stitches it to the skin. Ointment and an airtight dressing are applied to the insertion site. A chest X-ray is obtained.
- Pressure measurements are made at different times during the next 2 to 3 days. After they're all completed, the doctor removes the catheter.

What happens after the test?

A nurse will check on you regularly, keeping an eye on the site where the catheter was inserted for any signs of infection, such as redness, swelling, and discharge.

Does the test have risks?

- The test should be performed cautiously in a person with a heart block or an implanted pacemaker.
- The test can cause serious complications, such as a pulmonary embolism, pulmonary artery perforation, heart murmurs, blood clots, and irregular heartbeats.

What are the normal results?

The test records pressures within different parts of the heart. Normal readings are:
- Right atrium pressure: 1 to 6 millimeters of mercury
- Right ventricle pressure during contraction: 20 to 30 millimeters of mercury
- Right ventricle pressure at the end of relaxation: 5 millimeters of mercury
- Pulmonary artery pressure during contraction: 20 to 30 millimeters of mercury
- Pulmonary artery pressure during relaxation: about 10 millimeters of mercury
- Mean pulmonary artery pressure: less than 20 millimeters of mercury
- Pulmonary artery wedge pressure: 6 to 12 millimeters of mercury
- Left atrial pressure: about 10 millimeters of mercury.

Measurements of pressure in the arteries are made at different times during the next 2 to 3 days.

What do abnormal results mean?

Abnormally high pressure in the right atrium can indicate lung disease, failure of the right side of the heart, fluid overload, cardiac tamponade, tricuspid valve narrowing and insufficiency, or pulmonary high blood pressure. Abnormally high pressure in the right ventricle can be caused by pulmonary hypertension, narrowing of the pulmonic valve, right ventricular failure, severe inflammation of the heart, chronic heart failure, or ventricular septal defects.

An unusually high pulmonary artery pressure occurs in a left-to-right shunting (diversion) of blood within the heart, pulmonary high blood pressure or mitral stenosis, emphysema, a blood clot or fluid accumulation in the lungs, and left ventricular failure.

Elevated pulmonary artery wedge pressure can be caused by left ventricular failure, mitral valve narrowing and insufficiency, or cardiac tamponade.

BRAIN MONITORING

ELECTROENCEPHALOGRAPHY

Usually known by the abbreviation EEG, this test records the brain's electrical activity. It's performed by attaching electrodes to areas of the scalp. These electrodes record some of the brain's electrical activity and send this information to an electroencephalograph machine, which traces the brain waves on paper or a computer screen.

Why is this test done?

An electroencephalograph may be performed for the following reasons:
- To determine the presence and type of seizures
- To help diagnose brain abscesses and tumors
- To evaluate the brain's electrical activity in head injury, meningitis, encephalitis, mental retardation, and psychological disorders
- To confirm brain death.

*An electroencephalograph
can cause seizures if
a person already has
a seizure disorder.*

What should you know before the test?

▪ Don't drink caffeine-containing coffee, tea, colas, or other beverages beforehand. Otherwise, you can follow your usual diet.

▪ Thoroughly wash and dry your hair to remove hair sprays, creams, or oils.

▪ Tell the doctor or nurse if you take any medications — especially drugs for seizures, anxiety, insomnia, or depression. You may have to stop taking any of these medications for a day or two before the test.

▪ If you're going to have a "sleep electroencephalograph," you'll need to stay awake the night before the test. Just before the test, a nurse will give you a sedative to help you sleep during the test.

▪ You'll be asked to sign a form that gives your permission to do the test. Read the form carefully and ask questions if any portion of it isn't clear.

What happens during the test?

▪ During the test, you relax in a reclining chair or lie on a bed, and electrodes are attached to your scalp with a special paste. The electrodes don't cause any electric shocks.

▪ Before the recording procedure begins, close your eyes, relax, and remain still. Don't talk.

▪ The recording may be stopped now and then to let you rest or reposition yourself.

▪ After the initial recording, you may be tested under various stress-producing conditions to elicit patterns not observable while you're resting. For example, you may be asked to breathe deeply and rapidly for 3 minutes, which may elicit brain wave patterns typical of seizures or other problems. Or a bright light may be shone at you.

What happens after the test?

▪ The nurse will remove the electrode paste from your hair.

▪ If you received a sedative before the test, you'll feel drowsy afterward.

▪ The nurse will tell you when you can take any medications that were suspended for the test.

Does the test have risks?

▪ An electroencephalograph can cause seizures in a person with a seizure disorder. If a seizure occurs, the doctor will treat it right away.

What are the normal results?

An electroencephalograph records a portion of the brain's electrical activity as waves. Some of the waves are irregular, while others demonstrate frequent patterns. Among the basic waveforms are the alpha, beta, theta, and delta rhythms.

Alpha waves occur at a frequency of 8 to 12 cycles per second in a regular rhythm. They're present only when you're awake and alert but your eyes are closed. Usually, they disappear with visual activity or mental concentration.

Beta waves occur at a frequency of 13 to 30 cycles per second. They're generally associated with anxiety, depression, or the use of sedatives.

Theta waves occur at a frequency of 4 to 7 cycles per second. They're most common in children and young adults.

Delta waves occur at a frequency of 0.5 to 3.5 cycles per second. Normally, they occur only in young children and during sleep.

What do abnormal results mean?

Usually, about 100 pages of recording paper are evaluated, with particular attention paid to basic waveforms, symmetry of brain activity, brief bursts of energy, and responses to stimulation.

In seizure disorders, the electroencephalograph pattern may identify the specific type of seizure. In *absence seizures,* the electroencephalograph shows spikes and waves at a frequency of 3 cycles per second. In *generalized tonic-clonic* or *grand mal seizures*, it usually shows multiple, high-voltage, spiked waves in both hemispheres of the brain. In *complex partial seizures*, the electroencephalograph usually shows spiked waves in the affected region. And in *focal seizures*, it usually shows localized, spiked discharges.

In brain tumors or abscesses, the electroencephalograph may show slow waves (usually delta waves, but possibly beta waves). Generally, any condition that causes a diminishing level of consciousness alters the electroencephalograph pattern in proportion to the degree of consciousness lost. For example, if a person has meningitis or encephalitis, the electroencephalograph shows generalized, diffuse, and slow brain waves.

ELECTRICAL IMPULSES OF THE NERVOUS SYSTEM

A group of tests, which doctors call *evoked potential studies,* are used to measure the electrical activity of the central nervous system. They aid evaluation of visual and somatosensory pathways by measuring evoked potentials — the brain's electrical response to stimulation of the sensory organs or peripheral nerves.

The evoked potentials are recorded as electronic impulses by electrodes attached to the scalp and skin over various nerves. A computer separates these low-amplitude impulses from background brain wave activity and averages the signals from repeated stimuli. Testing may evaluate two forms of evoked potentials.

Visual evoked potentials, produced by exposing the eye to a rapidly reversing checkerboard pattern, help evaluate demyelinating diseases, injuries, and puzzling visual complaints.

Somatosensory evoked potentials, produced by electrically stimulating a peripheral sensory nerve, are used to diagnose peripheral nerve disease and locate brain and spinal cord tumors.

Why is this test done?

Evoked potential studies may be performed for the following reasons:
- To help diagnose brain and spinal cord tumors and abnormalities
- To check brain function
- To monitor comatose people and people under anesthesia
- To check on spinal cord function during spinal cord surgery
- To evaluate the brains of infants whose sensory systems can't be adequately assessed.

What should you know before the test?

- You'll learn about the test, including who will perform it, where it will take place, and that it usually lasts 45 to 60 minutes. During the test, you'll sit in a reclining chair or lay on a bed. If visual evoked potentials will be measured, electrodes will be attached to your scalp; if somatosensory evoked potentials will be measured, electrodes will be placed on your scalp, neck, lower back, wrist, knee, and ankle.
- Try to relax during the test. The electrodes won't hurt you.
- Remove all jewelry.

What happens during the test?

You lie in a reclining chair or on a bed and remain still and relax.

Visual evoked potentials

▪ You're placed 3 feet (1 meter) from the pattern-shift stimulator. Electrodes are attached to your scalp at different spots.

▪ As one eye is covered, you'll fix your gaze on a dot in the center of the screen.

▪ A checkerboard pattern is projected and then rapidly reversed or shifted 100 times, once or twice per second.

▪ A computer amplifies and averages the brain's response to each stimulus, and the results are plotted as a waveform.

▪ The procedure is repeated for the other eye.

Somatosensory evoked potentials

▪ Electrodes are attached to your skin over somatosensory pathways — typically the wrist, knee, and ankle to stimulate peripheral nerves. Other electrodes are placed on the scalp and other spots.

▪ Painless electrical stimulation is delivered to the peripheral nerve through the electrode. The intensity is adjusted to produce a minor muscle response such as a thumb twitch.

▪ Electrical stimuli are delivered 500 or more times, at a rate of 5 per second.

▪ A computer measures and averages the time it takes for the electrical current to reach the brain's cortex; the results, expressed in milliseconds, are recorded as waveforms.

▪ The test is repeated once to verify results; then the electrodes are repositioned and the entire procedure is repeated for the other side.

Painless electrical stimulation is delivered to the peripheral nerve — just enough to make a thumb twitch.

What are the normal results?

The test should reveal no abnormal waveforms.

What do abnormal results mean?

Abnormal results can occur in many conditions, such as multiple sclerosis, optic neuritis, retinopathies, amblyopia, sarcoidosis, Parkinson's disease, Huntington's disease, cervical spondylosis, brain tumors, Guillain-Barré syndrome, spinal cord injury, and others. However, the results of evoked potential studies alone can't confirm any of these diseases. Results must be interpreted in light of other tests.

Nerve conduction time: Clue to disease

Nerve conduction time is the speed at which nerves can transmit electrical messages from the body to the brain. Measuring nerve conduction time provides important information for diagnosing peripheral nerve injuries and diseases.

Performing the test

The doctor gives a person a mild electrical shock to stimulate a particular nerve. The shock is administered through the skin and underlying tissue. After each shock, a recording electrode that's placed a set distance from the site of the shock detects the response from the stimulated nerve. The lag between the shock and the response is measured. In peripheral nerve injuries and diseases, this lag time is abnormal.

NERVOUS SYSTEM MONITORING WITH ELECTROMYOGRAPHY

Electromyography, commonly abbreviated as EMG, is used to measure the electrical activity of certain skeletal muscle groups at rest and during voluntary contraction. In this test, the doctor inserts a needle electrode into a muscle and then measures the electrical discharge of the muscle, which is displayed electronically.

Why is this test done?

An electromyography may be performed for the following reasons:
- To help differentiate between primary muscle disorders, such as the muscular dystrophies, and secondary disorders
- To evaluate diseases characterized by degeneration of nerve tissue, such as amyotrophic lateral sclerosis
- To help diagnose neuromuscular disorders such as myasthenia gravis.

What should you know before the test?

- You'll learn about the test, including who will perform it, where it will take place, and its duration (1 hour). During the test, a needle will be inserted into selected muscles and you may feel some discomfort.
- Usually, you don't need to fast before the test. In some cases, cigarettes, coffee, tea, and cola may be restricted for 2 or 3 hours before the test.
- Tell the doctor or nurse if you're taking any medications.
- During the test, you may wear a hospital gown or any comfortable clothing that permits access to the muscles to be tested.
- You'll be asked to sign a form that gives your permission to do the test. Read the form carefully and ask questions if any portion of it isn't clear.

What happens during the test?

- You lie on a stretcher or bed or in a chair, depending on the muscles to be tested. Position your arm or leg so that the muscle to be tested is at rest.
- The doctor inserts the needle electrodes and places a metal plate under you. Then the muscle's electrical signal (called the *motor unit potential*) is recorded during rest and contraction.

• Frequently, the leadwires of the recorder are attached to an audio-amplifier so that the fluctuation of voltage within the muscle can be heard.

What happens after the test?
If you feel any pain, tell the nurse, who will apply warm compresses and give you pain medication.

Does the test have risks?
This procedure shouldn't be performed on a person with a bleeding disorder.

What are the normal results?
At rest, a normal muscle exhibits little electrical activity. During voluntary contraction, however, electrical activity increases markedly.

What do abnormal results mean?
Changes in electrical activity from the norm may indicate primary muscle diseases, such as the muscular dystrophies, amyotrophic lateral sclerosis, or myasthenia gravis.

Another test, called *nerve conduction time,* may be performed to help detect peripheral nerve disorders. (See *Nerve conduction time: Clue to disease.*)

FETAL MONITORING

EXTERNAL MONITORING OF THE FETUS

This painless test checks the health of the fetus. It can be performed before or during labor. This test doesn't harm the fetus in any way and doesn't interfere with normal labor.

During the test, the doctor positions an electronic device on the mother's abdomen, over the fetus. The device records the heart rate of the fetus and, during labor, the strength and frequency of contractions.

Why is this test done?

External monitoring of the fetus may be performed for the following reasons:

- To measure the heart rate of the fetus and the frequency of contractions
- To detect distress in the fetus
- To determine the need for internal fetal monitoring.

What should you know before the test?

- If this test is being done before labor, you should eat a meal just before it. Eating increases the fetus's activity and reduces the test time.
- You'll be asked to sign a form that gives your permission to do the test. Read the form carefully and ask questions if any portion of it isn't clear.

What happens during the test?

- You lie on the examining table with your abdomen exposed.
- The doctor or nurse feels your abdomen to identify the fetal chest area and locates the most distinct heart sounds. Then an electronic device called an *ultrasound transducer* is secured over this area with an elastic band or strap. The transducer directs sound waves toward the fetus. These sound waves have a pitch so high they can't be heard by human ears. When the sound waves reach the fetus, they rebound to the transducer, which sends them to a computer for interpretation and display.

Monitoring before labor

The doctor may repeat the test weekly, if needed.

Monitoring before labor with a nonstress test

- You hold the transducer in your hand and push it each time you feel the fetus move.
- If these movements don't rouse the fetus, the nurse may shake your abdomen and repeat the test.

Monitoring before labor with a stress test

- The test can be done in two ways: by administering a drug called *oxytocin* or by nipple stimulation.
- If you receive oxytocin, the test continues until three contractions occur within 10 minutes, each lasting longer than 45 seconds.
- If nipple stimulation is used instead, you'll be asked to rub one nipple with your fingers until a contraction begins. If a second contraction doesn't occur in 2 minutes, the nurse tells you to rub the

If you're being tested before labor begins, eat a meal first. It increases the baby's activity and reduces the test time.

nipple again. If contractions don't start within 15 minutes, you rub both nipples at the same time.

Monitoring during labor

The transducer is placed over the area of greatest uterine activity during contractions (usually the fundus).

Does the test have risks?

The stress test could cause fetal distress during oxytocin administration or nipple stimulation. In such cases, the test is discontinued and the doctor is notified.

What are the normal results?

The normal heart rate for a fetus ranges from 120 to 160 beats per minute. That's roughly double the normal rate for an adult. The heart rate for a fetus may normally differ from one minute to the next by 5 to 25 beats.

What do abnormal results mean?

A heart rate of less than 120 beats per minute may indicate a heart problem, poor position of the fetus, or an inadequate supply of oxygen. A slow heart rate may also be caused by drugs taken by the mother.

A heart rate of more than 160 beats per minute may be caused by drug use by the mother or her fever, rapid heart rate, or hyperthyroidism. It can also warn of inadequate oxygen for the fetus or signal a fetal infection or irregular heartbeat.

A fluctuation of less than 5 beats per minute may be due to an irregular heartbeat, an inadequate oxygen supply, an infection, or the mother's use of drugs. Accelerations of more than 25 beats per minute may signal lack of oxygen. They may precede or follow variable decelerations and may indicate a breech position.

The nonstress test can suggest problems that may be present at birth. The stress test can also suggest these problems. If it continues to be abnormal, internal fetal monitoring or a cesarean birth may be necessary.

The normal heart rate for a fetus ranges from 120 to 160 beats per minute. That's roughly double the normal adult rate.

INTERNAL MONITORING OF THE FETUS

This test, which is performed only during labor, accurately checks on the health of the fetus. Internal monitoring can be performed only after the membranes have ruptured and the cervix has dilated 1¼ inches (3 centimeters).

To perform the test, the doctor attaches a small electrode to the fetus's scalp. The electrode allows the doctor to directly monitor the heart rate of the fetus. (See *How internal fetal monitoring works*.)

Why is this test done?

Internal monitoring of the fetus may be performed for the following reasons:
- To check the heart rate of the fetus, especially for changes from beat to beat
- To measure the frequency and pressure of contractions, which allows doctors to monitor the progress of labor
- To check on the health of the fetus during labor and to determine if a cesarean section is necessary.

What should you know before the test?

- You may be told to expect mild discomfort when the uterine catheter and scalp electrode are inserted.
- You'll be asked to sign a form that gives your permission to do the test. Read the form carefully and ask questions if any portion of it isn't clear.

What happens during the test?

- As you lie on the examining table, the doctor examines your vagina. Breathe through your mouth and relax your abdominal muscles.
- After the vaginal exam, the doctor touches the scalp of the fetus, inserts a small plastic tube carrying the electrode and a wire into the cervix, and gently attaches the electrode to the fetal scalp. The doctor then removes the tube.
- The doctor attaches the wire to a transducer, which is strapped securely to your thigh. Another cable attaches the transducer to the fetal monitor. Then monitoring begins.
- If monitoring indicates a problem, you may receive intravenous fluids and oxygen and be turned on your side (preferably, your left). If these

How internal fetal monitoring works

To perform internal fetal monitoring, the doctor attaches an electrode to the scalp of the fetus. The electrode detects each beat of the fetal heart and sends this information to an amplifier.

Subsequently, a device called a *cardiotachometer* measures the intervals between heartbeats and creates a graph of the fetal heart rate. The graph or waveform appears on a monitor.

At the same time, a catheter within the uterus measures the frequency and pressure of uterine contractions. This information also appears as a waveform on the monitor.

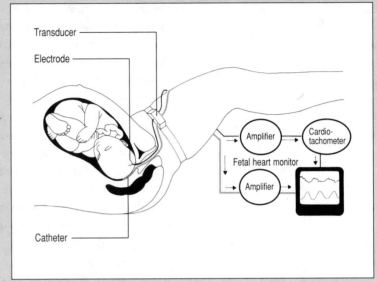

measures return heart rate patterns to normal, labor may continue. If abnormal patterns continue, a cesarean section may be necessary.

Does the test have risks?

- Internal fetal monitoring won't be performed if the doctor is unsure about the fetus's presenting part.
- The test also won't be done if the mother has cervical or vaginal herpes lesions.
- The test carries a slight risk to the mother with a perforated uterus or an infection. It also carries a slight risk to the fetus with a scalp abscess or a blood clot.

What are the normal results?

The normal heart rate for the fetus ranges from 120 to 160 beats per minute. This rate can normally vary by 5 to 25 beats per minute.

What do abnormal results mean?

A heart rate of less than 120 beats per minute may indicate a heart problem, malpositioned fetus, or an inadequate supply of oxygen. A slow heart rate may also be caused by drugs taken by the mother, such as Inderal or narcotic pain relievers.

A heart rate of more than 160 beats per minute may be caused by drug use by the mother or her fever, rapid heart rate, or hyperthyroidism. It can also warn of inadequate oxygen for the fetus or signal a fetal infection or irregular heartbeat.

A fluctuation of less than 5 beats per minute may be caused by an irregular heartbeat, an inadequate oxygen supply, an infection, or the mother's use of drugs.

A slowing of the fetal heart rate after a contraction begins, a lag time greater than 20 seconds, and a recovery time of more than 15 seconds may be related to a uterine or placental problem, a lack of adequate oxygen for the fetus, or acidosis. Recurrent and persistently late slowing of the heart rate usually indicates serious fetal distress.

Sudden, sharp drops in heart rate, if unrelated to contractions, are commonly related to cord compression. A severe drop in heart rate indicates fetal distress.

6

ENDOSCOPY:
Peering through
the Body's Passageways

RESPIRATORY SYSTEM

EXAMINATION OF THE LARYNX

Called *direct laryngoscopy,* this test detects problems in the larynx, the upper part of the windpipe that contains the vocal cords. The larynx is sometimes referred to as the voice box.

This test lets the doctor see the larynx by the use of a fiber-optic endoscope or laryngoscope passed through the mouth and pharynx to the larynx. The doctor will use it especially for children, for people with strong gag reflexes, for people who've had no response to short-term therapy to relieve symptoms, or for people with symptoms of pharyngeal or laryngeal disease. (See *Indirect laryngoscopy: A method of viewing the larynx.*)

Why is this test done?
Laryngoscopy may be performed for the following reasons:
- To detect lesions or strictures and to remove benign tumors or foreign bodies from the larynx
- To help the doctor diagnose laryngeal cancer
- To examine the larynx when indirect laryngoscopy is inadequate.

What should you know before the test?
- You'll be told to fast for 6 to 8 hours before the test.
- The test will be performed in a dark operating room.
- You'll be given a sedative to help you relax, medication to reduce secretions and, during the procedure, a general or local anesthetic. Be assured that this procedure won't obstruct your breathing.
- The nurse will ask you to sign a consent form.
- Just before the test, you'll be asked to remove any dentures, contact lenses, and jewelry and to empty your bladder.

What happens during the test?
- You lie on your back, with your arms at your sides, and are encouraged to breathe through your nose and relax.
- You're given a general anesthetic. Alternatively, your mouth and throat may be sprayed with a local anesthetic.

Indirect laryngoscopy: A method of viewing the larynx

This procedure is usually performed in the doctor's office. It allows the doctor to see the larynx, using a warm laryngeal mirror positioned at the back of the throat, a head mirror held in front of the mouth, and a light source.

Undergoing this test
You're asked to sit erect in a chair and stick your tongue out as far as possible. The tongue is grasped with a piece of gauze and held in place with a tongue depressor. If your gag reflex is sensitive, a local anesthetic may be sprayed on the pharyngeal wall. Then, the larynx is observed at rest and when you make a noise. Polyps may also be removed during this procedure.

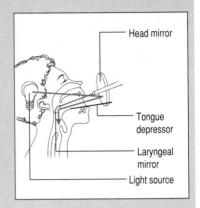

Head mirror

Tongue depressor

Laryngeal mirror

Light source

■ The laryngoscope is put through your mouth, the larynx is examined for abnormalities, and a specimen or secretions may be removed for further study. Minor surgery, such as removal of polyps or nodules, may be performed at this time.

What happens after the test?
■ The nurse may give you a soothing ice collar to minimize laryngeal swelling.
■ You'll be told to spit saliva into a basin, rather than swallow it, and to refrain from clearing your throat and coughing.
■ You'll be advised to avoid smoking until there's no evidence of complications.
■ The doctor will restrict food and fluids until your gag reflex returns (usually 2 hours). Then you may resume your usual diet, beginning with sips of water.
■ You may experience temporary loss of voice, hoarseness, or sore throat.

What are the normal results?
A normal larynx shows no evidence of inflammation, lesions, strictures, or foreign bodies.

What do abnormal results mean?

The combined results of direct laryngoscopy, a biopsy (removal and analysis of tissue), and radiography may indicate laryngeal cancer. Direct laryngoscopy may show benign lesions, strictures, or foreign bodies and, with a biopsy, may distinguish swelling of the larynx from a radiation reaction or tumor.

EXAMINATION OF THE LOWER AIRWAYS

A test called *bronchoscopy* is used to examine the lower airways. The doctor can see the larynx, windpipe, and bronchi through a flexible fiber-optic bronchoscope. A brush, biopsy forceps, or a catheter may be passed through the bronchoscope to withdraw specimens for a laboratory exam. (See *Undergoing bronchoscopy.*)

Why is this test done?

Bronchoscopy may be performed for the following reasons:
- To let the doctor visually examine a possible tumor, obstruction, secretion, bleeding, or foreign body
- To help the doctor diagnose lung cancer, tuberculosis, interstitial lung disease, or a fungal or parasitic lung infection
- To remove foreign bodies, malignant or benign tumors, mucus plugs, or excessive secretions from the tracheobronchial tree.

What should you know before the test?

- You'll be told to fast for 6 to 12 hours before the test.
- For the test, the room will be darkened, and the procedure will take 45 to 60 minutes. Results are usually available in 1 day. A tuberculosis report may take up to 6 weeks, however.
- Chest X-rays and blood studies will be performed before the bronchoscopy.
- You may receive an intravenous sedative to help you relax.
- If your test isn't being performed under general anesthesia, a local anesthetic will be sprayed into your nose and mouth to suppress the gag reflex. The spray has an unpleasant taste, and you may feel some discomfort during the procedure.

Undergoing bronchoscopy

In a bronchoscopy, the doctor inserts a flexible tube through a person's nostril into the bronchi. The bronchoscope, shown enlarged here, has four channels. Two channels (A) provide a light source. A third channel (B) allows the doctor to see. A fourth channel (C) allows the passage of medical instruments (to obtain a tissue sample for a biopsy, for instance) or medication.

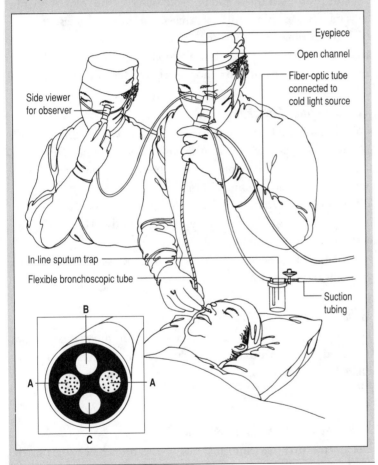

Side viewer for observer

Eyepiece

Open channel

Fiber-optic tube connected to cold light source

In-line sputum trap

Flexible bronchoscopic tube

Suction tubing

B

A   A

C

- Remember that your breathing won't be blocked during the procedure and oxygen will be administered through the bronchoscope.
- The nurse will ask you to sign a consent form and will check your history for hypersensitivity to anesthesia.
- Just before the test, you'll be asked to remove any dentures, hearing aids, or jewelry.

What happens during the test?

- You're asked to lie on an examining table or bed or to sit upright in a chair.
- The nurse urges you to remain relaxed, with your arms at your sides, and to breathe through your nose. Supplemental oxygen is available, if necessary.
- After the local anesthetic is sprayed into your throat and takes effect, a bronchoscope is introduced. The doctor inspects the anatomic structure of the windpipe and bronchi, observes the color of the mucous membrane lining, and notes masses or inflamed areas.
- The doctor may use biopsy forceps to remove a tissue specimen from a suspicious area, a bronchial brush to obtain cells from the surface of a lesion, or a suction device to remove foreign bodies or mucus plugs.

You may experience hoarseness, loss of voice, or sore throat after this test. These effects are only temporary.

What happens after the test?

- You'll rest in bed, and the nurse will instruct you to spit saliva into a basin rather than swallow it. Also, you'll have to refrain from clearing your throat and coughing, which might dislodge the clot at the biopsy site and cause hemorrhaging.
- The doctor will restrict food and fluids until your gag reflex returns (usually in 1 hour). Then you may resume your usual diet, beginning with sips of clear liquid or ice chips.
- Remember that hoarseness, loss of voice, and sore throat after this procedure are only temporary.

What are the normal results?

The windpipe normally consists of smooth muscle containing C-shaped rings of cartilage at regular intervals, and it's lined with a ciliated mucous membrane. The bronchi appear similar to the windpipe.

What do abnormal results mean?

The doctor may see abnormalities of the bronchial wall and the windpipe or find abnormal substances that require tissue and cell studies to confirm or eliminate a long list of diseases, including interstitial lung disease, bronchogenic cancer, tuberculosis, or other lung infections. Correlation of X-ray, bronchoscopic, and lab findings with the person's symptoms is essential.

EXAMINATION OF THE CHEST

Called *mediastinoscopy*, this test evaluates the lymph nodes and other structures in the chest. Using a device called an *exploring speculum* with a built-in fiber light and side slits, mediastinoscopy permits palpation and a biopsy (removal and analysis) of lymph node tissue in the chest. The doctor uses this surgical procedure when tests such as sputum cytology, lung scans, X-rays, and a bronchoscopic biopsy fail to confirm a diagnosis.

Why is this test done?
A mediastinoscopy may be performed for the following reasons:
- To help the doctor detect bronchogenic cancer, lymphoma (including Hodgkin's disease), and sarcoidosis
- To determine the stages of lung cancer.

What should you know before the test?
- You'll be told to fast after midnight before the test.
- You'll be given a general anesthetic, and the procedure will take approximately 1 hour.
- You may have temporary chest pain, tenderness at the incision site, or a sore throat (from intubation).
- A nurse will ask you to sign a consent form.
- You'll be given a sedative the night before the test and again before the procedure.

After a mediastinoscopy, you may experience chest pain, tenderness at the incision site, or a sore throat.

What happens during the test?
- After the endotracheal tube is in place, a small incision is made and the surgeon feels for the lymph nodes.
- The mediastinoscope is inserted, and tissue specimens are collected and sent to the lab for frozen section examination.
- If analysis confirms an operable, cancerous tumor, the doctor may do a thoracotomy and pneumonectomy immediately.

Does the test have risks?
Although complications are rare, the nurse will watch for signs of fever, fluid in the lungs, difficulty breathing, diminished breath sounds on the affected side, a rapid heartbeat, and high blood pressure.

What are the normal results?

Normally, lymph nodes appear as small, smooth, flat oval bodies of lymphoid tissue.

What do abnormal results mean?

Malignant lymph nodes usually indicate lung or esophageal cancer or lymphomas. The doctor uses information about the stage of lung cancer to plan therapy.

THORACOSCOPY

In this test, an endoscope is inserted directly into the chest wall to allow the doctor to examine the area around the lungs called the pleural space. It's used for both diagnostic and therapeutic purposes and can sometimes replace traditional open-chest surgery. Thoracoscopy reduces risk (by reducing the use of open-chest surgery) and postoperative pain, decreases surgical and anesthesia time, and allows faster recovery.

Thoracoscopy is used for both diagnostic and therapeutic purposes and can sometimes replace traditional open-chest surgery.

Why is this test done?

Thoracoscopy may be performed for the following reasons:
- To help the doctor diagnose pleural disease
- To obtain a biopsy specimen from the mediastinum
- To treat lung conditions, such as cysts, blebs (fluid-containing structures, similar to blisters), and fluid accumulation between the lung tissue and its lining
- To perform wedge resections.

What should you know before the test?

- The nurse will describe the procedure and remind you that, after the thoracoscopy, an open thoracotomy may be still be needed for a diagnosis or treatment and general anesthesia may be required.
- You'll be told not to eat or drink fluids for 10 to 12 hours before the procedure.
- You may be given preoperative tests (such as pulmonary function and coagulation tests, an electrocardiogram, and a chest X-ray), and you'll be asked to sign a consent form.

What happens during the test?

- After you're anesthetized, a tube is inserted, a small incision is made, and another tube with a lens is inserted.
- Two or three more small incisions are made, and more tubes are placed for the insertion of suctioning and dissection instruments.
- The camera lens and instruments are moved from site to site as needed.

What happens after the test?

- You'll be given pain relievers as needed.
- You'll have a chest tube and drainage system in place after surgery.

Does the test have risks?

- Complications, although rare, include possible hemorrhage, nerve injury, perforation of the diaphragm, air emboli, and tension pneumothorax.
- You won't be given a thoracoscopy if you have blood clotting problems or lesions near major blood vessels, if you've had previous thoracic surgery, or if you can't breathe adequately with one lung.

What are the normal results?

A normal pleural cavity contains a small amount of lubricating fluid that facilitates movement of the lung and chest wall. The layers of the lung sac are lesion-free and able to separate from each other.

What do abnormal results mean?

Lesions next to or involving the sac around the lungs or the wall between them can be seen and the doctor can take biopsies to reach a diagnosis and make decisions about treatment. After accumulated fluid is removed, sterile talc can be blown into the pleural space to promote healing and prevent future accumulations. Blebs may be removed to reduce the risk of lung collapse.

DIGESTIVE SYSTEM

EXAMINATION OF THE DIGESTIVE TRACT

This procedure's medical name is one of the longest words in the English language: *esophagogastroduodenoscopy*. In spite of its 26 letters, the word simply means a look at the lining of the upper digestive tract: the esophagus, stomach, and upper intestine. (See *The upper digestive tract*.)

During the test, the doctor can withdraw specimens for lab evaluation of abnormalities detected by X-rays. Also, it allows removal of foreign bodies by suction or forceps. The test eliminates the need for extensive exploratory surgery and can be used to detect small or surface lesions missed by X-rays.

Why is this test done?

The test may be performed for the following reasons:
- To help the doctor diagnose inflammatory disease, malignant and benign tumors, ulcers, Mallory-Weiss syndrome, and structural abnormalities (see *How a peptic ulcer forms and develops*, pages 204 and 205.)
- To evaluate the stomach and duodenum after surgery
- To obtain an emergency diagnosis of duodenal ulcer or esophageal injury such as that caused by swallowing chemicals.

What should you know before the test?

- You'll be told to fast for 6 to 12 hours before the test.
- The procedure takes about 30 minutes.
- If you require an emergency exam, your stomach contents will be withdrawn through a tube inserted through your nostril.
- A blood sample may be drawn before the procedure.
- Before the endoscope is inserted, you'll receive a sedative to help you relax, but you'll remain conscious. If the procedure is being done on an outpatient basis, you should arrange for transportation home.
- You'll be asked to sign a consent form.
- Just before the procedure, you'll be asked to remove any dentures, eyeglasses, jewelry, hairpins, combs, and constricting undergarments.

This procedure's medical name is one of the longest words in the English language: esophagogastroduodenoscopy. The exam simply looks at the lining of the upper digestive tract.

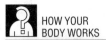

HOW YOUR BODY WORKS

The upper digestive tract

The digestive tract includes the mouth, pharynx, esophagus, stomach, small intestine (duodenum, jejunum, ileum), and large intestine (cecum, colon, rectum, anal canal). Throughout the digestive tract, peristalsis (muscle contraction) propels the food along. Sphincters close openings to prevent food from coming back up.

Saliva starts the work

Digestion begins in the mouth through chewing and the action of the enzyme amylase — secreted in saliva — which breaks down starches. Food is lubricated by the glycoprotein mucin, then swallowed as what doctors call a *bolus*. While the food is passing through the esophagus, it's also lubricated by mucous secretions. Digestion continues in the stomach through the action of glandular secretions.

The hormone gastrin, the most potent stimulus of gastric secretion, boosts the release of hydrochloric acid. In turn, the acid lowers the pH of the stomach's contents, converting secreted pepsinogen to pepsin. Pepsin begins breaking down protein into products ranging from large polypeptides to amino acids.

As the stomach churns

Through a churning motion, the stomach breaks food into tiny particles, mixes them with gastric juices, and pushes the mass toward the top of the intestine. Chyme (the liquid portion) enters the intestine in small amounts. Solid material remains in the stomach until it liquefies (usually 1 to 6 hours). Although limited amounts of water, alcohol, and certain drugs are absorbed in the stomach, chyme passes unabsorbed into the duodenum.

What happens during the test?

▪ A bitter-tasting local anesthetic is sprayed into your mouth and throat to calm the gag reflex and your tongue and throat may feel swollen, making swallowing seem difficult. Let the saliva drain from the side of your mouth. A suction machine may be used to remove saliva, if necessary.

▪ A mouth guard is inserted to protect your teeth and the endoscope, but it doesn't obstruct your breathing.

▪ You may experience pressure in your stomach as the endoscope is moved about and a feeling of fullness when air or carbon dioxide is pumped in. The air distends and flattens your stomach wall to help the doctor see.

▪ While you lie on your left side, the examiner guides the tip of the endoscope to the back of your throat and downward.

▪ A camera may be attached to the endoscope to photograph areas for later study, or a measuring tube may be passed through the endoscope to determine the size of a lesion.

▪ Biopsy forceps to obtain a tissue specimen for analysis or a cytology brush to obtain cells may also be passed through the scope.

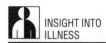

INSIGHT INTO
ILLNESS

How a peptic ulcer forms and develops

If you have one of the two peptic ulcer types — duodenal or gastric — this is how it forms and develops.

Duodenal ulcer

A duodenal ulcer may begin with increased stomach motility (movement), causing the stomach's contents to empty into the duodenum, the first section of intestine. The contents may move so rapidly that gastric acid hasn't yet been neutralized by the food it's digesting. Consequently, excessive acid goes to work eroding the duodenal lining. The result: inflammation and erosion. Duodenal ulcers usually affect the pylorus, the opening from the stomach.

Gastric ulcer

A gastric ulcer is probably not caused by excessive acid but by too little mucus production or a breakdown in the stomach's protective mucous membrane lining. This allows acid to permeate, inflame, and erode underlying tissues.

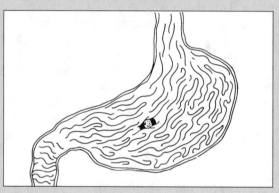

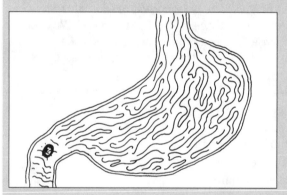

What happens after the test?

▪ The doctor will withhold food and fluids until your gag reflex returns — usually in 1 hour — then you may have fluids and a light meal.

▪ You may burp some of the pumped-in air and may have a sore throat for 3 or 4 days.

▪ If you feel soreness at the intravenous site, the nurse will apply warm soaks.

▪ If you're leaving the hospital, be sure to have transportation home. You shouldn't drive for 12 hours because you may be drowsy from sedation.

▪ Immediately report persistent difficulty in swallowing, pain, fever, black stools, or bloody vomit.

How erosion works

Once tissue is inflamed, the body responds by releasing histamine. Histamine, in turn, stimulates acid secretion, which increases the capillaries' permeability to proteins such as pepsin, leading to swelling of the mucous membranes and a possible obstruction.

Unchecked, the ulcer erodes the layers of the stomach lining, damaging blood vessels in the sub-mucous membranes and causing hemorrhage and shock. Further erosion into the muscularis and serosa causes perforation, peritonitis and, possibly, death.

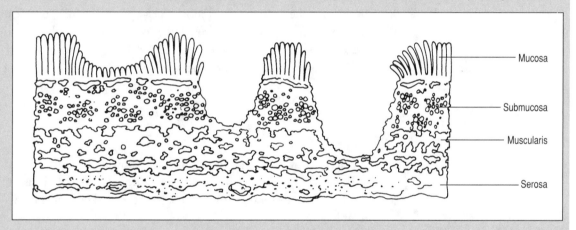

Does the test have risks?

▪ This procedure is generally safe, but can cause perforation of the esophagus, stomach, or duodenum, especially if the person undergoing the procedure is restless or uncooperative.

▪ This procedure won't be performed in people with conditions such as Zenker's diverticulum, a large aortic aneurysm, or someone with a recent ulcer perforation.

What are the normal results?

The smooth mucous membrane of the esophagus is normally yellow-pink and is marked by a fine vascular network. The healthy stomach shows an orange-red mucous membrane, and the duodenum is reddish and parts of it appear velvety.

What do abnormal results mean?

The test may reveal ulcers, benign or malignant tumors, and inflammatory disease, including esophagitis, gastritis, and duodenitis. It can discover functional and structural problems, but for some abnormalities, other tests are more accurate.

EXAMINATION OF THE LARGE INTESTINE

In this test, the doctor uses a flexible, fiber-optic endoscope to look at the lining of the large intestine. The medical name for this test is *colonoscopy.* (See *The lower digestive tract.*)

The doctor may use this procedure for people with histories of constipation or diarrhea, persistent rectal bleeding, or lower abdominal pain, or when the results of other tests are inconclusive.

Why is this test done?

A colonoscopy may be performed for the following reasons:
- To detect or evaluate inflammatory and ulcerative bowel disease
- To help the doctor diagnose colonic strictures and benign or malignant lesions
- To evaluate the colon after surgery for recurrence of polyps or malignant lesions.

What should you know before the test?

- You'll be told to take only clear liquids for 48 hours before the test.
- The test generally takes 30 to 60 minutes.
- The large intestine must be thoroughly cleaned to be clearly visible. You'll take a laxative or castor oil in the evening and an enema 3 to 4 hours before the test until the return is clear. Soapsuds enemas aren't used.
- You'll be given a sedative to help you relax about 30 minutes before the test.
- You'll be asked to sign a consent form.

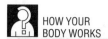
HOW YOUR
BODY WORKS

The lower digestive tract

Digestion and absorption occur in the lower digestive system, primarily in the small intestine, where millions of fingerlike villi increase the surface area.

Enzymes go to work

For digestion, the small intestine relies on the many enzymes produced by the pancreas or by the intestinal lining. Pancreatic enzymes empty into the intestine and begin digesting protein into amino acids, fat into fatty acids and glycerol, and starches into sugars. Intestinal enzymes convert protein to amino acids and digest complex sugars like glucose, fructose, and galactose.

Bile helps absorb vitamins

Bile also participates in digestion and absorption. After formation in the liver, bile is stored and concentrated in the gallbladder. It's released in response to a hormone secreted by the duodenum and is then emptied into the duodenum through the ampulla of Vater. Bile helps neutralize stomach acid and promotes the emulsification of fats and the absorption of the fat-soluble vitamins A, D, E, and K.

The large intestine plays its part

When food reaches the ileocecal valve and enters the large intestine (2 to 10 hours after eating), all its nutritional value has been absorbed. The first half of the large intestine absorbs water, sodium, and chloride, reducing bulk. The second half stores and further dehydrates the digestive material until defecation. The second half of the large intestine may also excrete water, potassium, and bicarbonate.

Bacteria finish the job

Bacteria in the colon putrefy undigested foods and synthesize vitamins K, B_{12}, B_2 (riboflavin), and B (thiamine). Then they produce gas, which helps propel feces toward the anus.

Intestinal gas may also be caused by swallowed air or diffusion of blood gases. Rectal distention by feces stimulates the defecation reflex, which is assisted by voluntary sphincter relaxation. Normal passage of feces through the large intestine takes 24 to 40 hours.

What happens during the test?

- You lie on your left side, with your knees flexed.
- The examiner tells you to breathe deeply and slowly through your mouth as the doctor palpates the mucous membrane of the anus and rectum and as the colonoscope is inserted.
- The colonoscope is well lubricated to ease its insertion. It initially feels cool, and you may feel an urge to defecate when it's inserted and advanced.
- Air may be pumped through the colonoscope to distend the intestinal wall and help the doctor see the lining and advance the instrument. Air normally escapes around the instrument, and you shouldn't attempt to control it.
- Suction may be used to remove blood or liquid feces that obscure the doctor's vision, but this won't cause discomfort.

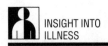

INSIGHT INTO
ILLNESS

Diverticula: A potentially dangerous development in the digestive tract wall

Diverticula are small pouches that form along the colon wall. They develop from a buildup of pressure that pushes the mucous layer out through a weakness in the layer of muscles around the colon.

As the illustration shows, a narrow neck connects a diverticulum to the intestinal lumen. To make things worse, fecal matter may accumulate within this pouch, cutting off its blood supply and leading to infection and inflammation.

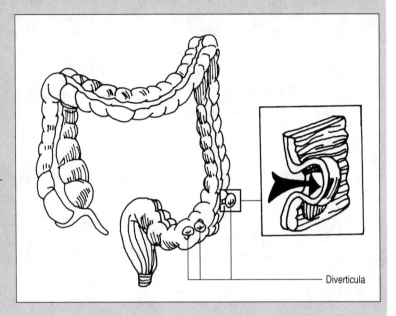

Diverticula

- A biopsy forceps or a cytology brush may be passed through the colonoscope to obtain specimens for blood and cell exams. An electrocautery snare may be used to remove polyps.

What happens after the test?
- If the examiner removes a tissue specimen, it will be sent immediately to the lab.
- After you've recovered from sedation, you may resume your usual diet.
- If a polyp has been removed, there may be some blood in your stools.

Does the test have risks?
- Colonoscopy is usually considered a safe procedure but can cause perforation of the large intestine, excessive bleeding, and retroperitoneal emphysema.
- The doctor won't use this procedure if you have some forms of bowel disease.

What are the normal results?

Normally, the large intestine beyond the colon appears light pink-or-ange and is marked by crescent-shaped folds and deep tubular pits. Blood vessels are visible beneath the intestinal mucous membrane, which glistens from mucus secretions.

What do abnormal results mean?

Visual examination of the large intestine, matched with blood and cell test results, may indicate proctitis, colitis, Crohn's disease, and malignant or benign lesions. Diverticular disease or the site of lower digestive tract bleeding can be detected through visual examination alone. (See *Diverticula: A potentially dangerous development in the digestive tract wall.*)

EXAMINATION OF THE LOWER INTESTINE

This procedure allows the doctor to look at the lining of the distal sigmoid colon, the rectum, and the anal canal. The doctor uses a proctoscope, a sigmoidoscope, and fingers to check for problems. The medical name for this test is *proctosigmoidoscopy.*

The test is usually done for people with lower abdominal pain, trouble with defecation, recent changes in bowel habits, or passage of mucus, blood, or pus.

Why is this test done?

Proctosigmoidoscopy may be performed for the following reasons:
- To help the doctor diagnose inflammatory, infectious, and ulcerative bowel disease
- To diagnose malignant and benign neoplasms
- To detect hemorrhoids, hypertrophic anal papilla, polyps, fissures, fistulas, and abscesses in the rectum and anal canal.

What should you know before the test?

- The test requires passage of two special instruments through the anus. It takes 15 to 30 minutes.
- You'll be told to take only clear liquids for 48 hours before the test, to avoid eating fruits and vegetables before the procedure, and to fast the morning of the procedure.
- Laxatives or an enema may be ordered to clear the intestine to give the doctor a better view.
- The nurse will ask you to sign a consent form and will check your history for barium tests within the past week because barium in the colon hinders accurate examination.

What happens during the test?

- You're secured to a tilting table that rotates into horizontal and vertical positions.
- The examiner's finger and the instrument are well lubricated to ease insertion, the instrument initially feels cool, and you may feel the urge to defecate when it's inserted and advanced.
- The instrument stretches your intestinal wall and causes brief muscle spasms or colicky lower abdominal pain.
- You should breathe deeply and slowly through your mouth to relax your abdominal muscles. This calms the urge to defecate and eases any discomfort.
- Air may be pumped through the endoscope into the intestine to distend its walls. This causes air to escape around the endoscope, but you shouldn't attempt to control it.
- A suction machine removes blood, mucus, or liquid feces that obscure the doctor's view, but it won't cause you discomfort.
- To obtain specimens from suspicious areas of the intestinal mucous membrane, a biopsy forceps, a cytology brush, or a culture swab is passed through the sigmoidoscope.
- Polyps may be removed for a histologic exam by insertion of an electrocautery snare through the sigmoidoscope.
- After the sigmoidoscope is withdrawn, the proctoscope is lubricated, and you're told that it's about to be inserted. Be assured that you'll experience less discomfort during passage of the proctoscope.
- If a biopsy (removal and analysis) of tissue from the anal canal is required, you're given a local anesthetic first.

Air may be pumped through the endoscope into the intestine to distend its walls. This causes air to escape around the endoscope, but you shouldn't attempt to control it.

What happens after the test?

- After the exam is completed, the proctoscope is withdrawn.
- If air was pumped into the intestine, you may pass gas.
- If a biopsy or polypectomy was performed, blood may appear in your stools.

Does the test have risks?

Possible complications of this procedure include rectal bleeding and, rarely, bowel perforation.

What are the normal results?

The mucous membrane of the sigmoid colon appears light pink-orange and is marked by crescent-shaped folds and deep tubular pits. The rectal mucous membrane is redder due to its rich vascular network and deepens to a purple hue. The lower two-thirds of the anus is lined with smooth gray-tan skin and joins with the hair-fringed perianal skin.

What do abnormal results mean?

The doctor can see and feel abnormalities of the anal canal and rectum, including internal and external hemorrhoids, anal fissures, anal fistulas, and abscesses. However, a biopsy, culture, and other lab tests are often necessary to detect various disorders.

REPRODUCTIVE SYSTEM

COLPOSCOPY

This test lights and magnifies the image of the vagina and cervix, letting the doctor see more than in a routine vaginal exam. The doctor uses a colposcope primarily to evaluate abnormal cells or grossly suspicious lesions and to examine the cervix and vagina after a positive Pap test. During the exam, a biopsy (removal and analysis of tissue) may be performed and photographs taken of suspicious lesions with the colposcope and its attachments.

Colposcopy provides more information than the doctor can obtain in a routine vaginal exam.

Why is this test done?

A colposcopy may be performed for the following reasons:

- To help the doctor confirm cervical cancer after a positive Pap test
- To evaluate vaginal or cervical lesions
- To monitor conservatively treated cervical intraepithelial neoplasia (a type of cancer)
- To monitor women whose mothers received the drug diethylstilbestrol (DES) during pregnancy.

What should you know before the test?

- You won't need to change your diet before the test.
- The test is safe and painless, and it takes 10 to 15 minutes.
- A biopsy may be performed at the time of the exam; this may cause minimal but easily controlled bleeding.

What happens during the test?

- You lie on the examining table with your feet in the stirrups and a drape over you.
- The examiner inserts the speculum and may take a specimen for a Pap test.
- The nurse may try to help you by telling you to breathe through your mouth and relax your abdominal muscles.
- After the cervix and vagina are examined, a biopsy is performed on areas that appear abnormal.

What happens after the test?

If a biopsy was done, you'll be told to abstain from intercourse and not to insert anything in your vagina (except a tampon) until healing of the biopsy site is confirmed.

Does the test have risks?

Risks include bleeding (especially during pregnancy) and infection.

What are the normal results?

Normally, cervical vessels show a network and hairpin capillary pattern. The surface contour is smooth and pink.

The nurse may try to help you relax by telling you to breathe through your mouth and concentrate on relaxing your abdominal muscles.

What do abnormal results mean?

The doctor may find abnormalities such as white areas or mosaic patterns. Other cell changes may suggest cancer or inflammatory changes (usually from infection), atrophic changes (usually from aging), and evidence of viruses.

LAPAROSCOPY

This test is used to detect abnormalities of the uterus, fallopian tubes, and ovaries. The doctor views the abdominal cavity by inserting a laparoscope (a small, fiber-optic telescope) through the abdominal wall.

This surgical technique may be used to detect abnormalities, such as cysts, adhesions, fibroids, and infection. It can also be used therapeutically to perform procedures such as the removal of adhesions, an ovarian biopsy (removal and analysis of tissue), tubal ligation, and the removal of foreign bodies.

Why is this test done?

Laparoscopy may be performed for the following reasons:
- To help the doctor identify the cause of pelvic pain
- To help detect endometriosis, ectopic pregnancy, or pelvic inflammatory disease
- To evaluate pelvic masses or the fallopian tubes of women who are infertile
- To determine the stage of a cancer.

Laparoscopy may be performed as part of treatment during such procedures as removal of adhesions or tubal ligation.

What should you know before the test?

- You'll be told to fast after midnight before the test or at least 8 hours before surgery.
- The test takes only 15 to 30 minutes.
- The nurse will tell you whether you'll receive a local or general anesthetic and whether the procedure will require overnight hospitalization.
- You may experience pain at the puncture site and in the shoulder.
- You'll be asked to sign a consent form.

What happens during the test?

- You're anesthetized and placed in the same position as for a Pap test — on your back with your feet in stirrups.
- The examiner puts a catheter in your bladder and then manually examines your pelvic area to detect any abnormalities that may interfere with the test.
- A tube that carries the biopsy instrument and the laparoscope is inserted into the peritoneal cavity. The examiner moves it to view the pelvis and abdomen and then may perform minor surgical procedures such as an ovarian biopsy.

What happens after the test?

- The nurse will help you walk as soon as possible after you recover from the anesthesia.
- You may resume your usual diet.
- The nurse may tell you to restrict activity for 2 to 7 days.
- Some abdominal and shoulder pain is normal and should disappear within 24 to 36 hours. You may be given a mild pain reliever.

Does the test have risks?

- Potential risks of laparoscopy include a punctured visceral organ that can bleed or spill intestinal contents into the peritoneum.
- The doctor won't use laparoscopy for people with advanced abdominal wall cancer, advanced respiratory or cardiovascular disease, intestinal obstruction, a palpable abdominal mass, a large abdominal hernia, chronic tuberculosis, or a history of peritonitis.

What are the normal results?

The uterus and fallopian tubes are normal in size and shape, free of adhesions, and motile. The ovaries are normal in size and shape; cysts and endometriosis are absent. Dye injected through the cervix flows freely.

What do abnormal results mean?

The doctor can see such abnormalities as ovarian cysts, adhesions, endometriosis, and fibroids.

SKELETAL SYSTEM

EXAMINATION OF A JOINT

This test, which is also called *arthroscopy,* is a visual exam of the interior of a joint (most often the knee) with a specially designed fiber-optic endoscope called an *arthroscope.* This endoscope is inserted through a tube that has been inserted into the joint cavity. (See *Points about joints,* page 216.)

Diagnosis by arthroscopy is highly accurate; in fact, the accuracy rate of this procedure is about 98%. During arthroscopy the doctor may also perform surgery or a biopsy (removal and analysis of tissue). Usually, a local anesthetic is used. The procedure may be performed under spinal or general anesthesia, especially if surgery is anticipated.

A camera may be attached to the arthroscope to photograph the inside of a joint for later study.

Why is this test done?
Arthroscopy may be performed for the following reasons:
- To detect and diagnose joint disorders
- To monitor disease progression
- To perform joint surgery
- To help the doctor monitor the effectiveness of therapy.

What should you know before the test?
- If surgery or other treatment is anticipated, it may be done during arthroscopy.
- You'll be told to fast after midnight before the procedure.
- If local anesthesia is to be used, you may feel brief discomfort from the injection and the pressure of the tourniquet on your leg.
- A nurse will ask you to sign a consent form.
- Just before the procedure, the nurse may shave the area of the joint and then give you a sedative to relax you for the procedure.

What happens during the test?
Although techniques vary depending on the surgeon, the following knee arthroscopy procedure is typical:
- After you lie on the operating table, an inflatable tourniquet is placed around your leg but not tightened.

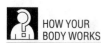

Points about joints

Joints are made of two bones joined in various ways. Like bones, the joints' structures differ according to their function.

Synovial joints
Also known as *diarthroses,* these joints are the most common type. They allow angular and circular movement. To achieve freedom of movement, synovial joints have special characteristics: the bones' two contact surfaces have a smooth covering, called *articular cartilage,* that acts as a cushion. As the contact surfaces glide on each other, a fibrous capsule holds them together. The synovial membrane lines the space between the contact surfaces and secretes a clear viscous fluid called *synovial fluid,* which lubricates joint movements.

Fibrous joints
Fibrous joints, called *synarthroses,* allow only a slight range of motion and provide stability when a tight connection is necessary, as in the sutures joining the bones of your skull.

Cartilaginous joints
Cartilaginous joints, called *amphiarthroses,* allow limited movement such as between the vertebrae of your spine.

- Your leg is scrubbed according to standard surgical procedure, and a waterproof stockinette is applied.
- Your leg is elevated and wrapped from toes to lower thigh with an elastic bandage to drain as much blood from the leg as possible.
- The tourniquet is inflated and the elastic bandage removed so the local anesthetic can be given.
- If the procedure is being performed under a local anesthetic, you feel a thumping sensation when a tube containing a sharp instrument is inserted into the capsule of your knee joint. The sharp instrument is removed and the arthroscope is inserted through this tube.
- Instruments are changed, depending on the procedure.
- After a visual exam, the doctor may perform a synovial biopsy or surgery on the knee joint.

What happens after the test?
- The arthroscope is removed, the joint is irrigated by way of the tube, the tube is removed, and gentle pressure is applied to the knee to remove the normal saline solution.
- The incision site is dressed.
- You may walk as soon as you're fully awake but should avoid excessive use of the joint for a few days.
- You may resume your usual diet.

Does the test have risks?
- Complications are rare, but may include infection, swelling, synovial rupture, blood clots, numbness, and joint injury.
- The doctor won't use arthroscopy for a person with flexibility of less than 50 degrees, or for a person with local skin or wound infections.

What are the normal results?
Normally, joints are smooth and snug, cartilage appears smooth and white, and ligaments and tendons appear cablelike and silvery.

What do abnormal results mean?
An arthroscopic exam can reveal diseased tissue, ligaments, and cartilage. The doctor can see cysts and evidence of diseases such as synovitis, rheumatoid and degenerative arthritis, and foreign bodies associated with gout and other disorders.

BIOPSIES:
Checking for Cancer

RESPIRATORY SYSTEM

LUNG BIOPSY

This test checks the condition of the lungs after X-rays or bronchoscopy fail to identify the cause of a respiratory illness. (See *Common tissue biopsies.*)

A specimen of lung tissue is extracted by closed or open technique for a lab exam. Closed technique, performed under local anesthesia, includes both needle and transbronchial biopsies. Open technique is done under general anesthesia in the operating room.

The doctor chooses needle biopsy when the suspect lesion is readily accessible or when it originates in the lung's functional tissue, is confined to it, or is affixed to the chest wall. Needle biopsy provides a much smaller specimen than the open technique.

Transbronchial biopsy, the removal of multiple specimens through a fiber-optic bronchoscope, may be the doctor's choice for people with widespread lung disease or tumors or when the person's poor health rules out an open biopsy.

Open biopsy is used to study a well-defined lesion that may require surgery.

Why is this test done?

A lung biopsy is performed to confirm a diagnosis of widespread lung disease and lesions.

What should you know before the test?

- You'll be asked to fast after midnight before the procedure. (You may be permitted to have clear liquids the morning of the test.)
- A chest X-ray and blood studies will be done before the biopsy.
- The procedure takes 30 to 60 minutes, and test results should be available in a few days.
- The nurse will ask you to sign a consent form.
- You'll be given a mild sedative 30 minutes before the biopsy to help you relax. You'll receive a local anesthetic, but you feel a sharp, passing pain when the biopsy needle touches the lung.

Common tissue biopsies

BIOPSY TYPE AND TARGET TISSUE	EQUIPMENT
Excision Surgical removal of an entire lesion from any tissue; may require only a local anesthetic	**Scalpel** 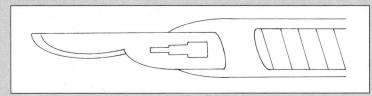
Shaving Tissue shaved from a raised surface lesion on the skin	**Scalpel** 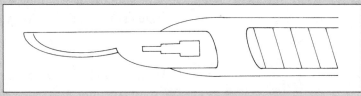
Needle Removal of a core of tissue from bone, bone marrow, breast, lung, pleura, lymph node, liver, kidney, prostate, synovial membrane, thyroid	**Cutting needle** 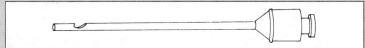
Aspiration Removal of a tissue sample from bone marrow or breast	**Flexible or fine aspiration needle, needle guide, and aspiration syringe** 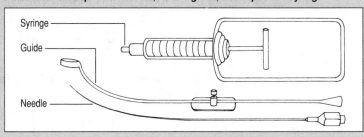
Punch incision Removal of a tissue specimen from core of lesion in skin or cervix	**Punch** 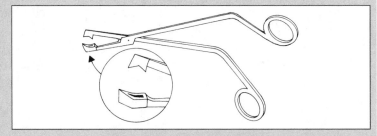

What happens during the test?

■ After the biopsy site is selected, lead markers are placed on your skin and X-rays are made to verify their correct placement.

■ You're in a sitting position, with your arms folded on a table in front of you. You're told to hold this position, to remain as still as possible, and to refrain from coughing.

■ Using a needle, the doctor anesthetizes the intercostal muscles and parietal pleura, makes a small incision with a scalpel, and introduces the biopsy needle through the incision, chest wall, and lung lining into the tumor or the pulmonary tissue.

■ When the needle is in the tumor or pulmonary tissue, the specimen is obtained and the needle is withdrawn.

■ Because coughing or movement during biopsy can cause tearing of the lung by the biopsy needle, the nurse helps to keep you calm and still.

What happens after the test?

■ A nurse will press on the biopsy site to stop the bleeding and will apply a small bandage.

■ You'll be given another X-ray immediately after the biopsy is completed.

■ You may resume your normal diet.

Does the test have risks?

You won't be given a needle biopsy if you have emphysema, blood clotting problems, or some forms of heart disease.

What are the normal results?

Normal pulmonary tissue shows uniform texture of the alveolar (air-sac) ducts, alveolar walls, bronchioles, and small vessels.

What do abnormal results mean?

Microscopic exam of a pulmonary tissue specimen can reveal abnormal cells and supplements the results of other lab tests to confirm cancer or lung disease.

PLEURAL BIOPSY

This test permits a microscopic exam of pleural tissue, the sac that covers your lungs. Tissue is removed by a needle biopsy or open biopsy.

Needle pleural biopsy is performed under local anesthesia. It usually follows thoracentesis (aspiration of pleural fluid), which is performed to determine the cause of excess fluid in the sacs that cover the lung.

Open pleural biopsy lets the doctor see the pleura and the underlying lung. It's performed in the operating room.

Why is this test done?

A pleural biopsy may be performed for the following reasons:
- To help the doctor differentiate between nonmalignant and malignant disease
- To diagnose viral, fungal, or parasitic disease and collagen vascular disease of the pleura.

What should you know before the test?

- The needle biopsy takes 30 to 45 minutes to perform, although the needle remains in the pleura for less than 1 minute.
- Blood studies will precede the biopsy, and chest X-rays will be taken before and after the biopsy.
- The nurse will ask you to sign a consent form.
- You'll receive a local anesthetic and should feel little pain.

What happens during the test?

- You're seated on the side of the bed, with your feet resting on a stool and your arms supported by a table. You'll hold this position and remain still during the biopsy.
- The local anesthetic is administered.
- The doctor inserts a needle into the pleura, withdraws a specimen, and sends it to the lab.

What happens after the test?

- The nurse will clean the skin around the biopsy site and apply an adhesive bandage.
- You'll have another chest X-ray immediately after the biopsy.

You're seated on the side of the bed, with your feet resting on a stool and your arms supported by a table. You'll hold this position and remain still during the biopsy.

Does the test have risks?

You won't be given a pleural biopsy if you have a severe bleeding disorder.

What are the normal results?

The normal pleura consists primarily of cells, flattened in a uniform layer.

What do abnormal results mean?

Microscopic exam of the tissue specimen can show malignant disease, tuberculosis, or viral, fungal, parasitic, or collagen vascular disease.

DIGESTIVE SYSTEM

SMALL INTESTINE BIOPSY

The doctor performs this test to find out what may be causing poor absorption in the intestine or diarrhea. It produces larger specimens than endoscopic biopsy and allows removal of tissue from areas beyond an endoscope's reach.

In this method, several similar types of capsules are swallowed and guided to the bowel for tissue collection. A mercury-weighted bag is attached to one end of each capsule, and a thin polyethylene tube is attached to the other end. Once the bag, capsule, and tube are in place in the small bowel, suction in the tube draws the mucous membrane into the capsule and closes it, cutting off the piece of tissue within. This is an invasive procedure, but it causes little pain and complications are rare.

Why is this test done?

This biopsy is performed to help diagnose diseases of the intestine.

What should you know before the test?

- You'll be told to restrict food and fluids for at least 8 hours before the test. Aspirin and anticoagulants (blood-thinning drugs) will be withheld before the test.
- The procedure takes 45 to 60 minutes but causes little discomfort.
- The nurse will ask you to sign a consent form.
- You'll undergo a blood coagulation test before the biopsy.

What happens during the test?

- The doctor moistens the tube, capsule, and bag to ease its progress.
- The back of your throat is sprayed with a local anesthetic to decrease gagging.
- As you sit upright, the capsule is placed in your throat, and you're asked to flex you neck and swallow as the tube is advanced.
- You lie on your right side, and then the tube is advanced again. The tube's position is checked by fluoroscopy or the doctor pushes air through the tube and listens with a stethoscope for air to enter the stomach.
- Next, the tube is advanced, bit by bit, to pass the capsule through the opening between the stomach and the intestine. (The nurse may talk to you about food to stimulate your stomach and help the biopsy capsule move into your intestine.)
- When fluoroscopy confirms that the capsule has passed into your intestine, you're kept on your right side to allow the capsule to move into the second and third portions of the small bowel.
- You may hold the tube loosely to one side of your mouth if it makes you more comfortable.
- The capsule position is checked again by fluoroscopy. When the capsule is in a site the doctor has chosen, the biopsy sample can be taken.
- You lie on your back so the capsule's position can be checked again, and then the specimen is removed and sent to the lab.

While you're lying there, waiting for the test to finish, the nurse may start talking about food. The idea is to stimulate your stomach to help the biopsy capsule move into your intestine.

What happens after the test?

You can resume your normal diet.

Does the test have risks?

The biopsy won't be performed on a person who's uncooperative or who's taking aspirin or anticoagulants. It also shouldn't be performed on people with uncontrolled clotting disorders.

What are the normal results?

A normal biopsy sample consists of fingerlike villi, crypts, columnar epithelial cells, and round cells.

What do abnormal results mean?

Small intestine tissue that reveals microscopic changes in cell structure may indicate disorders called *Whipple's disease, abetalipoproteinemia, lymphoma, lymphangiectasia,* and *eosinophilic enteritis.* It may also show parasitic infections, vitamin B_{12} deficiency, and malnutrition. Such disorders require further studies.

LIVER BIOPSY

This test is used to diagnose liver disorders. Using a needle inserted through your chest, the doctor removes a core of liver tissue for microscopic analysis. This procedure is performed under local or general anesthesia. Findings may help the doctor identify liver disorders after ultrasound, a computed tomography scan (commonly called a CAT scan), and other tests have failed to detect them.

Why is this test done?

This biopsy is performed to diagnose liver tissue disease, cancer, and infections.

What should you know before the test?

- You'll be told to restrict food and fluids for 4 to 8 hours before the test.
- The biopsy needle remains in the liver about 1 second, the entire procedure takes about 10 to 15 minutes, and test results are usually available in 1 day.
- The nurse will ask you to sign a consent form.
- The nurse will check your history to see if you have any hypersensitivity to the local anesthetic and to verify that you've undergone blood-clotting tests.
- You should empty your bladder just before the test.
- You may receive a local anesthetic. If so, you may experience pain similar to that of a punch in your right shoulder as the biopsy needle passes the phrenic nerve.

What happens during the test?

- You lie on your back, with your right hand under your head. Maintain this position and remain as still as possible during the procedure.
- The doctor feels around for your liver, selects the biopsy site, marks it, and injects the anesthetic.
- After the needle is inserted into your chest, the doctor asks you to take a deep breath, exhale, and hold your breath as you finish exhaling to prevent any movement of the chest wall.
- As you hold your breath, the biopsy needle is quickly inserted into the liver and withdrawn in 1 second.
- After the needle is withdrawn, you can breathe normally.

What happens after the test?

- You'll be told to lie on your right side for 2 hours, with a small pillow or sandbag under your shoulder to provide extra pressure. The nurse will suggest bed rest for the next 24 hours.
- If you feel pain, which may persist for several hours after the test, you may be given a pain reliever.
- You can resume your normal diet.

Does the test have risks?

You won't be given a liver biopsy if your blood doesn't clot quickly enough or if you have any of several lung, bile duct, liver, or blood diseases.

What are the normal results?

The normal liver consists of sheets of cells supported by a framework.

What do abnormal results mean?

An exam of the liver tissue may show widespread disease, such as cirrhosis or hepatitis, or infections such as tuberculosis. The test can show malignant tumors or nonmalignant lesions that require further studies.

After the test, you'll be told to lie on your right side for 2 hours, with a small pillow or sandbag under your shoulder to provide extra pressure.

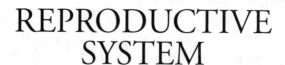

REPRODUCTIVE SYSTEM

BREAST BIOPSY

This test permits microscopic examination of a breast tissue specimen. Once mammography, thermography, and X-rays indicate the presence of breast masses, the biopsy can confirm or rule out cancer. Tissue is removed by a needle biopsy or open biopsy.

Needle biopsy or fine needle biopsy provides a core of tissue or fluid, but is used only for fluid-filled cysts and advanced cancerous lesions. Both needle methods have limited diagnostic value because of the small and perhaps unrepresentative specimens they provide.

Open biopsy provides a complete tissue specimen, which can be sectioned to allow more accurate evaluation. All three techniques require only a local anesthetic and can often be performed without an overnight stay in the hospital. However, open biopsy may require a general anesthetic if the woman is fearful or uncooperative.

Why is this test done?

A breast biopsy is done to help the doctor differentiate between benign and malignant breast tumors.

What should you know before the test?

- The doctor or nurse will want to discuss your medical history, including when you first noticed a lump, whether you have any pain, a change in the lump's size, or any link to your menstrual cycle. The nurse will ask about nipple discharge and nipple or skin changes, such as the characteristic "orange-peel" skin that may indicate an underlying inflammatory carcinoma. He or she will point out that breast masses don't always indicate cancer. (See *Collecting nipple discharge for lab study*.)
- If you're going to receive a local anesthetic, you won't need to change your diet or any medications before the test.
- If you're going to receive a general anesthetic, you'll be told to fast from midnight before the test until after the biopsy.

- The biopsy will take 15 to 30 minutes. Pretest studies, such as blood tests, urine tests, and chest X-rays, may be required.
- You'll be asked to sign a consent form.

What happens during the test?

Needle biopsy

- You're asked to undress to the waist, sit with your hands at your sides, and remain still.
- The biopsy site is cleaned, a local anesthetic is administered, and the needle is inserted into the lump.
- Fluid is withdrawn from the breast, put into a tube, and sent to the lab. (With fine-needle aspiration, a slide is made and viewed immediately under a microscope.)
- The nurse puts pressure on the biopsy site and, after bleeding stops, applies a bandage.
- Because breast fluid aspiration isn't diagnostically accurate, some doctors aspirate fluid only from cysts. If such fluid is clear yellow and the mass disappears, the aspiration procedure is both diagnostic and therapeutic. If the needle draws no fluid or if the cyst comes back two or three times, the doctor will order an open biopsy.

Open biopsy

- After you're given a general or local anesthetic, an incision is made in the breast to expose the lump.
- The examiner may then cut out a portion of tissue or remove the entire mass. If the mass is small and appears benign, it's usually removed. If it's larger or appears cancerous, a specimen is usually taken before the mass is removed.
- The specimen is sent to the lab.
- The incision is stitched, and an adhesive bandage is applied.

What happens after the test?

- If you received a local anesthetic during a needle or open biopsy, the nurse will watch your progress for a while before you can resume your normal activities.
- If you feel pain, you'll be given pain relievers.
- If you received a general anesthetic, you may remain in the hospital for at least 12 hours.

Collecting nipple discharge for lab study

Nipple discharge occurs normally during lactation. However, when this discharge occurs even though you're not breast-feeding a baby or occurs without breast masses or other signs of breast cancer, a lab study of the discharge can help find its cause. (If there were signs of breast cancer, the doctor would do a breast biopsy and other tests.)

Preparing the specimen

To prepare for taking the discharge specimen, the nurse will wash your nipple and pat it dry. Then, she will show you how to "milk" the breast to express the fluid. You'll discard the first drop and collect the next drop by moving a labeled glass slide across your nipple. (If a larger specimen is required, you'll need to collect it with a breast pump.)

What are the normal results?

Normally, breast tissue consists of cellular and noncellular connective tissue, fat lobules, and various milk ducts. It's pink, more fatty than fibrous, and shows no abnormal development of cells or tissue.

What do abnormal results mean?

Abnormal breast tissue may exhibit a wide range of malignant or benign abnormalities. Breast tumors are common in women and account for 32% of female cancers. Such tumors are rare in men (0.2% of male cancers).

If the biopsy confirms cancer, you'll need follow-up tests, including X-rays, blood studies, bone scans, and urinalysis, to determine appropriate treatment.

PROSTATE BIOPSY

This test uses a needle to withdraw a tissue specimen from the prostate. The doctor may chose to insert the needle through the perineal skin between the scrotum and the anus, through the rectum, or through the urethra. Tissue withdrawn by a needle is examined through a microscope.

Why is this test done?

A prostate biopsy may be performed for the following reasons:
- To confirm or rule out a diagnosis of prostate cancer
- To determine the cause of prostate enlargement.

What should you know before the test?

- You'll receive a local anesthetic, and the procedure takes less than 30 minutes.
- You'll be asked to sign a consent form.
- The nurse will check your history for hypersensitivity to the anesthetic or to other drugs.
- For a transrectal approach, you'll be given enemas until the return is clear. Your skin will be cleaned with an antibacterial agent to minimize the risk of infection.

- Just before the biopsy, you'll be given a sedative to make you more comfortable.
- You'll be told to remain still during the procedure and to follow instructions.

What happens during the test?
Perineal approach
- You lie on your left side with your knees to your chest or on your back with your knees up.
- You're given a local anesthetic; then a small incision is made.
- The examiner immobilizes the prostate by inserting a finger into the rectum and introduces the biopsy needle into a prostate lobe. The procedure is repeated several times for specimens, which are sent to the lab for analysis.

Transrectal approach
- This approach may be used without an anesthetic.
- You lie on the examining table on your left side.
- A biopsy needle is guided into the prostate, and you may feel pain as the needle enters and withdraws tissue.

Transurethral approach
- An endoscopic instrument is passed through the urethra, allowing the doctor a direct view of the prostate and passage of a cutting loop. The loop is rotated to obtain tissue and then withdrawn.
- After this procedure, you may remain in the hospital for 12 hours or more.

Does the test have risks?
Complications may include transient, painless passage of blood in the urine and bleeding into the prostatic urethra and bladder.

What are the normal results?
Normally, the prostate gland consists of a thin, fibrous capsule surrounding the stroma, which is made up of elastic and connective tissues and smooth-muscle fibers. The epithelial glands, found in these tissues and muscle fibers, drain into the chief excreting ducts.

What do abnormal results mean?
A microscopic exam can confirm cancer. Further tests, including bone scans, a bone marrow biopsy, and blood tests, identify the ex-

tent of the cancer. Blood tests can tell whether the cancer is confined to the prostate. In that case, radical surgery and irradiation, although controversial, can provide a high cure rate. If discovery of cancer is delayed, treatment requires estrogen therapy, as growth of the tumor depends on secretion of testosterone.

An exam can also detect benign prostate enlargement, prostatitis, tuberculosis, lymphomas, and rectal or bladder carcinomas.

CERVICAL BIOPSY

In this test, the doctor obtains a cervical tissue specimen for microscopic study. Sharp forceps are used to remove tissue, usually several specimens from all areas with abnormal tissue or from other sites around the cervical circumference.

Doctors use this procedure for women with suspicious cervical lesions, and usually time it for one week after menstruation. Biopsy sites are selected by looking at the cervix with a colposcope — called *direct visualization,* the most accurate method — or by staining normal tissue with a dye that doesn't color abnormal tissue (called *Schiller's test*).

Why is this test done?
A cervical biopsy may be performed for the following reasons:
- To help the doctor evaluate suspicious cervical lesions
- To diagnose cervical cancer.

What should you know before the test?
- The test takes about 15 minutes, and you may experience mild discomfort during and after the biopsy.
- If you're an outpatient, you should have someone accompany you home after the biopsy.
- You'll be asked to sign a consent form.
- Just before the biopsy, you'll be asked to empty your bladder.

What happens during the test?
- You lie on an examining table with your feet in the stirrups, as you would for a Pap test.

- The nurse urges you to relax as the unlubricated speculum is inserted.

Direct visualization
- The colposcope is inserted through the speculum; the biopsy site is located and cleaned.
- The biopsy forceps are then inserted through the speculum or the colposcope, and tissue is removed from any lesion or from selected sites.

Schiller's test
- An applicator stick saturated with iodine solution is inserted through the speculum. This stains the cervix to identify lesions for biopsy.
- Samples of the unstained tissue are removed and set to the lab.

After the test, you must avoid strenuous exercise for 8 to 24 hours.

What happens after the test?
- You'll be told to avoid strenuous exercise for 8 to 24 hours after the biopsy and encouraged to rest briefly before leaving the office.
- If a tampon was inserted after the biopsy, you should leave it in place for 8 to 24 hours. Some bleeding may occur, but you should report any bleeding that is heavier than your menstrual flow. The nurse will warn you to avoid using additional tampons, which can irritate the cervix and provoke bleeding.
- You should avoid douching and intercourse for 2 weeks, or as directed by your doctor.
- A foul-smelling, gray-green vaginal discharge is normal for several days after biopsy and may persist for 3 weeks.

What are the normal results?
Normal cervical tissue is composed of several kinds of cells, loose connective tissue, and smooth-muscle fibers, with no dysplasia or abnormal cell growth.

What do abnormal results mean?
A microscopic exam of a cervical tissue specimen is used to identify abnormal cells. Results may help to differentiate between cancer that develops in the cervical tissue and cancer that originates in other body organs and spreads to the cervix.

SKELETAL SYSTEM

BONE BIOPSY

This test permits microscopic exam of a bone specimen. The doctor uses a bone biopsy for people with bone pain and tenderness. If a bone scan, a computed tomography scan (commonly called a CAT scan), an X-ray, or arteriography reveals a mass or deformity, this test may be ordered.

During the test, a piece or core of bone is removed, either by a special drill needle using a local anesthetic or by surgical excision using a general anesthetic. Excision provides a larger specimen than a drill biopsy and permits immediate surgical treatment if quick analysis of the specimen reveals cancer.

A piece or core of bone is removed, either by a special drill needle or by surgery. Surgical excision provides a larger specimen than drill biopsy and permits immediate treatment.

Why is this test done?

A bone biopsy is performed to help the doctor distinguish between benign and malignant bone tumors.

What should you know before the test?

- For a drill biopsy, you won't need to change your diet before the test. For an open biopsy, you must fast overnight before the test.
- For a drill biopsy, you'll receive a local anesthetic but will still experience discomfort and pressure when the biopsy needle enters the bone.
- You'll be asked to sign a consent form.

What happens during the test?

Drill biopsy

- After the site is shaved and cleaned, you're given a local anesthetic.
- A special drill forces the needle into the bone and withdraws the bone sample. You're asked to hold very still during the procedure.

Open biopsy

- You're put under general anesthesia.
- An incision is made, and a piece of bone is removed and sent to the lab immediately for analysis. Further surgery can then be performed, depending on the findings.

What happens after the test?
Drill biopsy
The nurse will put pressure on the site with a sterile gauze pad. When the bleeding stops, the nurse will apply a topical antiseptic (povidone-iodine ointment) and an adhesive bandage or other sterile covering to close the wound and prevent infection.

Both types
- If you experience pain after the procedure, you'll be given pain killers. You'll also be monitored for signs of bone infection, such as fever, headache, pain on movement, and redness or abscess near the biopsy site.
- You may resume your normal diet.

Does the test have risks?
Possible complications include bone fracture, damage to surrounding tissue, and osteomyelitis (a bone infection).

What are the normal results?
Normal bone tissue consists of fibers of collagen and bone tissue.

What do abnormal results mean?
A bone specimen exam can reveal benign or malignant tumors. Most malignant tumors spread to bone through the blood and lymph systems from the breast, lungs, prostate, thyroid, or kidneys.

BONE MARROW ASPIRATION AND BIOPSY

This test permits microscopic examination of a bone marrow specimen. It gives the doctor reliable diagnostic information about blood disorders.

Marrow may be removed by aspiration or a needle biopsy under local anesthesia. In aspiration biopsy, a fluid specimen is removed from the bone marrow. In a needle biopsy, a core of marrow cells (not fluid) is removed. These methods are often used together to obtain the best possible marrow specimens.

Red marrow, which constitutes about 50% of an adult's marrow, actively produces red blood cells; yellow marrow contains fat cells and connective tissue and is inactive, but it can become active in response to the body's needs.

Why is this test done?

A bone marrow biopsy may be performed for the following reasons:
- To help the doctor diagnose blood diseases and anemias
- To diagnose primary and cancerous tumors
- To determine the cause of infection
- To help the doctor evaluate the stage of a disease such as Hodgkin's disease
- To evaluate the effectiveness of chemotherapy and other treatments.

What should you know before the test?

- You won't need to change your diet before the test.
- The biopsy usually takes only 5 to 10 minutes. Test results are generally available in 1 day.
- More than one bone marrow specimen may be required and a blood sample will be collected before biopsy for lab testing.
- The nurse will ask you to sign a consent form.
- You'll be told which biopsy site will be used — the sternum, anterior or posterior iliac crest, vertebral spinous process, rib, or tibia.
- You'll be given a local anesthetic but will feel pressure on insertion of the biopsy needle and a brief, pulling pain on removal of the marrow.
- You'll be given a mild sedative 1 hour before the test.

What happens during the test?

- The nurse positions you and urges you to remain as still as possible.
- The nurse may talk quietly to you during the procedure, describing what's being done and answering any questions.
- After the skin over the biopsy site is prepared and the area is draped, the local anesthetic is injected.
- The doctor inserts the needle and removes a bone marrow specimen. In an aspiration biopsy, slides are prepared for immediate analysis. In a needle biopsy, a specimen is taken from the marrow cavity and sent to the lab.

To obtain the best possible marrow specimens, the doctor may use two different methods — aspiration and needle biopsy — concurrently.

What happens after the test?

- The nurse will apply pressure to the site for 5 minutes or so.
- If an adequate marrow specimen hasn't been obtained on the first attempt at aspiration, the needle may be repositioned within the marrow cavity or may be removed and reinserted in another site within the anesthetized area. If the second attempt fails, a needle biopsy may follow the aspiration biopsy.

Does the test have risks?

- Bone marrow biopsy isn't used in people with severe bleeding disorders.
- Bleeding and infection may be caused by bone marrow biopsy at any site, but the most serious complications occur at the sternum. Such complications are rare but include puncture of the heart and major vessels causing severe hemorrhage.

What are the normal results?

Yellow marrow contains fat cells and connective tissue, Red marrow contains blood-making cells, fat cells, and connective tissue. An adult has a large blood-making capacity. An infant's marrow is mainly red, reflecting a small capacity.

What do abnormal results mean?

Microscopic examination of a bone marrow specimen can be used to detect myelofibrosis, granulomas, lymphoma, or cancer. Blood analysis, including cell counts, can alert the doctor to a wide range of disorders. Some of them are iron deficiency, anemias of blood disorders, infectious mononucleosis, and several kinds of leukemia.

*J*OINT BIOPSY

In this test, the doctor obtains a tissue specimen from the synovial membrane that lines a joint. The doctor uses a needle to remove a tissue specimen for a microscopic exam of the thin lining of a joint capsule. In a large joint, such as the knee, preliminary arthroscopy can help the doctor select the biopsy site. Joint biopsy is performed when analysis of synovial fluid — a viscous, lubricating fluid contained within the synovial membrane — doesn't yield answers.

Why is this test done?

A joint biopsy may be performed for the following reasons:

- To diagnose gout, pseudogout, bacterial infections and lesions, and granulomatous infections
- To help the doctor diagnose lupus, rheumatoid arthritis, or Reiter's disease
- To monitor joint problems.

What should you know before the test?

- You won't need to change your diet before the test.
- You'll be given a local anesthetic to minimize discomfort, but you'll experience brief pain when the needle enters the joint.
- The procedure takes about 30 minutes, and test results are usually available in 1 or 2 days.
- You'll be asked to sign a consent form.
- The nurse will tell you which site has been chosen for the biopsy — the knee (most common), elbow, wrist, ankle, or shoulder. Usually, the most painful joint is selected.
- You'll be given a sedative to help you relax.

What happens during the test?

- The nurse puts you in position, cleans the biopsy site, and drapes the area.
- The local anesthetic is injected into the joint space; then the tube to guide the needle is forcefully thrust into the joint space.
- The biopsy needle is inserted through the tube, and a tissue segment is cut off and removed.

What happens after the test?

- A pressure bandage is applied to the incision.
- If you feel pain, you'll be given pain relievers.
- The nurse will urge you to rest the joint for 1 day before resuming normal activity.

Does the test have any risks?

Complications include infection and bleeding into the joint, but these are rare.

The nurse will tell you which site has been chosen for the biopsy — the knee, elbow, wrist, ankle, or shoulder. Usually, the most painful joint is selected.

What are the normal results?

The synovial membrane surface should be relatively smooth, except for the fingerlike villi, folds, and fat pads that project into the joint cavity. The membrane tissue produces synovial fluid and contains a capillary network, lymphatic vessels, and a few nerve fibers.

What do abnormal results mean?

A microscopic exam of synovial tissue can diagnose a long list of diseases, including gout, pseudogout, tuberculosis, sarcoidosis, amyloidosis, synovial tumors, or synovial malignancy (rare). Such an examination can also aid the diagnosis of rheumatoid arthritis.

OTHER BIOPSIES

THYROID BIOPSY

This test permits microscopic examination of a thyroid tissue specimen. The doctor uses this procedure for people with thyroid enlargement or nodules, breathing and swallowing difficulties, vocal cord paralysis, weight loss, and a sensation of fullness in the neck. It's commonly performed when noninvasive tests (tests that don't enter the body), such as thyroid ultrasound and scans, are abnormal or inconclusive.

Thyroid tissue may be obtained from your neck with a hollow needle under local anesthesia or during an open (surgical) biopsy under general anesthesia. An open biopsy provides more information than a needle biopsy. It also permits a direct exam and immediate excision of suspicious tissue.

Why is this test done?

A thyroid biopsy may be performed for the following reasons:
- To help the doctor differentiate between benign and malignant thyroid disease
- To help diagnose Hashimoto's thyroiditis, subacute granulomatous thyroiditis, hyperthyroidism, and nontoxic nodular goiter.

What should you know before the test?

- You won't need to change your diet before the test (unless you're to be given a general anesthetic).
- The test takes 15 to 30 minutes, and results should be available in 1 day.
- The nurse will ask you to sign a consent form and will check your history for hypersensitivity to anesthetics or pain relievers.
- You'll receive a local anesthetic to minimize pain during the procedure, but you may experience some pressure when the specimen is withdrawn.
- You may have a sore throat the day after the test.
- You'll be given a sedative 15 minutes before the biopsy.

What happens during the test?

- For a needle biopsy, you lie on your back, with a pillow under your shoulder blades and your head back.
- As the examiner prepares to inject the local anesthetic, you're warned not to swallow.
- The examiner withdraws a specimen with a needle and sends it to the lab.

After the test, you'll have to avoid straining the biopsy site by putting both hands behind your neck when you sit up.

What happens after the test?

- The nurse will apply pressure to the biopsy site to stop bleeding, and then apply a bandage.
- You'll be told to avoid straining the biopsy site by putting both hands behind your neck when you sit up.

What are the normal results?

A microscopic exam of normal tissue shows fibrous networks dividing the gland.

What do abnormal results mean?

Malignant tumors appear as well-encapsulated, solitary nodules of uniform, but abnormal, structure. The test may also show benign tumors and patterns that indicate diseases such as thyroiditis and hyperthyroidism. Because thyroid cancers are frequently small and scattered, a negative report doesn't rule out cancer.

LYMPH NODE BIOPSY

This test allows microscopic study of lymph node tissue. The doctor surgically removes an active lymph node or uses a needle to withdraw a nodal specimen for microscopic exam. Both techniques usually use a local anesthetic and sample the superficial nodes in the cervical, collarbone, armpit, or groin region. Surgery is preferred because it yields a larger specimen. (See *The lymphatic system*, page 240.)

Lymph nodes swell during infection, but when they're enlarged for a long time and accompanied by other symptoms, the doctor may look for diseases such as chronic lymphatic leukemia, Hodgkin's disease, infectious mononucleosis, and rheumatoid arthritis.

A complete blood count, liver function studies, liver and spleen scans, and X-rays usually precede this test.

Why is this test done?
A lymph node biopsy may be performed for the following reasons:
- To find the cause of lymph node enlargement
- To distinguish between benign and malignant lymph node tumors
- To help the doctor determine the stage of a spreading cancer.

What should you know before the test?
- If you're to have a surgical biopsy, you'll be told to eat nothing after midnight before the test and to drink only clear liquids on the morning of the test. If a general anesthetic is needed for deeper nodes, you must also restrict fluids.
- For a needle biopsy, you won't need to change your diet before the test.
- The procedure takes 15 to 30 minutes, and the analysis takes 1 day to complete.
- The nurse will ask you to sign a consent form.
- If you receive a local anesthetic, you may experience discomfort during the injection.

What happens during the test?
Excisional biopsy
- The nurse prepares the skin over the biopsy site and drapes the area.
- The doctor makes an incision, removes an entire node, and sends it to the lab.

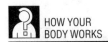

HOW YOUR
BODY WORKS

The lymphatic system

The lymphatic system is a network of capillary and venous channels. It returns excess interstitial (between-the-cells) fluids and proteins to the blood. The diagram below shows the main lymph nodes (glands) that are found throughout your body.

Cell wars

Bacteria from local tissue infection usually enter the bloodstream through the lymphatic system. When it's healthy, however, the lymphatic system provides a strong defense against bacteria and viruses. Before lymph reenters the bloodstream, afferent lymphatic vessels transport it to lymph nodes — clusters of lymphatic tissues throughout the body — where numerous lymphocytes destroy microorganisms and foreign particles.

Foreign particles that escape the lymphatic system are destroyed by white blood cells in the spleen, liver, and bone marrow.

The spleen is a germ trap

As blood circulates through the body, it flows into the spleen, where it's filtered. There, residing lymphocytes ingest abnormal or foreign cells while normal cells pass through. Bacteria that accompany digested food particles into the portal vein — which supplies the liver — are ingested by reticulum cells. Likewise, white blood cells formed in the bone marrow protect the body from invading bacteria.

Macrophages form still another defense system. These white cells in the tissues, lymph nodes, and red bone marrow migrate to inflamed areas and destroy infective particles.

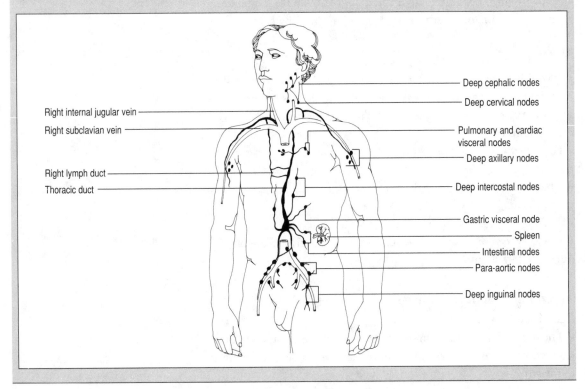

Needle biopsy

- After preparing the biopsy site and administering a local anesthetic, the doctor grasps the node between thumb and forefinger, inserts the needle directly into the node, and obtains a small core specimen.
- The needle is removed, and the specimen is sent to the lab.

What happens after the test?

- Pressure is put on the biopsy site to control bleeding, and an adhesive bandage is applied.
- You may resume your usual diet.

What are the normal results?

The normal lymph node is encapsulated by connective tissue and is divided into smaller lobes by tissue strands.

What do abnormal results mean?

A microscopic exam of the tissue specimen distinguishes between malignant and nonmalignant causes of lymph node enlargement. Lymphatic malignancy accounts for up to 5% of all cancers and is slightly more prevalent in males than in females. Hodgkin's disease, a lymphoma affecting the entire lymph system, is the leading cancer affecting adolescents and young adults.

SKIN BIOPSY

This type of biopsy provides a sample of skin for microscopic study. The doctor removes a small piece of tissue, under local anesthesia, from a lesion suspected of cancer or other problems. One of three techniques may be used: shave biopsy, punch biopsy, or excision biopsy. A shave biopsy cuts the lesion above the skin line, which allows further biopsy at the site. A punch biopsy removes an oval core from the center of a lesion. An excision biopsy removes the entire lesion. (See *How biopsies are obtained from different skin layers*, page 242.)

Lesions suspected of cancer usually have changed color, size, or appearance or fail to heal properly after injury.

How biopsies are obtained from different skin layers

Epidermal tissue specimens are generally removed by a shave biopsy. Both epidermal and dermal specimens may be obtained by a punch biopsy. Subcutaneous tissue specimens are removed by excision.

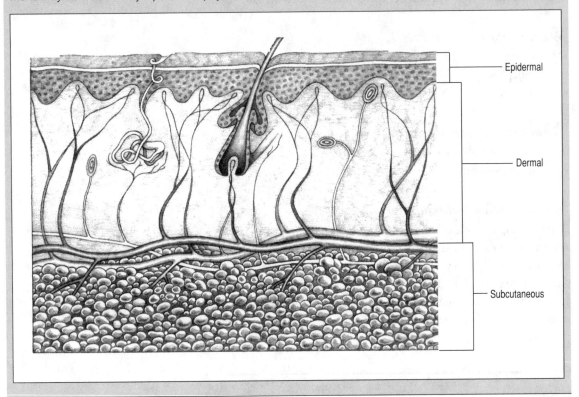

Epidermal

Dermal

Subcutaneous

Why is this test done?

A skin biopsy may be performed for the following reasons:
- To help the doctor differentiate between cancerous cells and benign growths
- To diagnose chronic bacterial or fungal skin infections.

What should you know before the test?

- You won't need to change your diet before the test.
- You'll receive a local anesthetic to minimize pain; the biopsy takes about 15 minutes, and test results are usually available in 1 day.
- The nurse will ask you to sign a consent form and will check your history for hypersensitivity to the local anesthetic.

What happens during the test?

You're given a local anesthetic.

Shave biopsy

- The protruding growth is cut off at the skin line with a scalpel and sent to the lab.
- The nurse applies pressure to the area to stop the bleeding.

Punch biopsy

The skin surrounding the lesion is pulled taut, and the doctor firmly applies the punch to the lesion and rotates it to obtain a tissue specimen. The plug is lifted with forceps or a needle and is cut off as deeply into the fat layer as possible.

Excision biopsy

The doctor uses a scalpel to totally cut out the lesion. The incision is made as wide and as deep as necessary.

What happens after the test?

- The nurse applies pressure to the site to stop the bleeding. The wound is stitched closed. If the incision is large, a skin graft may be required.
- If you have pain, the nurse will give you pain relievers.
- If you have stitches, keep the area clean and as dry as possible. Facial stitches will be removed in 3 to 5 days; trunk stitches, in 7 to 14 days.
- If you have adhesive strips, leave them in place for 14 to 21 days.

What are the normal results?

Normal skin consists of the epidermis and fibrous connective tissue (dermis).

What do abnormal results mean?

A microscopic exam of the tissue specimen may reveal a benign or malignant lesion. Malignant tumors include basal cell carcinoma, squamous cell carcinoma, and malignant melanoma. Benign growths include cysts, warts, moles, and several kinds of fibroid growths. Cultures can be used to detect chronic bacterial and fungal infections.

KIDNEY BIOPSY

In this test, doctor uses a needle to withdraw a core of kidney tissue for an exam. Also called *percutaneous renal biopsy*, this procedure may be performed during investigation of a long list of disorders. Non-invasive tests (those that don't enter the body), especially renal ultrasound and a computed tomography scan (commonly called a CAT scan), have replaced a kidney biopsy in many hospitals. (See *Urinary tract brush biopsy*.)

Why is this test done?

The kidney biopsy may be performed for the following reasons:
- To help the doctor diagnose kidney disease
- To monitor progression of kidney disease and to check the effectiveness of treatment.

What should you know before the test?

- You'll be asked to fast for 8 hours before the test.
- Blood and urine specimens are collected and tested before the biopsy.
- The doctor may schedule other tests, such as intravenous pyelography, ultrasonography, or an erect film of the abdomen, to help determine the biopsy site.
- The procedure takes only 15 minutes, and the needle is in the kidney for just a few seconds.
- The nurse will ask you to sign a consent form.
- You'll be given a mild sedative 30 minutes to 1 hour before the biopsy to help you relax.

What happens during the test?

- You're given a local anesthetic, but you may experience a pinching pain when the needle is inserted through your back into the kidney.
- You lie on a firm surface, with a sandbag beneath your abdomen.
- The nurse asks you to take a deep breath while your kidney is being felt by the doctor.
- The nurse asks you to hold your breath and remain immobile as the needle for the anesthetic is inserted through the back muscles and into the kidney.

The procedure takes only 15 minutes and the needle is in the kidney for just a few seconds.

Urinary tract brush biopsy

If the doctor says that X-rays show a lesion in your urinary tract, he or she may want to get a tissue specimen to analyze. The method called a *brush biopsy* is used to get the sample of cells. It's not used if you have a urinary tract infection or an obstruction at or below the biopsy site.

To prepare for the test, the nurse will check to be sure you're not sensitive to the dye that will be used in the test, or to the general, local, or spinal anesthetic that may be used. The nurse will also ask about sensitivity to any iodine-containing foods such as shellfish.

How the test is done
Just before the biopsy procedure, you'll be given a sedative and an anesthetic. You may feel some discomfort, but the procedure will be finished in 30 to 60 minutes, and follows these steps:
- You lie on your back.
- Using a cystoscope, the doctor passes a guide wire up the ureter and passes a urethral catheter over the guide wire.
- A dye is sent through the catheter. The doctor uses a fluoroscope to guide the catheter to a position next to the lesion.

- The dye is washed out with normal saline solution to prevent cell distortions.
- A nylon or steel brush is passed up the catheter and the lesion is brushed. This procedure is repeated at least six times, using a new brush each time.
- As each brush is removed from the catheter, a Pap smear is made, and the brush tip is cut off and placed in formalin for 1 hour. The biopsy material is then removed from the brush tip for a lab exam.
- When the last brush is withdrawn, the catheter is irrigated with normal saline solution to remove additional cells. These cells are also sent for examination.

Because brush biopsy may cause such complications as perforation, hemorrhage, infection, or spread of the dye, the nurse will watch for any abnormal reactions and report them to the doctor.

How results are interpreted
The lab can tell the difference between malignant and benign lesions, which may appear the same on X-rays.

- After the needle is in position, you're asked to hold your breath and remain as still as possible while the needle is withdrawn.
- After a small incision is made in the anesthetized skin, you're asked to hold your breath and remain still while the doctor inserts a needle with stylet.
- You're asked to breathe deeply again, and then hold still while the tissue specimen is withdrawn.
- If an adequate tissue specimen has not been obtained, the procedure is repeated immediately.

What happens after the test?
- The nurse will apply pressure to the biopsy site for 3 to 5 minutes to stop superficial bleeding, and then will apply a bandage.

- You'll be told to lie flat on your back without moving for at least 12 hours to prevent bleeding.
- You'll be encouraged to drink fluids to minimize colic and obstruction from blood clotting.
- You may resume a normal diet.

Does the test have risks?

- You shouldn't undergo a kidney biopsy if you have severe disorders, such as kidney cancer, bleeding disorders, very high blood pressure, or only one kidney.
- Complications of the biopsy may include bleeding, a hematoma, an arteriovenous fistula, and infection.

What are the normal results?

Normally, a section of kidney tissue shows the organ's cells and healthy tissues and structure.

What do abnormal results mean?

A microscopic exam of kidney tissue can reveal cancer or other kidney disease.

$$\boxed{8}$$

VISION &
HEARING TESTS:
Evaluating Sight & Sound

EYES & VISION

*E*YE EXAM WITH AN OPHTHALMOSCOPE

The doctor uses a special viewing instrument called an *ophthalmo-scope* to examine the back of your eye and check the optic disk, the retina and its blood vessels, and the macula. In contrast, an eye exam with a special viewing instrument called a *slit lamp* looks at the front of the eye. (See *A look at your eyes.*)

The ophthalmoscope itself is a small, hand-held instrument. It has a light source, a viewing device, a reflecting device to channel light into the person's eyes, and lenses to correct any inherent refractive error in the person's or doctor's eyes.

Why is this test done?

This eye exam may be performed to detect and evaluate problems at the back of the eye.

What should you know before the test?

- This test usually less than 5 minutes.
- You may receive eyedrops to dilate your pupils for better viewing, but you'll feel no discomfort during the test. Tell the doctor or nurse if you've ever had a bad reaction to eyedrops or if you have glaucoma.

What happens during the test?

- You sit upright in the exam chair. The doctor dims the room lights to keep reflections from interfering with the exam.
- The doctor sits about 2 feet (60 centimeters) away from you and slightly to your right. The exam usually begins with your right eye.
- Look straight ahead at some object during the full exam as the doctor checks the structures at the back of each eye.

What happens after the test?

If you received eyedrops, your near vision will be blurred for up to 2 hours. Your eyes may be sensitive to light for a while.

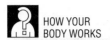

HOW YOUR
BODY WORKS

A look at your eyes

Called by poets the "windows of the soul," the eyes can express sadness, surprise, and a range of other emotions. For doctors and scientists, the organ of vision is a delicate, complex structure that has three layers.

Outer layer
The cornea and sclera make up the outermost layer of the eye. The cornea lies at the front of the eye. A transparent structure, the cornea bends light rays that enter the eye and helps to focus the images on the retina. Adjoining the cornea is the sclera, an opaque, white, fibrous coat covering the posterior five- sixths of the eye, through which nerves and blood vessels pass to penetrate the eye's interior.

Middle layer
The middle layer, known as the *uveal tract,* consists of the iris, the ciliary body, and the choroid. The colored iris has muscle fibers that regulate the light admitted to the eye's interior through the pupil, the circular opening. Behind the iris lies a transparent lens that can change its shape to focus light rays on the retina. The ciliary body permits flexibility of the lens for clearer vision. The choroid supplies blood to the retina and conducts blood and nerve impulses to the front of the eye.

Inner layer
The third layer of the eye, the retina, consists of a complicated network of the visual cells called *rods* and *cones,* and other nerve cells lined with pigment epithelium. At the back of the retina lies the fovea. Composed entirely of cones, the fovea is the area of most acute vision.

Chambers and their fluids
The anterior, or front, chamber of the eye, which is situated behind the cornea and in front of the iris and lens, is filled with aqueous humor. This fluid nourishes the internal parts of the eye and maintains constant pressure within the eyeball.

The vitreous cavity is surrounded by the retina and the optic nerve and makes up four-fifths of the back of the eye. It's filled with vitreous humor — a clear, gelatinous substance. Vitreous humor helps maintain the transparency and shape of the eye.

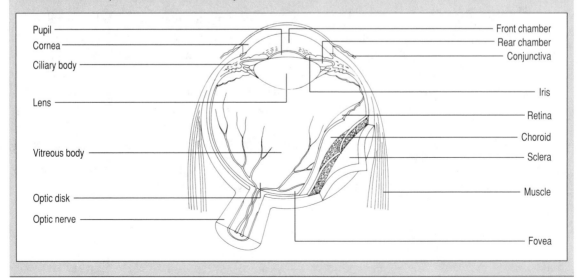

Pupil
Cornea
Ciliary body
Lens
Vitreous body
Optic disk
Optic nerve

Front chamber
Rear chamber
Conjunctiva
Iris
Retina
Choroid
Sclera
Muscle
Fovea

Does the test have risks?

Eyedrops shouldn't be used during the test if the person is allergic to them or has glaucoma.

What are the normal results?

The exam should show a normal optic disk, retina, macula, and other structures.

What do abnormal results mean?

The exam can identify corneal lesions, dense opacities of the aqueous or vitreous humor (such as from blood infiltration), cataracts, or a detached retina. It can also show changes characteristic of many eye diseases, such as glaucoma, optic neuritis, atrophy of the optic nerve, and inflammatory disease of the optic disk, retina, or uvea.

The exam shows the damaging effects of other diseases on the eye. High blood pressure causes spasms, hardening, and eventual blockage of the retina's blood vessels, leading to retinal swelling and hemorrhage. Diabetes may produce retinal fibroses, patches of white exudate, and tiny aneurysms (bulges) in retinal blood vessels.

EYE EXAM WITH A SLIT LAMP

Made up of a special lighting system and a binocular microscope, a slit lamp helps an eye doctor examine the front structures of the eye. Specifically, the doctor looks at the eyelids, eyelashes, conjunctiva, sclera, cornea, anterior chamber, iris, lens, and vitreous face of the eye. In contrast, an eye exam with a special viewing instrument called an *ophthalmoscope* looks at the back of the eye.

Why is this test done?

This type of eye exam may be performed to detect and evaluate problems at the front of the eye.

What should you know before the test?

- The test takes 5 to 10 minutes and requires that you remain still. The test is painless.
- Tell the doctor or nurse if you've ever had a bad reaction to eyedrops or if you have glaucoma.
- If you wear contact lenses, you'll remove them for the test (unless the test is being performed to evaluate the fit of the lens).

What happens during the test?

- You sit in the examining chair with both feet on the floor, your chin on the rest, and your forehead against the support bar. You may receive eyedrops. The doctor dims the lights in the room.
- The doctor examines the eyes starting with the lids and lashes and progressing to the vitreous face. In some cases, a special camera may be attached to the slit lamp to photograph portions of the eye.

What happens after the test?

If you received eyedrops, your near vision will be blurred for up to 2 hours. Your eyes may be sensitive to light for a while.

Does the test have risks?

Eyedrops shouldn't be used during the test if a person is allergic to them. They should also not be used in a person with glaucoma.

What are the normal results?

The exam should reveal no abnormalities in the front of the eye.

What do abnormal results mean?

The exam may detect corneal abrasions and ulcers, lens opacities, inflammation of the iris, and conjunctivitis, as well as irregularly shaped corneas. Some abnormal findings may indicate impending disorders. For example, early-stage lens opacities may signal the development of cataracts.

VISUAL ACUITY TESTS

These tests evaluate your distance and near vision. In a distance vision test, you read letters on a standardized chart, commonly called a *Snellen chart,* from a distance of 20 feet (6 meters). Charts showing the letter E in various positions and sizes are used for young children and other people who can't read. The smaller the symbol you can identify, the sharper your distance vision.

Near or reading vision may be tested as well, using a standardized card such as the Jaeger card, which has print samples in different sizes.

The Snellen test should be performed on all people with eye complaints. Near-vision testing is routine for people with eyestrain or reading difficulty and for everyone over age 40.

Why are these tests done?
Visual acuity tests may be performed for the following reasons:
- To test distance and near vision
- To check for vision problems.

What should you know before the tests?
If you wear glasses, you'll be reminded to bring them with you for the tests.

What happens during the tests?
The doctor checks distance and near vision.

Checking distance vision
- You sit 20 feet (6 meters) away from the eye chart. If you're wearing glasses, remove them so your uncorrected vision can be tested first.
- You cover one eye and are asked to read the smallest line of letters you can see on the chart. Try to read a line even if you can't see it clearly because intelligent guesses usually mean you can recognize some of the symbols' details.
- Next, cover the other eye and repeat the test.
- If you wear glasses, your corrected vision is tested using the same procedure.

Checking near vision

- Remove your glasses and cover one eye. The examiner asks you to read the Jaeger card at your customary reading distance.
- After testing one eye, the examiner tests the other. If you wear glasses, your corrected vision is also tested.

What are the normal results?

Most charts for distance vision are read at 20 feet (6 meters). If your vision is normal, you have 20/20 vision. This means that the smallest symbol you can identify at 20 feet (6 meters) is the same symbol that a person with normal vision can identify at the same distance. A person may have better-than-normal vision. For example, a person with 20/15 vision can read at 20 feet what a person with normal vision can see at 15 feet (4.5 meters).

Normal near vision is usually recorded as 14/14 because standard test charts, such as the Jaeger card, are generally held 14 inches (35 centimeters) from a person's eyes.

A normal or better-than-normal vision test doesn't necessarily indicate normal vision, however. For example, a vision problem may be present if a person consistently misses the letters on one side of all the lines. Such a finding indicates the need for further tests.

What do abnormal results mean?

If you can't read the 20/20 line on the Snellen chart, you don't have normal distance vision. (See *Sight and the aging process.*) If you can read the 20/40 line, for instance, your vision is less than normal. In this case, you would read at 20 feet what a person with normal vision would read at 40 feet (12 meters). A person who has 20/200 vision in the better corrected eye is considered legally blind.

The Jaeger card test can identify poor near vision. A result, for instance, of 14/20 means that the person can read at 14 inches what a person with normal vision can read at 20 inches (50 centimeters).

A person with less-than-normal vision needs further tests to tell if the problem results from an injury or illness or indicates the need for corrective lenses.

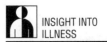

INSIGHT INTO ILLNESS

Sight and the aging process

The lens of the eye normally becomes less elastic as we age. This loss of elasticity hampers the ability of the lens to change its shape. As a consequence, vision often gets worse from adolescence into adulthood.

Presbyopia

A condition called *presbyopia*, or poor near vision, occurs in many middle-age people. It can be helped by wearing reading glasses.

Severe vision loss

Later in life, more serious conditions can develop. Eye tissue may become damaged and severely limit vision, especially if a person has a chronic illness, such as diabetes. Another serious condition, cataracts, often strikes elderly people. In this illness, one or both lenses become clouded and surgery may be necessary.

EARS & HEARING

BALANCE AND COORDINATION TESTS

A person who complains of dizziness or a loss of balance may undergo these screening tests. The tests evaluate balance and coordination as a person performs various movements with the eyes open and closed.

Why are these tests done?

Balance and coordination tests may be performed for the following reasons:

- To help identify vestibular or brain disorders affecting the entire body (balance tests)
- To help identify vestibular or brain disorders affecting the arms (coordination tests).

What should you know before the tests?

- You'll learn about the tests, including who will perform them, where they will take place, and their duration. There's little danger of falling during the test.
- The doctor will check your physical condition, which will influence your ability to do the tests.
- Tell the doctor or nurse if you recently drank alcohol or took sedatives or tranquilizers.

What happens during the tests?

Testing balance

You're asked to perform as many of the following movements as possible:

- Stand with your feet together, arms at your sides, and eyes open for 20 seconds. Try to maintain this position for another 20 seconds with your eyes closed.
- Stand on one foot for 5 seconds, then on the other foot for 5 seconds. Next, repeat the procedure with your eyes closed.
- Stand heel to toe for 20 seconds with your eyes opened. Then try to maintain the position with your eyes closed for another 20 seconds.
- Walk forward and backward in a straight line, heel to toe, first with your eyes open, and then with them closed.

Testing coordination
- Sit and face the examiner, who holds out his or her index finger at your shoulder level.
- Touch the examiner's finger with your right index finger.
- Lower your arm and close your eyes. Try to touch the examiner's finger again.
- Next, repeat the entire maneuver using your left index finger.

Do the tests have risks?
When checking balance, the examiner will stand close to you to catch you if you start to fall.

What are the normal results?
A healthy person maintains balance with the eyes open and closed and can also touch the examiner's finger with the eyes open and closed.

What do abnormal results mean?
The tests can identify a vestibular lesion, which can cause swaying or falling when the person's eyes are closed. A brain lesion causes swaying or falling when eyes are open or closed.

EAR EXAM WITH AN OTOSCOPE

This test inspects the ear canal and eardrum using a hand-held instrument called an *otoscope*. (See *A look inside your ear,* page 256.) It's a basic part of any ear exam and should be performed before other ear tests. A doctor, a nurse, or an audiologist can perform this test.

Why is this test done?
An otoscopic exam may be performed for the following reasons:
- To detect foreign bodies, impacted wax, narrowing, or other problems in the ear canal
- To detect a problem in the middle ear, such as an infection or a perforated eardrum.

What should you know before the test?
This test is usually painless and takes less than 5 minutes.

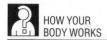

HOW YOUR BODY WORKS

A look inside your ear

The ear has three parts: external, middle, and inner. Each of these parts is necessary for hearing.

External ear: Passageway for sound
The external ear consists of the auricle or pinna (the visible part) and the ear canal. These structures direct and send sound toward the eardrum. The ear canal also serves as a resonating tube, amplifying sound. The eardrum, also called the *tympanic membrane,* divides the external and middle parts of the ear.

Middle ear: The body's smallest bones within
The middle ear is a small air space that contains the body's smallest bones (ossicles): the malleus ("hammer"), the incus ("anvil"), and the stapes ("stirrups"). By their delicate vibrations, they transmit sound from the eardrum to the inner ear through a membrane called the *oval window.*

Inner ear: A sea of sound
The inner ear contains tiny organs for hearing. It also controls our sense of balance. The temporal bone surrounds and protects these interconnected, fluid-filled structures.

The organ for hearing is the cochlea. A coiled, snail-shaped tube, the cochlea contains fluid that's set in motion by the vibrations of the three tiny middle ear bones. The cochlear duct contains the organ of Corti, where sensitive hair cells convert fluid disturbances into nerve impulses. These impulses travel along the eighth cranial nerve to the brain for interpretation.

The vestibular organs, such as the semicircular canals, control balance. Changes in body position disturb the fluid in these canals and stimulate vestibular hair cells. These hair cells dispatch messages to the brain, enabling muscles to respond to position changes.

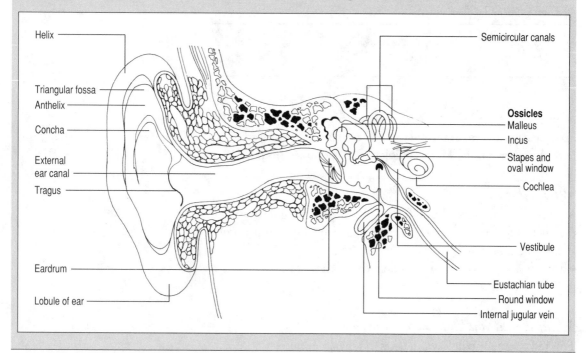

What happens during the test?

- You sit in a chair and the examiner pulls your ear upward and backward to straighten the canal, which makes insertion of the otoscope easier.
- The examiner looks through the otoscope's lens and check for redness, swelling, discharge, foreign bodies, or scaling in the canal.
- Then the examiner gently advances the instrument until the eardrum is visible, checks its color and contours, and looks for any perforation. You should hold still throughout this procedure.

Does the test have risks?

- The otoscope could irritate the ear canal, especially if it's infected.
- The eardrum could be damaged or perforated if the otoscope is inserted too far or if the person moves abruptly during the exam.

What are the normal results?

The test should show no problems in the external and middle ear. The eardrum should look thin, translucent, shiny, and intact.

What do abnormal results mean?

Scarring, discoloration, or retraction or bulging of the eardrum indicates an infection or other problem.

Hearing Test with an Audiometer

Usually performed by an audiologist, this test helps to determine the presence and degree of a hearing loss. It gives a record of the thresholds (the softest sounds) at which a person can hear a set of test tones introduced through headphones or a bone conduction (sound) vibrator.

During the test, a person will hear tones at octave frequencies between 125 and 8,000 Hertz to obtain air conduction thresholds and at frequencies between 250 and 4,000 Hertz to obtain bone conduction thresholds.

Comparison of air and bone conduction thresholds can suggest a conductive, sensorineural, or mixed hearing loss. (See *Three types of hearing loss.*) Because the test does not indicate the cause of the loss, further tests of hearing and balance as well as X-rays may be needed.

Three types of hearing loss

A hearing loss may be caused by injury or disease in any part of the ear. Doctors usually classify this loss as conductive, sensorineural, or mixed.

Conductive hearing loss

This type of hearing loss results from impaired sound transmission through the external or middle portions of the ear. These portions conduct sound vibrations to the inner ear, where the sensorineural system begins.

A conductive hearing loss may be caused by impacted wax, a perforated eardrum, a middle ear infection, or a condition called *otosclerosis*. In otosclerosis, new abnormal bone grows around the stapes, the smallest bone in the body. This new bone cements the stapes, preventing it from vibrating and sending sound to the inner ear.

Sensorineural hearing loss

A problem in the inner ear, the eighth cranial nerve, or other nerve pathways to the brain causes a sensorineural loss. The cause may be Ménière's disease, certain drugs, labyrinthitis, tumors, or MS.

Mixed hearing loss

A mixed loss is a combination problem: part conductive and part sensorineural.

Checking hearing in school children

Screening programs in nursery and elementary schools try to find children with hearing deficits. Finding such children early can avoid later problems with language development and general learning. Screening tests, performed by a nurse or audiologist and graded *pass* or *fail,* simply point out a problem and identify the need for more precise testing.

Who should be checked?

The American Speech-Language-Hearing Association recommends yearly hearing checks for all children from preschool to grade 3. This age-group has a high rate of hearing loss.

The association also recommends testing children with:
- speech or language problems
- learning difficulties or special needs
- classroom behavior problems, such as a lack of attention to the teacher or to classmates, unusual visual alertness, or confusion
- allergies or repeated colds or earaches
- recent placement in a new school.

Why is this test done?

A hearing test with an audiometer may be performed for the following reasons:
- To determine the presence, type, and degree of hearing loss
- To check communication abilities and rehabilitation needs.

What should you know before the test?

- The test will take about 20 minutes. You and the audiologist may sit, facing each other, in a quiet room. Or, you may sit in a separate, soundproof booth.
- Just before the test, remove any jewelry or apparel that obstructs proper headphone placement.

What happens during the test?

- The audiologist checks your ear canal for impacted wax.
- Next, the audiologist presses a finger on each ear to rule out possible closure of the ear canal under pressure from the headphones. The headphones are positioned properly and the headband is tightened.
- Each ear will be checked, beginning with the ear with the better hearing (if this is known). You'll hear tones that vary in loudness and should raise your hand (or press the response button) each time you hear a tone. Respond even if the tone is very faint.

Air conduction test

- The audiologist sends a medium-pitched tone to one of your ears and reduces its loudness until you can no longer hear it. Next, the audiologist slowly increases the loudness until you can hear the tone again. Signal each time you hear the tone.
- After testing your hearing at one pitch, the audiologist changes the tone to another pitch and again varies the loudness. Altogether, the audiologist will check your hearing at seven different pitches, from very low to very high.
- After checking one ear, the audiologist repeats the test on the other ear.

Bone conduction test

- The audiologist removes the headphones and places a special vibrator on the bone behind one of your ears.
- Signal each time you hear a tone.

What happens after the test?

If test results are inconsistent, you'll need additional tests.

What are the normal results?

The normal range of hearing is 0 to 25 decibels for adults and 0 to 15 decibels for children. (See *Checking hearing in school children.*)

What do abnormal results mean?

The test indicates the degree of hearing loss. The relationship between threshold responses for air and bone conduction tones determines the type of hearing loss. In a sensorineural loss, both thresholds are depressed. In a conductive loss, air thresholds are depressed, but bone thresholds are unchanged. In a mixed hearing loss, both thresholds are abnormal, with air conduction more depressed than bone conduction.

HEARING TESTS WITH A TUNING FORK

Tuning fork tests are quick, valuable tools for detecting hearing loss and obtaining preliminary information as to its type. (See *Hearing tests: Identifying pitch and loudness.*) There are three tuning fork tests: the Weber, the Rinne, and the Schwabach.

- The *Weber test* determines whether a person perceives the tone of the tuning fork in one ear or both.
- The *Rinne test* compares air and bone conduction in both ears. (See *Two pathways of hearing,* page 260.)
- The *Schwabach test* compares the person's bone conduction with that of the examiner, who is assumed to have normal hearing.

Results of these tests aren't definite. If test results indicate that the person may have a hearing problem, he or she will have to undergo another hearing test, this time with an audiometer.

Why are these tests done?

Tuning forks tests may be performed for the following reasons:
- To check for a hearing loss
- To help distinguish different types of hearing loss.

What should you know before the tests?

These tests are painless and take only a few minutes. Your concentration and prompt responses are essential for accurate testing.

Hearing tests: Identifying pitch and loudness

Hearing tests check a person's ability to identify sounds at different pitches and loudness levels.

Pitch

The highness or the lowness of a sound, pitch is usually called *frequency.* Measured in units known as *Hertz,* frequency is the number of times a sound vibrates in a second. Although our ears can detect frequencies of 20 to 20,000 Hertz, those between 500 and 2,000 Hertz are the most important. They're the frequencies of normal conversations in a quiet place.

Loudness

The volume of a sound — its loudness — is usually called *intensity.* It's measured in units known as *decibels.* One decibel is roughly the smallest difference in loudness that the human ear can detect. A faint whisper registers 10 to 15 decibels, whereas a normal conversation registers 50 to 60. A shout reaches 70 to 80 decibels. Louder sounds, such as a jet engine or amplified rock music, can damage hearing temporarily or even permanently.

Two pathways of hearing

Sound reaches the organ of hearing, the cochlea in the inner ear, by two routes. It can reach the cochlea by air conduction or bone conduction.

called the *malleus* (or hammer), the *incus* (anvil), and the *stapes* (stirrups) vibrate. As they vibrate, these bones send sound to the inner ear.

By air

In this pathway, sound travels from outside the body into the air-filled corridor called the *ear canal*. After crossing the eardrum, it passes through the air-filled spaces of the middle ear, where three tiny bones

By bone

In this pathway, sound travels from outside the body by conduction through surrounding bone structures and directly to the inner ear, thereby bypassing the ear canal and the middle ear.

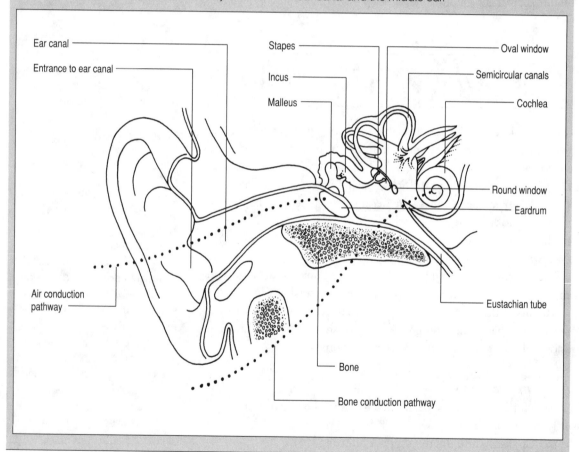

Undergoing the Weber test

This illustration shows a person undergoing the Weber tuning fork test to detect hearing loss. The base of a vibrating tuning fork is placed on the person's forehead. If the tone is louder in one ear than the other, then the person may have a conductive hearing loss in that ear.

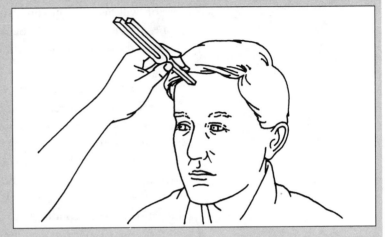

What happens during the tests?

Use hand signals to indicate whether a tone is louder in your right ear or left ear and also when you stop hearing the tone.

Weber test

- The examiner vibrates the tuning fork and places its base on the middle of your forehead. (See *Undergoing the Weber test.*)
- The examiner asks you if the tone is louder in your left ear or your right ear or if it's equally loud in both.

Rinne test

- The examiner vibrates the tuning fork and places its base on a bone behind your ear.
- Then the examiner moves the tuning fork next to your ear canal and asks which location has the louder or longer sound. After you answer, the examiner repeats the test on the other ear.

Schwabach test

- The examiner again vibrates the tuning fork, places its base on a bone behind your ear, and asks if you hear the tone. If you do, the examiner immediately places the tuning fork behind his or her ear and listens for the tone.
- The examiner alternates the tuning fork between the two of you until one of you stops hearing the sound.
- The examiner repeats the test on the other ear.

What are the normal results?

A person with normal hearing will respond to the Weber test by hearing the same tone equally loud in both ears. In the Rinne test, the person will hear the air-conducted tone louder or longer than the bone-conducted tone. In the Schwabach test, the person will hear the tone for the same duration as the examiner.

What do abnormal results mean?

In the Weber test, lateralization of the tone to one ear suggests a conductive loss on that side or a sensorineural loss on the other side. If a person's hearing loss is in one ear, the Weber test may suggest the type of loss. If a person's hearing loss is in both ears, the test may help to identify the ear with the better bone conduction.

In the Rinne test, hearing the bone-conducted tone louder or longer than the air-conducted tone indicates a conductive loss. With a hearing loss in one ear, the tone may be louder when conducted by bone, but in the opposite ear. A sensorineural loss is indicated when the sound is louder by air conduction.

In the Schwabach test, hearing the tone longer than the examiner suggests a conductive loss; conversely, a shorter duration indicates a sensorineural loss.

9

SPECIAL FUNCTION TESTS:
Evaluating the Body's Responses

DIGESTION & EXCRETION

Acid perfusion test

Also called the *Bernstein test,* the acid perfusion test evaluates the competence of the lower esophageal sphincter (the valve that prevents acidic stomach juices from backing up the esophagus and irritating it). In some cases, the pyloric sphincter, which prevents backflow of bile salts, may be similarly evaluated. Esophageal irritation causes burning pains above the stomach or behind the breastbone, which radiate to the back or the arms. This test distinguishes chest pains caused by digestive tract problems from those caused by heart problems. To perform this test, the doctor delivers different liquids into the esophagus through a tube.

The acid perfusion test distinguishes chest pains caused by digestive tract problems from those caused by heart problems.

Why is this test done?
The acid perfusion test may be performed to distinguish chest pains caused by esophagitis from those caused by heart disease.

What should you know before the test?
▪ This test usually lasts about 1 hour. It involves passing a tube through your nose into the esophagus, during which you may feel discomfort, a desire to cough, or a gagging sensation.
▪ Follow these restrictions: no antacids for 24 hours before the test, no food for 12 hours, and no fluids or smoking for 8 hours.

What happens during the test?
▪ After you're seated, the doctor inserts a thin tube through your nose into your stomach — a distance of about 12 inches (30 centimeters).
▪ The doctor attaches a syringe to the tube and draws up some of the stomach contents. Next, the doctor pulls the tube back into the esophagus and delivers liquids through it. Tell the doctor if you feel any pain or a burning sensation.
▪ The doctor removes the tube.

What happens after the test?

- If you feel stomach pain or burning, the nurse will give you an antacid. If you have a sore throat, the nurse will give you lozenges.
- You may resume your usual diet and any medications withheld for the test.

Does the test have risks?

- The test shouldn't be done if a person has recently had a heart attack or has a history of esophageal varices, heart failure, or other heart diseases.
- The test can cause severe coughing if the catheter enters the windpipe instead of the esophagus.
- An irregular heartbeat can develop during insertion of the catheter.

What are the normal results?

Absence of pain or burning is the normal result.

What do abnormal results mean?

Pain or burning during the test indicates esophagitis.

CYSTOMETRY

This test checks the bladder's neuromuscular function. Because cystometry results can be ambiguous, additional tests, such as cystourethrography and intravenous pyelography, may be necessary.

Why is this test done?

Cystometry may be performed for the following reasons:
- To evaluate detrusor muscle function and tone (the detrusor muscle surrounds the bladder and on contraction serves to expel urine)
- To help determine the cause of a bladder problem.

What should you know before the test?

- The test usually lasts about 40 minutes unless additional tests are ordered.
- You should urinate just before the procedure.

- You'll feel a strong urge to urinate during the test and may feel embarrassed or uncomfortable.
- You'll be asked to sign a form that gives your permission to do the test. Read the form carefully and ask questions if any portion of it isn't clear.

What happens during the test?

- You lie on your back on the examining table.
- The doctor inserts a thin catheter through the urethra into the bladder to measure residual urine level.
- To test the bladder's response to thermal sensation, the doctor puts a small amount of liquid into your bladder. Tell the doctor if you feel the need to urinate or if you feel nauseated, flushed, or uncomfortable.
- Next, the doctor connects the catheter to the cystometer and puts more fluid or a gas into the bladder. Let the doctor know when you *first* feel an urge to void and then when you feel you *must* urinate.
- When the bladder reaches its full capacity, you're asked to urinate so that the full bladder pressure can be measured. The bladder is then drained and, if no additional tests are required, the catheter is removed.

What happens after the test?

- Take a sitz bath or warm tub bath if you feel discomfort.
- You may have some blood in your urine. If you still have it after urinating three times, tell the doctor or nurse.

Does the test have risks?

Cystometry shouldn't be performed if a person has a urinary tract infection.

What are the normal results?

The test should show no abnormal pressures, volumes, or sensations. The bladder should be able to hold about a pint of fluid.

What do abnormal results mean?

The test can identify a condition called *neurogenic bladder,* in which a lesion in the nervous system affects urination.

> *When the bladder reaches its full capacity, you're asked to urinate so that the full bladder pressure can be measured.*

ESOPHAGEAL ACIDITY TEST

This test checks the function of the lower esophageal sphincter — the circular band of muscles that tightens to prevent the backward flow of acidic digestive juices from the stomach into the esophagus. When this muscle doesn't function as it should, the esophagus becomes inflamed, causing heartburn.

The test measures the pH, or the level of acidity, within the esophagus using an electrode attached to a catheter.

Why is this test done?

The esophageal acidity test may be performed for the following reasons:
- To check the competence of the lower esophageal sphincter
- To evaluate complaints of persistent heartburn.

What should you know before the test?

- You'll learn about the test, including who will perform it, where it will take place, and its duration (about 45 minutes). During the test, a tube will be passed through your mouth into your stomach and you may experience slight discomfort, a desire to cough, or a gagging sensation.
- The doctor may tell you not to take medications, such as antacids or drugs for ulcers, for 24 hours before the test.
- You'll probably be told that you must fast and refrain from smoking after midnight before the test.

What happens during the test?

- The doctor inserts a catheter into your mouth. Swallow when it reaches the back of your throat.
- Using the catheter, the doctor positions the pH electrode at the lower esophageal sphincter. You're asked to bear down as if you're trying to have a bowel movement or to lift your legs. After you do, the doctor measures the pH in the esophagus.
- If the pH is normal, the doctor moves the catheter into your stomach and instills a solution to help fill the stomach. To test sphincter function, the doctor raises the catheter and asks you to perform the same movements again.

When the lower esophageal sphincter fails to tighten and hold back stomach acid, your esophagus becomes inflamed, causing heartburn.

What happens after the test?

- You may resume your usual diet and restart any medications that were withheld for the test.
- Tell the nurse if you have a sore throat. You can have lozenges.

Does the test have risks?

- The test can cause severe coughing if the catheter enters the windpipe instead of the esophagus.
- An irregular heartbeat can develop during the insertion of the catheter.

What are the normal results?

The pH of the esophagus normally exceeds 5.0.

What do abnormal results mean?

A severely acid pH of 1.5 to 2.0 indicates backward flow of digestive juices because the lower esophageal sphincter doesn't tighten sufficiently. Additional tests, such as a barium swallow, are necessary.

D-XYLOSE ABSORPTION TEST

This test evaluates people who have symptoms of malabsorption, such as weight loss, malnutrition, weakness, and diarrhea. The test uses a sugar called *D-xylose* that's absorbed in the small intestine, passed through the liver without being metabolized, and excreted in the urine. Because it is absorbed in the small intestine without being digested, measurement of D-xylose in the urine and blood indicates the absorptive capacity of the small intestine.

Why is this test done?

The D-xylose absorption test may be performed to help diagnose malabsorption and identify its cause.

What should you know before the test?

- You must fast overnight before the test and will have to fast and remain in bed during the test.
- Several blood samples will be taken during the test. You may feel some discomfort from the needle punctures and the pressure of the tourniquet.
- Your urine will be collected for a 5- or 24-hour period.
- Don't take any aspirin before the test.

What happens during the test?

- During the test period, you need to stay in bed. You won't be able to eat or drink anything (other than the D-xylose).
- The nurse inserts a needle into a vein in your arm and collects a blood sample. The nurse also collects a urine sample.
- You receive a small amount of D-xylose dissolved in 8 ounces (240 milliliters) of water, followed by an additional 8 ounces of water.
- The nurse collects a blood sample 2 hours later and also collects all urine during the 5 or 24 hours after D-xylose ingestion.

What happens after the test?

- You may have an upset stomach or mild diarrhea.
- You may resume your usual diet.

What are the normal results?

The normal results vary by a person's age:
- Children: more than 30 milligrams of D-xylose per deciliter of blood in 1 hour; urine, 16% to 33% of ingested D-xylose excreted in 5 hours
- Adults under age 65: 25 to 40 milligrams of D-xylose per deciliter of blood in 2 hours; urine, more than 4 grams excreted in 5 hours
- Adults over age 65: 25 to 40 milligrams of D-xylose per deciliter of blood in 2 hours; urine, more than 3.5 grams excreted in 5 hours and more than 5 grams excreted in 24 hours.

What do abnormal results mean?

Low blood and urine D-xylose levels are usually caused by malabsorption disorders, such as sprue and celiac disease. However, low levels may also be caused by enteritis, Whipple's disease, multiple jejunal diverticula, myxedema, rheumatoid arthritis, alcoholism, severe heart failure, and fluid in the abdomen.

EXTERNAL SPHINCTER ELECTROMYOGRAPHY

This test determines how well the bladder and urinary sphincter muscles work together. The urinary sphincter is a ringlike band of muscles that constricts around the urethra and helps to control urination.

External sphincter electromyography measures the electrical activity of the external urinary sphincter using skin electrodes or other devices.

The test is done primarily for people who have lost control over their urination. Often, a person who is given this test will also undergo cystometry and voiding urethrography tests.

Loss of control over urination is the primary reason for performing external sphincter electromyography.

Why is this test done?

External sphincter electromyography may be performed for the following reasons:
- To check the neuromuscular function of the external urinary sphincter
- To check the functional balance between bladder and sphincter muscle activity.

What should you know before the test?
- This test usually lasts 30 to 60 minutes.
- When a man is being tested, the nurse may shave hair from a small area behind the scrotum. When a woman is being tested, the nurse may shave a small area around the urethra.

What happens during the test?
- As you lie on the examining table, the nurse applies electrode paste and tapes the electrodes in place.
- After electrode placement, the recording starts. You're asked to alternately relax and tighten the sphincter.
- When sufficient data have been recorded, the nurse removes the electrodes gently and cleans and dries the area.

What happens after the test?
- Tell the doctor or nurse if you feel pain or observe any blood during urination.
- Take a warm bath and drink plenty of fluids.

Does the test have risks?

The test can irritate the urethra, producing painful and frequent urination and blood in the urine.

What are the normal results?

The test shows increased muscle activity when the person tightens the external urinary sphincter and decreased muscle activity when he or she relaxes it.

What do abnormal results mean?

Failure of the sphincter to relax or increased muscle activity during urination suggests a disorder, such as neurogenic bladder, spinal cord injury, multiple sclerosis, Parkinson's disease, or stress incontinence.

*U*RINE FLOW TEST

This simple test uses a device called a *uroflowmeter* to detect and evaluate an abnormal pattern of urination. The uroflowmeter is contained in a funnel into which the person urinates. This device records flow patterns and measures the volume of urine voided per second, time of measurable urine flow, and total voiding time, including any interruptions.

Why is this test done?

The urine flow test may be performed for the following reasons:
- To evaluate bladder function
- To indicate a blockage of the bladder outlet.

What should you know before the test?

- This test usually lasts 10 to 15 minutes.
- Don't urinate for several hours before the test and drink plenty of fluids so you'll have a full bladder and a strong urge to void.
- You'll have complete privacy during the test.

What happens during the test?

- Remain still while urinating and don't strain.
- Push the flowmeter start button, count for 5 seconds, and urinate. When you're finished, count for 5 seconds and push the button again.

What are the normal results?

Normal flow rates depend on the person's age and sex and the volume of urine voided.

What do abnormal results mean?

This test can detect reduced resistance in the urethra, stress incontinence, bladder outlet obstruction, or poor tone of the detrusor muscle.

MISCELLANEOUS TESTS

COLD STIMULATION TEST FOR RAYNAUD'S SYNDROME

This test helps the doctor to detect Raynaud's syndrome, a circulatory disorder that affects the fingers and occasionally the toes (see *What Raynaud's syndrome feels like*). This test works by recording temperature changes in the fingers before and after they're put into ice water.

Why is this test done?

The cold stimulation test is performed to detect Raynaud's syndrome.

What should you know before the test?

- This test usually lasts 20 to 40 minutes. You may feel uncomfortable when your hands are briefly immersed in ice water.
- During the test, remove your watch and other jewelry from your wrists. Try to relax.

What happens during the test?

- The nurse tapes a temperature-measuring device to each of your fingers and records the temperature.
- Submerge your hands in the ice water for 20 seconds. After you remove them, the nurse records the temperature of your fingers immediately and every 5 minutes thereafter until the temperature returns to the pretest level.

Does the test have risks?

The cold stimulation test shouldn't be done if a person has gangrene or open, infected wounds on the fingers.

What are the normal results?

Normally, the temperature of the fingers returns to the pretest level within 15 minutes.

What do abnormal results mean?

If the temperature of the fingers takes longer than 20 minutes to return to the pretest level, the person may have Raynaud's syndrome.

What Raynaud's syndrome feels like

Raynaud's syndrome causes episodes during which the small arteries in the hands and sometimes the feet tighten. As a consequence, not enough blood reaches the fingers or toes, which may become pale and feel numb or tingling. Stress or exposure to cold temperatures brings on this reaction.

Who's at risk?
Raynaud's syndrome afflicts women five times more often than men. For the most part, it first strikes between the late teens and age 40.

DEXAMETHASONE SUPPRESSION TEST

In this test, the doctor measures hormone levels to screen for depression or for Cushing's syndrome, a disorder in which excessive steroid hormones appear in the blood. During the test, a person takes the drug dexamethasone, which reduces steroid hormones in healthy people. However, the drug fails to lower steroid levels in people with Cushing's syndrome or some forms of depression.

Why is this test done?

The dexamethasone suppression test may be performed for the following reasons:

- To diagnose Cushing's syndrome
- To help diagnose depression.

What should you know before the test?
- Don't eat or drink fluids for 12 hours before the test.
- Tell the doctor or nurse if you're taking any medications that may affect the test. Many drugs, including steroids, oral contraceptives, lithium, methadone, aspirin, diuretics, and morphine, can't be taken after midnight on the night before the test.
- After you receive dexamethasone, two blood samples will be taken during the test. You may feel some discomfort from the needle punctures and the pressure of the tourniquet.

What happens during the test?
- You receive a small dose of dexamethasone at 11 p.m.
- The next day, the nurse takes blood samples at 4 p.m. and 11 p.m.

What happens after the test?
If swelling develops at the needle puncture site, warm soaks may be applied to ease discomfort.

What are the normal results?
A blood cortisol level of 5 or more micrograms per deciliter indicates failure of dexamethasone suppression.

What do abnormal results mean?
A normal result doesn't rule out depression, but an abnormal result strengthens the diagnosis. An abnormal result occurs in people with Cushing's syndrome, severe stress, and depression that's likely to respond to treatment with antidepressant drugs.

A normal result doesn't rule out depression, but an abnormal result strengthens the diagnosis.

PULMONARY FUNCTION TESTS

Pulmonary function tests evaluate the amount of air a person is able to breathe in and out of the lungs. A device called a *spirometer* measures the amount of air entering and leaving the lungs.

These tests are performed on people with suspected lung problems.

Why are these tests done?

Pulmonary function tests may be performed for the following reasons:
- To determine the cause of shortness of breath
- To determine if a lung problem is caused by an obstructive disease (which blocks the breathing passageways) or a restrictive disease (which hinders the expansion of the lungs)
- To check the effectiveness of treatments for breathing problems
- To evaluate a person's breathing before surgery.

What should you know before the tests?

- Before the tests, you'll be shown how to use a spirometer.
- Eat only a light meal before the tests. If you're a smoker, you won't be able to smoke for 4 to 6 hours before the tests.
- The accuracy of the tests depends on your cooperation. The tests are painless and you will be allowed time to rest between each test.
- Just before the tests, you should urinate and loosen tight clothing. If you wear dentures, you can keep them in during the tests to help form a seal around the mouthpiece.
- You'll need to wear a noseclip for some of the tests.

What happens during the tests?

- To measure *tidal volume,* you breathe normally into the mouthpiece 10 times.
- To measure *expiratory reserve volume,* you breathe normally for several breaths and then exhale as completely as possible.
- To measure *vital capacity,* you inhale as deeply as possible and exhale into the mouthpiece as completely as possible, three times. The test result showing the largest volume is used.
- To measure *inspiratory capacity,* you breathe normally for several breaths and then inhale as deeply as possible.
- To measure *functional residual capacity,* you breathe normally into a spirometer that contains an inert gas (usually helium or nitrogen) in a known volume of air. After a few breaths, the concentration of inert gas in the spirometer and in the lungs reaches equilibrium. The point of equilibrium and the concentration of gas in the spirometer is recorded.
- To measure *thoracic gas volume,* you're put into an airtight box and asked to breathe through a tube. At the end of an exhalation, the tube is blocked and you're asked to pant.
- To measure *forced vital capacity* and *forced expiratory volume,* you inhale as slowly and deeply as possible and then exhale into the mouthpiece as quickly and completely as possible, three times.

To measure what doctors call vital capacity, you inhale as deeply as possible and exhale into the mouthpiece as completely as possible, three times.

- To measure *maximal voluntary ventilation,* you breathe into the mouthpiece as quickly and deeply as possible for 15 seconds.
- To measure *diffusing capacity for carbon monoxide,* you inhale a gas mixture and then hold your breath for 10 seconds before exhaling.

What happens after the tests?

You can resume your usual diet and daily activities.

Do the tests have risks?

Pulmonary function tests shouldn't be done if a person has chest pains (angina), has had a recent heart attack, or has a severe heart problem.

What are the normal results?

The normal results depend on a person's age, height, weight, and sex and are often expressed as a percentage. The following results are normal:
- Tidal volume: 5 to 7 milliliters per kilogram of body weight
- Expiratory reserve volume: 25% of vital capacity
- Inspiratory capacity: 75% of vital capacity
- Forced expiratory volume: 83% of vital capacity after 1 second, 94% after 2 seconds, and 97% after 3 seconds.

What do abnormal results mean?

Usually, results are considered abnormal if they're less than 80% of normal results. Abnormal results can suggest a number of obstructive lung diseases, such as emphysema and chronic bronchitis, and restrictive diseases, such as pulmonary fibrosis.

TENSILON TEST

A doctor performs this test to help determine the cause of muscle weakness. The test is named after the drug Tensilon (also known as *edrophonium),* a rapid-acting drug that improves muscle strength.

Why is this test done?

The Tensilon test may be performed for the following reasons:
- To help diagnose myasthenia gravis, a disorder marked by faulty transmission of impulses from nerves to muscles, leading to muscular weakness
- To tell the difference between myasthenic and cholinergic crises; a myasthenic crisis may occur in people with myasthenia gravis and is marked by difficulty in breathing; a cholinergic crisis is similar but results from drugs used to treat myasthenia gravis
- To monitor oral cholinesterase therapy.

What should you know before the test?

- You won't have to restrict food or fluids beforehand.
- You'll be asked if you're taking any medications that affect muscle function, if you're receiving anticholinesterase therapy, or if you have drug hypersensitivities or respiratory disease.
- The test usually lasts 15 to 30 minutes. During the test, a small tube will be inserted into a vein in your arm and the drug Tensilon will be given periodically. You'll be asked to make repetitive muscle movements.
- Tensilon may produce some unpleasant effects, but someone will be with you at all times during the test and any reactions will quickly disappear.
- To ensure accuracy, the test may be repeated several times.

After you take Tensilon, you're asked to perform repetitive muscle movements, such as opening and closing your eyes and crossing and uncrossing your legs.

What happens during the test?

- The nurse inserts an intravenous line.
- The doctor may initially give a small dose of Tensilon and ask you to do various exercises, such as counting to 100 until your voice diminishes or holding your arms above your shoulders until they drop. When the muscles are fatigued, the doctor injects the rest of the Tensilon.
- After Tensilon is administered, you're asked to perform repetitive muscle movements, such as opening and closing your eyes and crossing and uncrossing your legs. The test may be repeated.

What happens after the test?

The nurse will remove the intravenous line and will check on you.

Does the test have risks?

▪ Because Tensilon may cause side effects, the doctor may choose not to perform this test in people with very low blood pressure, a slow heart rate, or a blockage in the intestine or urinary tract.

▪ People with respiratory ailments such as asthma should receive the drug atropine during the test to minimize the side effects of Tensilon.

What are the normal results?

People who don't have myasthenia gravis usually develop small muscle contractions in response to Tensilon.

What do abnormal results mean?

If a person has myasthenia gravis, muscle strength should improve within 30 seconds after administration of Tensilon. All people with myasthenia gravis show improved strength in this test; some, however, respond only slightly and may have to undergo a repeat test to confirm the diagnosis.

People in myasthenic crisis show brief improvement in muscle strength after Tensilon administration. Those in cholinergic crisis may experience greater weakness.

10

BLOOD CELL & CLOTTING TESTS:
Screening for Blood Diseases

BLOOD CELL COUNTS

RED BLOOD CELL COUNT

A red blood cell count is part of a group of tests known as the *complete blood count.* The most vital role of red blood cells is carrying oxygen from the lungs to other tissues and carrying waste gases from other tissues to the lungs for expulsion from the body. The red blood cell count is used to find out how many red blood cells are in a sample of blood. (See *Blood: Its vital functions*, page 282.)

Why is this test done?
A red blood cell count may be performed for the following reasons:
- To find out the number and sizes of red blood cells
- To evaluate the protein content and condition of red blood cells
- To support other tests for diagnosing blood problems.

What should you know before the test?
- You don't need to change your diet before the test.
- You may feel slight discomfort from the tourniquet pressure and the needle puncture.
- Drawing a blood sample takes less than 3 minutes.

What happens during the test?
- A nurse or medical technician inserts a needle into a vein, usually in your forearm. A blood sample is collected in a tube, which is then sent to a lab for testing.
- When a young child has this test, a small amount of blood is taken from the finger or earlobe.

What happens after the test?
If swelling develops at the needle puncture site, warm soaks are applied to the area to ease discomfort.

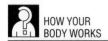

HOW YOUR
BODY WORKS

Blood: Its vital functions

Blood is a fluid tissue that performs many vital functions as it circulates through the body. Most important is its ability to transport oxygen from the lungs to other body tissues and to return carbon dioxide from the tissues to the lungs to be exhaled.

Other functions performed by the blood include coagulation (clotting), which stops bleeding and helps heal injuries; regulation of body temperature; maintenance of acid-base and fluid balances in the body; movement of nutrients and hormones to body tissues; and disposal of wastes through the kidneys, lungs, and skin.

Characteristics of blood

Blood is three times thicker than water, tastes slightly salty, and is slightly alkaline, or basic, the opposite of acidic. Oxygen-rich blood flows through the body in vessels called *arteries*; oxygen-depleted blood is carried away from the organs and tissues in vessels called *veins.* Blood in the arteries is bright red; oxygen-poor blood in the veins is dark red.

Components of blood

Blood has two major components: plasma, which is the clear, straw-colored liquid portion, and the formed elements — red blood cells, white blood cells, and platelets — which help in clotting.

Red blood cells are also known as *erythrocytes* and *red corpuscles.* Red blood cells carry oxygen from the lungs to the tissues and carbon dioxide from the tissues back to the lungs to be exhaled. The white blood cells, which are also called *leukocytes,* help the body fight infection. Blood also contains several important forms of protein.

What are the normal results?

Normal red blood cell counts vary, depending on the type of sample and on the person's age and sex:

- Men: 4.2 to 5.4 million red blood cells per microliter of blood
- Women: 3.6 to 5.0 million red blood cells per microliter of blood
- Children: 4.6 to 4.8 million red blood cells per microliter of blood
- Full-term infants: 4.4 to 5.8 million red blood cells per microliter of blood at birth, decreasing to 3 to 3.8 million at age 2 months and increasing slowly thereafter.

Normal counts may be higher in people living at high altitudes.

What do abnormal results mean?

An elevated red blood cell count may indicate polycythemia. A depressed count may indicate anemia, fluid overload, or severe bleeding. Further blood tests are needed to confirm a diagnosis.

HEMATOCRIT

This test measures the percentage of red blood cells, or *hematocrit*, in a blood sample. For example, 40% hematocrit means there are 40 milliliters of red blood cells in a 100-milliliter sample.

Why is this test done?
A hematocrit test may be performed for the following reasons:
- To help diagnose blood disorders, such as polycythemia, anemia, or abnormal hydration
- To calculate the volume and concentration of blood particles.

What should you know before the test?
- You don't need to change your diet before the test.
- A small blood sample is required for this test.

What happens during the test?
- A nurse or medical technician cleans your fingertip and then punctures it with a small lancet.
- A blood sample is drawn into a small device called a *capillary tube.*
- The tube is sealed and then placed in a centrifuge to separate the red hematocrit from the clear portion of the blood.
- A small amount of blood may be taken from the finger or earlobe of a small child.

What happens after the test?
If swelling develops at the needle puncture site, warm soaks are applied to the area to ease discomfort.

What are the normal results?
Hematocrit is usually measured electronically. Normal levels vary, depending on the type of sample, the lab procedure, and the person's sex and age. (See *Hematocrit values throughout the lifespan,* page 284.)

What do abnormal results mean?
Low hematocrit suggests anemia or massive blood loss. High hematocrit indicates a problem due to blood loss or dehydration.

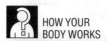

HOW YOUR
BODY WORKS

Hematocrit values throughout the lifespan

Hematocrit test results show the percentage of packed red blood cells in a whole blood sample. Values vary with a person's age. The values shown below are normal for the age-groups shown.

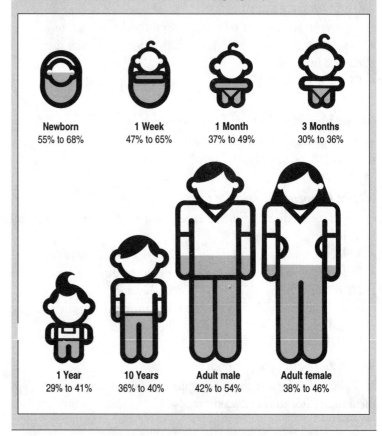

Newborn
55% to 68%

1 Week
47% to 65%

1 Month
37% to 49%

3 Months
30% to 36%

1 Year
29% to 41%

10 Years
36% to 40%

Adult male
42% to 54%

Adult female
38% to 46%

RED CELL INDICES

The red cell indices are calculated using the results of the red blood cell count, hematocrit, and total hemoglobin tests. These indices provide important information about the size, hemoglobin level, and hemoglobin weight of an average red cell.

Why is this test done?

Red cell indices are calculated to help diagnose anemia.

What should you know before the test?

- This test requires a blood sample, which takes less than 3 minutes to collect.
- You may feel slight discomfort from the needle puncture and tourniquet pressure.

What happens during the test?

A nurse or medical technician inserts a needle into a vein, usually in your forearm. A blood sample is collected in a tube, which is then sent to a lab for testing.

What happens after the test?

If swelling develops at the needle puncture site, warm soaks are applied to the area to ease discomfort.

What are the normal results?

The indices tested include mean corpuscular volume, mean corpuscular hemoglobin, and mean corpuscular hemoglobin concentration.

Mean corpuscular volume, the ratio of hematocrit to the red blood cell count, expresses the average size of the red blood cells and indicates whether they're microcytic (undersized), macrocytic (oversized), or normocytic (normal). Mean corpuscular hemoglobin gives the weight of hemoglobin (a type of protein) in an average red cell. Mean corpuscular hemoglobin concentration, the ratio of hemoglobin weight to hematocrit, defines the level of hemoglobin in 100 milliliters of packed red cells. It helps distinguish normochromic (normally colored) red cells from hypochromic (paler) red cells.

The range of normal red cell indices is as follows:

- Mean corpuscular volume: 84 to 99 cubic microns
- Mean corpuscular hemoglobin: 26 to 32 picograms
- Mean corpuscular hemoglobin concentration: 30% to 36%.

What do abnormal results mean?

Low mean corpuscular volume and mean corpuscular hemoglobin concentration can indicate iron deficiency anemia, pyridoxine-responsive anemia, or thalassemia. A high mean corpuscular volume suggests macrocytic anemias.

ERYTHROCYTE SEDIMENTATION RATE

This test measures the rate at which erythrocytes (red blood cells) settle in a blood sample during a specified time period. The erythrocyte sedimentation rate is a sensitive but nonspecific test that's frequently the earliest indicator of disease when other tests or physical signs are normal. The erythrocyte sedimentation rate commonly increases greatly in widespread inflammatory disorders; elevations may be prolonged in localized inflammation or cancer.

A change in the erythrocyte sedimentation rate is frequently the first indicator of disease.

Why is this test done?

The erythrocyte sedimentation rate may be measured for the following reasons:
- To evaluate the condition of red blood cells
- To monitor inflammatory or malignant disease
- To aid detection and diagnosis of such diseases as tuberculosis and connective tissue disease.

What should you know before the test?

- This test requires a blood sample, which takes less than 3 minutes to collect.
- You may feel slight discomfort from the needle puncture and tourniquet pressure.
- You don't need to change your diet before the test.

What happens during the test?

A nurse or medical technician inserts a needle into a vein, usually in your forearm. A blood sample is collected in a tube, which is then sent to a lab for testing.

What happens after the test?

If swelling develops at the needle puncture site, warm soaks are applied to the area to ease discomfort.

What are the normal results?

Normal sedimentation rates range from 0 to 20 millimeters per hour. The rates gradually increase with age.

What do abnormal results mean?

The erythrocyte sedimentation rate increases in pregnancy, anemia, acute or chronic inflammation, tuberculosis, rheumatic fever, rheumatoid arthritis, and some cancers.

Polycythemia, sickle cell anemia, hyperviscosity, and low plasma fibrinogen or globulin levels tend to slow the erythrocyte sedimentation rate.

*R*ETICULOCYTE COUNT

Reticulocytes are immature red blood cells. They're generally larger than mature red blood cells. In this test, reticulocytes in a blood sample are counted. The number of reticulocytes is then expressed as a percentage of the total red cell count. Because only a small blood sample is used, the test result may be imprecise. Therefore, the reticulocyte count is compared with red blood cell count or hematocrit test results.

Why is this test done?

A reticulocyte count may be performed for the following reasons:
- To detect anemia or to monitor its treatment
- To distinguish between types of anemias
- To help assess blood loss or the bone marrow's response to anemia.

What should you know before the test?

- You don't need to change your diet before the test.
- This test requires a blood sample, which takes less than 3 minutes to collect.
- You may feel slight discomfort from the needle puncture and tourniquet pressure.

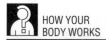
HOW YOUR
BODY WORKS

Understanding bone marrow's role

Bone marrow is soft tissue that is found mostly in the cavities of long bones, such as the femur, or thigh bone; humerous, or upper arm bone; and sternum, or upper chest bones.

Blood from bones
Marrow produces the body's blood cells. Just before a person's birth, the marrow of all bones produces red blood cells. The amount of blood-producing marrow decreases as a person grows; by adulthood, the marrow of the sternum and ribs and of the vertebrae (backbone) and pelvis (hips) produces most red cells. Red blood cell production decreases with advancing age.

Bone marrow is either red or yellow. Red marrow, which is found mostly in the spongy tissue at the ends of bones, produces red blood cells, white blood cells, and platelets, which help the blood clot after injury. Yellow marrow, which replaces red marrow as the patient ages, is mostly inactive. It lies in the spongy tissue at the ends of a bone and in a canal that runs through the center of the bone.

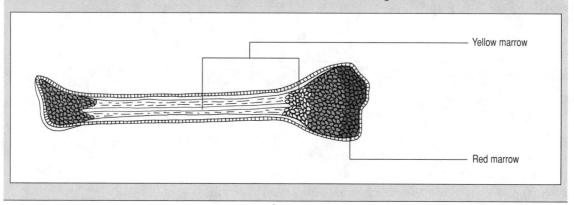
Yellow marrow

Red marrow

- Medications that may affect test results are withheld before this test, whenever possible.

What happens during the test?
- A nurse or medical technician inserts a needle into a vein, usually in your forearm. A blood sample is collected in a tube, which is then sent to a lab for testing.
- A small amount of blood is taken from the finger or earlobe when an infant or child is tested.

What happens after the test?
- If swelling develops at the needle puncture site, warm soaks are applied to the area to ease discomfort.
- You may resume taking medications that were withheld before the test.

- If the results of your test show an abnormal reticulocyte count, it may be repeated to detect trends or changes.

What are the normal results?

Reticulocytes compose 0.5% to 2% of the total red blood cell count. In infants the normal reticulocyte count ranges from 2% to 6% at birth, decreasing to adult levels in 1 to 2 weeks.

What do abnormal results mean?

A low reticulocyte count indicates hypoplastic or pernicious anemia.

A high reticulocyte count may occur after therapy for iron deficiency anemia or pernicious anemia. An increased reticulocyte count also may indicate hemolysis (red blood cell rupture) or a bone marrow response to anemia due to blood loss. (See *Understanding bone marrow's role*.)

TOTAL HEMOGLOBIN

Hemoglobin is a type of protein in red blood cells. Its purpose is to carry oxygen in the blood. The total hemoglobin test is used to measure the amount of hemoglobin per deciliter (100 milliliters) of whole blood. It's usually part of a complete blood count. Hemoglobin concentration correlates closely with the red blood cell count.

Why is this test done?

A total hemoglobin test may be performed for the following reasons:
- To detect anemia or polycythemia or to assess your response to treatment for these disorders
- To help the doctor calculate additional information for a complete blood count.

What should you know before the test?

- You don't need to change your diet before the test.
- This test requires a blood sample, which takes less than 3 minutes to collect.
- You may feel slight discomfort from the needle puncture and tourniquet pressure.

What happens during the test?

■ A nurse or medical technician inserts a needle into a vein, usually in your forearm. A blood sample is collected in a tube, which is then sent to a lab for testing.

■ A small amount of blood is taken from the finger or earlobe when a young child is tested.

What happens after the test?

If swelling develops at the needle puncture site, warm soaks are applied to the area to ease discomfort.

What are the normal results?

Hemoglobin concentration varies, depending on the type of sample drawn (capillary blood samples for infants and venous blood samples for all others) and on the person's age and sex. (See *Hemoglobin values throughout the lifespan.*)

What do abnormal results mean?

Low hemoglobin concentration may indicate anemia, recent hemorrhage, or fluid retention. All three cause hemodilution.

Elevated hemoglobin suggests hemoconcentration from polycythemia or dehydration.

HEMOGLOBIN COMPONENTS

This test separates and measures normal and some abnormal forms of hemoglobin in the blood. In this test, a blood sample is placed on a material that allows it to separate into a series of distinctly pigmented bands. Results are compared with those of a normal sample.

Why is this test done?

Hemoglobin components may be tested for the following reasons:

■ To calculate the different components of hemoglobin

■ To aid the diagnosis of thalassemia.

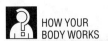

HOW YOUR
BODY WORKS

Hemoglobin values throughout the lifespan

Hemoglobin test results show the amount of hemoglobin in a person's blood. The results are expressed in grams of hemoglobin per deciliter of whole blood. Hemoglobin values vary with a person's age. For example, the normal hemoglobin range for an adult woman is 12 to 16 grams of hemoglobin for each deciliter of blood in her body.

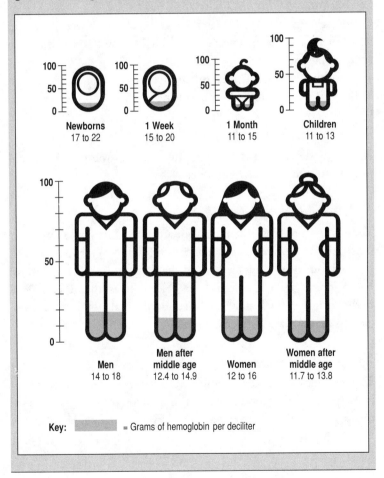

Newborns
17 to 22

1 Week
15 to 20

1 Month
11 to 15

Children
11 to 13

Men
14 to 18

Men after middle age
12.4 to 14.9

Women
12 to 16

Women after middle age
11.7 to 13.8

Key: = Grams of hemoglobin per deciliter

What should you know before the test?

- You don't need to change your diet before the test.
- This test requires a blood sample, which takes less than 3 minutes to collect.
- You may feel slight discomfort from the needle puncture and tourniquet pressure.
- The nurse or technician checks your history for blood transfusions within the past 4 months.

What happens during the test?

- A nurse or medical technician inserts a needle into a vein, usually in your forearm. A blood sample is collected in a tube, which is then sent to a lab for testing.
- When the test is performed on an infant or child, a small amount of blood is taken from the finger or earlobe.

What happens after the test?

If swelling develops at the needle puncture site, warm soaks are applied to the area to ease discomfort.

What are the normal results?

Various components of hemoglobin are labeled hemoglobin A, hemoglobin A_2, hemoglobin S, hemoglobin F, and so forth. In adults, hemoglobin A accounts for more than 95% of all hemoglobins; hemoglobin A_2, 2% to 3%; and hemoglobin F, less than 1%. In newborns, hemoglobin F normally accounts for half the total. Hemoglobins A and C are normally absent.

What do abnormal results mean?

This test allows identification of various types of hemoglobin. Certain types may indicate various hemolytic diseases — such as thalassemia — which are characterized by ruptured red blood cells.

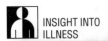

INSIGHT INTO
ILLNESS

Who inherits sickle cell anemia?

The most serious risk of inheriting this disorder occurs when both parents have sickle cell anemia (figure 1). Childbearing — if possible at all — is dangerous for the mother, and all offspring will have sickle cell anemia.

When one parent has sickle cell anemia and one does not (figure 2), all offspring will be carriers of sickle cell anemia. This means they carry and can pass on to their children a trait for the disorder, yet show no outward signs of the illness themselves.

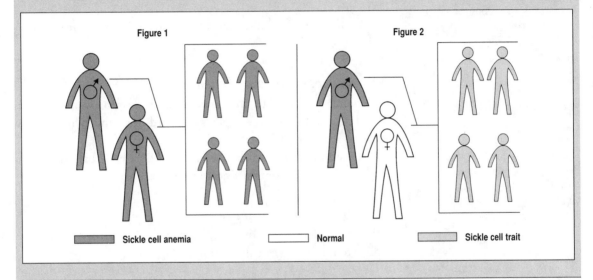

SICKLE CELL TEST

Also known as the *hemoglobin S test*, this test detects *sickle cells* in the bloodstream. These are severely deformed, rigid red blood cells that may slow blood flow. Sickle cell disease almost exclusively affects people with African ancestry. It affects 0.2% of African Americans. (See *Who inherits sickle cell anemia?*)

Although this test is useful as a rapid screening procedure, the results may not be accurate. The hemoglobin component test is performed to confirm the diagnosis if the presence of hemoglobin S is strongly suspected. (See *Prenatal test for sickle cell anemia,* page 294.)

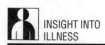

INSIGHT INTO
ILLNESS

Prenatal test for sickle cell anemia

When both parents of a developing fetus are suspected carriers of sickle cell trait, a reliable test is now available that can detect whether the fetus has the sickle cell trait or the disease. Many major medical centers throughout the United States perform the test. Also, any doctor can request the fetal sickle cell test if both parents are suspected carriers.

An opportunity for counseling
The test requires a blood sample from both parents and an amniotic fluid sample. About 1 week is required to complete the test, which can generally be performed between the 14th and 18th weeks of pregnancy. This provides an opportunity for the parents to seek genetic counseling if the disorder is suspected.

Why is this test done?

The sickle cell test may be performed to identify sickle cell disease and sickle cell trait.

What should you know before the test?

- You don't need to restrict food or fluids before the test.
- The nurse or technician checks your history for blood transfusions within the past 3 months.
- This test requires a blood sample, which takes less than 3 minutes to collect.
- You may feel slight discomfort from the needle puncture and tourniquet pressure.

What happens during the test?

- A nurse or medical technician inserts a needle into a vein, usually in your forearm. A blood sample is collected in a tube, which is then sent to a lab for testing.
- When the test is performed on an infant or child, a small amount of blood is taken from the finger or earlobe.

What happens after the test?

If swelling develops at the needle puncture site, warm soaks are applied to the area to ease discomfort.

What are the normal results?

Results of this test are reported as positive or negative. A normal or negative result suggests the absence of hemoglobin S.

What do abnormal results mean?

A positive result may indicate the presence of sickle cells, but the hemoglobin component test is needed to further diagnose the sickling tendency. Rarely, in the absence of hemoglobin S, other abnormal hemoglobins may cause sickling.

HEINZ BODIES

Heinz bodies are particles of damaged hemoglobin that accumulate on red blood cell membranes. Although Heinz bodies are removed from red blood cells by the spleen, they can cause hemolysis (red blood cell destruction) and are a major cause of hemolytic anemias.

Why is this test done?

This test may be performed to determine the cause of anemia.

What should you know before the test?

- You don't need to change your diet before the test.
- This test requires a blood sample, which takes less than 3 minutes to collect.
- You may feel slight discomfort from the needle puncture and tourniquet pressure.
- Whenever possible, medications that may affect test results are withheld before the test.

What happens during the test?

A nurse or medical technician inserts a needle into a vein, usually in your forearm. A blood sample is collected in a tube, which is then sent to a lab for testing.

What happens after the test?

- If swelling develops at the needle puncture site, warm soaks are applied to the area to ease discomfort.
- You may resume taking medications that were withheld before the test.

What are the normal results?

A negative test result indicates an absence of Heinz bodies.

What do abnormal results mean?

A positive test result signifies the presence of Heinz bodies. This may indicate an inherited red cell enzyme deficiency, the presence of unstable hemoglobins, thalassemia, or drug-induced red cell injury. Heinz bodies may also be present after spleen surgery.

IRON AND IRON-BINDING CAPACITY

A necessary nutrient, iron is found in many foods. (See *Choosing iron-rich foods*.) After dietary iron is absorbed by the intestine, it's distributed to the liver and other areas of the body for synthesis, storage, and transport. Iron is essential to the formation and function of hemoglobin, the oxygen-transporting element of blood. This test measures the amount of iron in a blood sample.

In the bloodstream, iron is bound to a protein called *transferrin*. The second phase of this test, iron-binding capacity, measures the amount of iron that would occur in the blood if the transferrin were completely saturated with iron. (See *The iron path*, page 298.)

You need iron in your diet to be healthy. This test checks the amount of iron in a blood sample.

Why is this test done?
Iron and iron-binding capacity may be determined for the following reasons:
- To evaluate the body's capacity to store iron
- To estimate total iron storage
- To aid diagnosis of hemochromatosis
- To help distinguish iron deficiency anemia from anemia of chronic disease
- To help evaluate a person's nutrition status.

What should you know before the test?
- You don't need to change your diet before the test.
- This test requires a blood sample, which takes less than 3 minutes to collect.
- You may feel slight discomfort from the needle puncture and tourniquet pressure.
- The nurse or medical technician will check your drug history for the use of any medications that may affect test results. Usually these drugs are withheld before the test.

What happens during the test?
A nurse or medical technician inserts a needle into a vein, usually in your forearm. A blood sample is collected in a tube, which is then sent to a lab for testing.

SELF-HELP

Choosing iron-rich foods

Doctors recommend 18 milligrams of iron a day for women age 50 and under and 10 milligrams a day for men and women over age 50. Consult the following list to find the foods highest in iron.

Food	Quantity	Iron content (milligrams)
Oysters	3 ounces	13.2
Beef liver	3 ounces	7.5
Prune juice	½ cup	5.2
Clams	2 ounces	4.2
Walnuts	½ cup	3.75
Ground beef	3 ounces	3.0
Chickpeas	½ cup	3.0
Bran flakes	½ cup	2.8
Pork roast	3 ounces	2.7
Cashew nuts	½ cup	2.65
Shrimp	3 ounces	2.6
Raisins	½ cup	2.55
Sardines	3 ounces	2.5
Spinach	½ cup	2.4
Lima beans	½ cup	2.3
Kidney beans	½ cup	2.2
Turkey, dark meat	3 ounces	2.0
Prunes	½ cup	1.9
Roast beef	3 ounces	1.8
Green peas	½ cup	1.5
Peanuts	½ cup	1.5
Potato	1	1.1
Sweet potato	½ cup	1.0
Green beans	½ cup	1.0
Egg	1	1.0

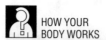

HOW YOUR
BODY WORKS

The iron path

Iron from the food you eat is absorbed and is oxidated, or gains oxygen, in the bowel. Next, it circulates to the bone marrow for hemoglobin production and to all iron-hungry body cells. In the spleen, iron is recycled back to the bone marrow or into storage. Storage areas in the liver, spleen, bone marrow, and reticuloendothelial system hold iron as ferritin until the body needs it. The body conserves iron, losing small amounts through skin, feces, urine, and menstrual blood. Normal iron metabolism is essential for red cell function.

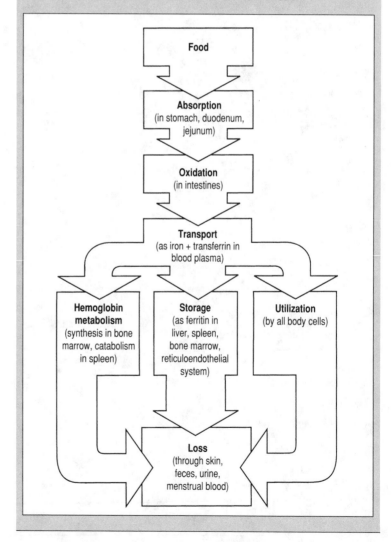

What happens after the test?

- If swelling develops at the needle puncture site, warm soaks are applied to the area to ease discomfort.
- You may resume taking medications that were withheld before the test.

What are the normal results?

Normal iron and iron-binding capacity levels are as follows:

	IRON (micrograms per deciliter)	IRON-BINDING CAPACITY (micrograms per deciliter)	PERCENT SATURATION
Men	70 to 150	300 to 400	20 to 50
Women	80 to 150	300 to 450	20 to 50

What do abnormal results mean?

In iron deficiency, iron levels decrease and iron-binding capacity increases. In people with chronic inflammations (such as rheumatoid arthritis), iron levels may be low in the presence of adequate body stores, but iron-binding capacity may be unchanged or may decrease.

Iron overload may not change iron levels until relatively late in a condition. But, in general, iron increases and iron-binding capacity remains the same.

FERRITIN

A major iron-storage protein, ferritin normally appears in small quantities in the blood. In a healthy adult, the ferritin level is directly related to the amount of available iron that's stored in the body.

Why is this test done?

Ferritin levels may be determined for the following reasons:

- To screen for iron deficiency and iron overload
- To measure iron storage

- To distinguish between iron deficiency (a condition of low iron storage) and chronic inflammation (a condition of normal storage).

What should you know before the test?

- You don't need to change your diet before this test.
- This test requires a blood sample, which takes less than 3 minutes to collect.
- You may feel slight discomfort from the needle puncture and tourniquet pressure.
- A nurse or medical technician checks your history for any transfusion within the last 4 months.

What happens during the test?

A nurse or medical technician inserts a needle into a vein, usually in your forearm. A blood sample is collected in a tube, which is then sent to a lab for testing.

What happens after the test?

If swelling develops at the needle puncture site, warm soaks are applied to the area to ease discomfort.

What are the normal results?

Normal ferritin levels vary with age and within wide ranges, as follows:
- Newborns: 25 to 200 nanograms of ferritin per milliliter of blood
- 1 month: 200 to 600 nanograms
- 2 to 5 months: 50 to 200 nanograms
- 6 months to 15 years: 7 to 140 nanograms
- Men: 20 to 300 nanograms
- Women: 20 to 120 nanograms.

What do abnormal results mean?

High ferritin levels may indicate acute or chronic liver disease, iron overload, leukemia, infection or inflammation, Hodgkin's disease, or chronic anemias. In these disorders, iron reserves in the bone marrow may be normal or significantly increased. Ferritin levels are characteristically normal or slightly elevated in a person with chronic kidney disease.

Low ferritin levels indicate chronic iron deficiency.

WHITE BLOOD CELL COUNT

A white blood cell count is also called a *leukocyte count*. It's part of a complete blood count. This test finds out how many white cells are in a small blood sample.

White blood cell counts may vary by as much as 2,000 on any given day, due to strenuous exercise, stress, or digestion. White blood cells help the body fight infection. The number of white blood cells may increase or decrease significantly in certain diseases, but as a diagnostic tool, the white blood cell count is useful only when a person's white cell differential and health status are considered. (See *Surround and destroy: How white blood cells fight foreign particles,* page 302.)

Why is this test done?

A white blood cell count may be performed for the following reasons:
- To detect an infection or inflammation
- To determine the need for further tests, such as the white blood cell differential or bone marrow biopsy
- To monitor a person's response to cancer therapy.

What should you know before the test?

- You should avoid strenuous exercise for 24 hours before the test. Also avoid eating a heavy meal before the test.
- This test requires a blood sample, which takes less than 3 minutes to collect.
- You may feel slight discomfort from the needle puncture and tourniquet pressure.
- If you're being treated for an infection, this test will be repeated to monitor your progress.
- Certain medications, including antibiotics, drugs for seizures, thyroid hormone antagonists, and nonsteroidal anti-inflammatory agents (such as ibuprofen) may interfere with the test results.

What happens during the test?

A nurse or medical technician inserts a needle into a vein, usually in your forearm. A blood sample is collected in a tube, which is then sent to a lab for testing.

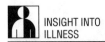

**INSIGHT INTO
ILLNESS**

Surround and destroy: How white blood cells fight foreign particles

In response to infection, white blood cells rush to the site of inflammation. There, phagocytosis occurs — the bacteria or other foreign particles that cause infection are engulfed and destroyed.

First, disease-fighting antibodies coat the bacteria (phase 1). Next, the white blood cell surrounds the bacteria with pseudopods, which are footlike extensions (phase 2). The foreign particles are destroyed by digestion in the white blood cell (phase 3). Finally, the white blood cell releases the digested debris (phase 4) and continues to fight infection.

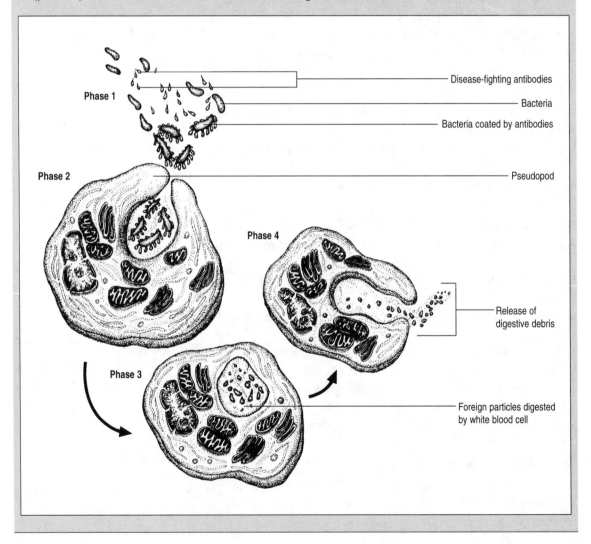

What happens after the test?

- If swelling develops at the needle puncture site, warm soaks are applied to the area to ease discomfort.
- You may resume activity that was restricted before the test.
- If test results show that you have severe leukopenia, you may have little or no resistance to infection and will need protective isolation.

What are the normal results?

Normal white blood cell counts range from 4,000 to 10,000 white blood cells per cubic millimeter of whole blood.

What do abnormal results mean?

An elevated white blood cell count, which doctors call *leukocytosis*, often indicates infection, such as an abscess, meningitis, appendicitis, or tonsillitis. A high count also may be caused by leukemia or by dead tissue from burns, heart attack, or gangrene.

A low white blood cell count — or leukopenia — indicates bone marrow problems. This may be caused by viral infections or from toxic reactions to poisons. Leukopenia characteristically accompanies the flu, typhoid fever, measles, infectious hepatitis, mononucleosis, and rubella.

WHITE BLOOD CELL DIFFERENTIAL

White blood cells, also called *leukocytes*, are classified into five major types: neutrophils, eosinophils, basophils, lymphocytes, and monocytes. The white blood cell differential is used to evaluate the distribution of these various leukocytes in the blood. It also tells the doctor about the structure of these cells. The information is used in evaluating the immune system.

Why is this test done?

A white blood cell differential test may be performed for the following reasons:

- To evaluate the immune system and the body's capacity to resist and overcome infection
- To detect and identify various types of leukemia

- To determine the stage and severity of an infection
- To detect and assess allergic reactions
- To detect parasitic infections.

What should you know before the test?

- You don't need to restrict food or fluids, but you should refrain from strenuous exercise for 24 hours before the test.
- This test requires a blood sample, which takes less than 3 minutes to collect.
- You may feel slight discomfort from the needle puncture and tourniquet pressure.
- The nurse or medical technician will check your drug history for the use of any medications that may affect test results. Usually these drugs are withheld for a period before the test.

What happens during the test?

A nurse or medical technician inserts a needle into a vein, usually in your forearm. A blood sample is collected in a tube, which is then sent to a lab for testing.

What happens after the test?

- If swelling develops at the needle puncture site, warm soaks are applied to the area to ease discomfort.
- An eosinophil count may be ordered as a follow-up test if a high or low eosinophil level is reported.

What are the normal results?

The chart below provides relative levels for the five types of white blood cells classified in the differential:

Types of cells	Adults	Boys ages 6 to 18	Girls ages 6 to 18
Neutrophils	47.6% to 76.8%	38.5% to 71.5%	41.9% to 76.5%
Lymphocytes	16.2% to 43%	19.4% to 51.4%	16.3% to 46.7%
Monocytes	0.6% to 9.6%	1.1% to 11.6%	0.9% to 9.9%
Eosinophils	0.3% to 7%	1% to 8.1%	0.8% to 8.3%
Basophils	0.3% to 2%	0.25% to 1.3%	0.3% to 1.4%

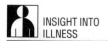
INSIGHT INTO
ILLNESS

How diseases affect white blood cell count

White blood cells are classified into five major types: neutrophils, eosinophils, basophils, lymphocytes, and monocytes. Changes in the levels of these blood cell types, as revealed by lab tests, provide evidence for a wide range of diseases and other conditions.

CELL TYPE	INCREASED BY	DECREASED BY
Neutrophils 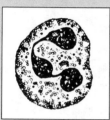	▪ Infections: osteomyelitis, otitis media, salpingitis, blood poisoning, gonorrhea, endocarditis, smallpox, chickenpox, herpes, Rocky Mountain spotted fever ▪ Localized tissue death due to heart attack, burns, carcinoma ▪ Metabolic disorders: diabetic acidosis, eclampsia, uremia, thyrotoxicosis ▪ Stress response due to acute hemorrhage, surgery, excessive exercise, emotional distress, third trimester of pregnancy, childbirth ▪ Inflammatory disease: rheumatic fever, rheumatoid arthritis, acute gout, vasculitis and myositis	▪ Bone marrow depression due to radiation or cytotoxic drugs ▪ Infections: typhoid, tularemia, brucellosis, hepatitis, flu, measles, German measles, mumps, infectious mononucleosis ▪ Hypersplenism: liver disease and storage diseases ▪ Collagen vascular disease such as lupus ▪ Deficiency of folic acid or vitamin B_{12}
Eosinophils 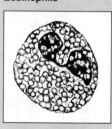	▪ Allergic disorders: asthma, hay fever, food or drug sensitivity, serum sickness, angioneurotic edema ▪ Parasitic infections: trichinosis, hookworm, roundworm, amebiasis ▪ Skin diseases: eczema, pemphigus, psoriasis, dermatitis herpes ▪ Cancers: chronic myelocytic leukemia, Hodgkin's disease, spread and deterioration of solid tumors ▪ Miscellaneous: collagen vascular disease, adrenocortical hypofunction, ulcerative colitis, polyarteritis nodosa, postsplenectomy, pernicious anemia, scarlet fever, excessive exercise	▪ Stress response due to injury, shock, burns, surgery, mental distress ▪ Cushing's syndrome

(continued)

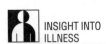

INSIGHT INTO
ILLNESS

How diseases affect white blood cell count *(continued)*

CELL TYPE	INCREASED BY	DECREASED BY
Basophils 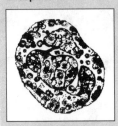	▪ Chronic myelocytic leukemia, polycythemia vera, some chronic hemolytic anemias, Hodgkin's disease, systemic mastocytosis, myxedema, ulcerative colitis, chronic hypersensitivity states, and nephrosis	▪ Hyperthyroidism, ovulation, pregnancy, stress
Lymphocytes 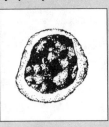	▪ Infections: pertussis, brucellosis, syphilis, tuberculosis, hepatitis, infectious mononucleosis, mumps, German measles, cytomegalovirus ▪ Other: thyrotoxicosis, hypoadrenalism, ulcerative colitis, immune diseases, lymphocytic leukemia	▪ Severe debilitating illness, such as congestive heart failure, kidney failure, advanced tuberculosis ▪ Defective lymphatic circulation, high levels of adrenal corticosteroids, immunodeficiency due to immunosuppressives
Monocytes 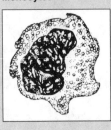	▪ Infections: subacute bacterial endocarditis, tuberculosis, hepatitis, malaria, Rocky Mountain spotted fever ▪ Collagen vascular disease: lupus, rheumatoid arthritis, polyarteritis nodosa ▪ Carcinomas, monocytic leukemia, lymphomas	▪ Immunosuppression

For an accurate diagnosis, the doctor will interpret differential test results in relation to the total white blood cell count. (See *Interpreting the white blood cell differential.*)

What do abnormal results mean?

Abnormal differential patterns provide evidence for a wide range of diseases and conditions. For example, high levels of some leukocytes are associated with various allergic diseases and reactions to parasites. (See *How diseases affect white blood cell count,* pages 305 and 306.)

BLOOD CLOTTING TESTS

BLEEDING TIME

This test measures the duration of bleeding after a small skin incision. Bleeding time depends on the elasticity of the blood vessel wall and on the number and effectiveness of platelets, which are small, disk-like structures in the blood that help blood coagulate (clot). (See *Birth of a blood clot,* page 308.)

Bleeding time may be measured by one of four methods doctors call *Duke, Ivy, template,* or *modified template.* The template methods are the most accurate because the incision size is standardized. Although this test is usually performed on a person with a personal or family history of bleeding disorders, it's also useful for screening before surgery, along with a platelet count.

Why is this test done?

Bleeding time may be determined for the following reasons:
- To measure the time required to form a clot and stop bleeding
- To assess the platelet response and constriction of blood vessels after an injury
- To detect platelet function disorders.

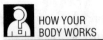

HOW YOUR
BODY WORKS

Birth of a blood clot

When hemorrhage (bleeding) occurs with an injury, platelets gather at the site of injury, releasing platelet factors. These factors combine with other plasma factors to convert prothrombin to thrombin. Then thrombin converts fibrinogen to fibrin, the essential part of the clot.

BLOOD CLOT FORMATION

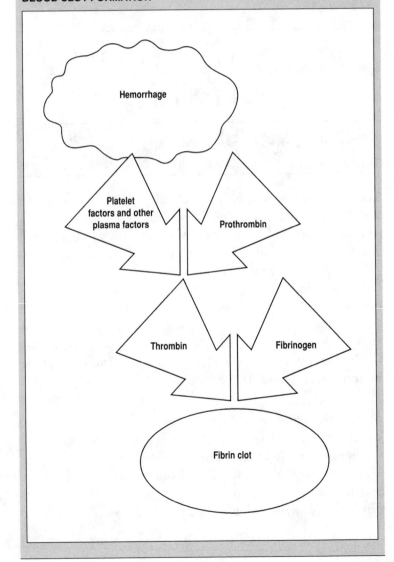

What should you know before the test?

- You don't need to change your diet before the test.
- This test requires small incisions on your forearm or earlobe. You may feel some discomfort from the incisions, the antiseptic, and the tightness of the blood pressure cuff. The test takes only 10 to 20 minutes to perform. The incisions will leave small scars that are barely visible when healed.
- The nurse or technician checks your history for recent use of drugs that prolong bleeding time. If you use such medications and are being tested to identify a suspected bleeding disorder, the test may be postponed and the drugs discontinued. If the test is part of preparation before surgery, it proceeds as scheduled.

A test for bleeding time may be performed before surgery to ward off potential problems.

What happens during the test?

- *Template and modified template methods*: A nurse or medical technician inflates a blood pressure cuff on your upper arm and applies a template to your forearm. For the template method, a lancet is used to make two small incisions. For the modified template method, a spring-loaded blade is used to make the incisions. The nurse gently blots drops of blood every 30 seconds until the bleeding stops in both cuts. The average bleeding time of the two cuts is calculated.
- *Ivy method:* After applying the pressure cuff, the nurse makes three small punctures, then follows a similar blotting and calculation technique.
- *Duke method:* Your shoulder is draped with a towel and a small puncture is made in your earlobe. The blotting and recording procedure is the same.

What happens after the test?

- If you have a bleeding tendency (due to hemophilia, for example), a pressure bandage is placed over the incision for 24 to 48 hours and it is checked regularly.
- If you don't have a bleeding tendency, the incision is dressed.
- You may resume taking medications that were discontinued before the test.

Does the test have risks?

- This test is usually not recommended for a person whose platelet count is less than 75,000 cells per cubic millimeter.
- If bleeding doesn't slow down after 15 minutes, the test is discontinued.

What are the normal results?

The normal range of bleeding time is from 2 to 8 minutes in the template method; from 2 to 10 minutes in the modified template method; from 1 to 7 minutes in the Ivy method; and from 1 to 3 minutes in the Duke method.

What do abnormal results mean?

Prolonged bleeding time may indicate blood disorders, such as Hodgkin's disease, acute leukemia, disseminated intravascular coagulation, hemolytic disease of the newborn, Schönlein-Henoch purpura, severe liver disease such as cirrhosis, or severe deficiency of factors I, II, V, VII, VIII, IX, or XI.

Prolonged bleeding time in a person with a normal platelet count suggests a platelet function disorder and requires more investigation.

PLATELET COUNT

Platelets, or thrombocytes, are the smallest formed elements in blood. They promote blood clotting after an injury. A platelet count is one of the most important blood tests done.

Why is this test done?

A platelet count may be performed for the following reasons:

- To determine if blood clots normally
- To evaluate platelet production
- To assess the effects of chemotherapy or radiation therapy on platelet production
- To diagnose and monitor a severe increase or decrease in platelet count.

What should you know before the test?

- You don't need to change your diet before the test.
- This test requires a blood sample, which takes less than 3 minutes to collect.
- You may feel slight discomfort from the needle puncture and tourniquet pressure.
- The nurse or medical technician will check your drug history for the use of any medications that may affect test results. Usually these drugs are withheld for a period before the test.

What happens during the test?

The nurse or medical technician inserts a needle into a vein, usually in your forearm. A blood sample is collected in a tube, which is then sent to a lab for testing.

What happens after the test?

If swelling develops at the needle puncture site, warm soaks are applied to the area to ease discomfort.

What are the normal results?

Normal platelet counts range from 130,000 to 370,000 platelets per cubic millimeter of whole blood.

What do abnormal results mean?

Thrombocytopenia (a low platelet count) can be caused by bone marrow problems, such as cancer, leukemia, or infection; folic acid or vitamin B_{12} deficiency; pooling of platelets in an enlarged spleen; increased platelet destruction due to drugs or immune disorders; or mechanical injury to platelets. A platelet count that falls below 50,000 can cause spontaneous bleeding. When it drops below 5,000, fatal central nervous system bleeding or massive gastrointestinal hemorrhage is possible.

Thrombocytosis (a high platelet count) can be caused by severe bleeding, infections, cancer, iron deficiency anemia, and recent surgery, pregnancy, or spleen removal. A high count also can be caused by inflammatory disorders.

A platelet count is one of the most important blood tests.

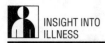

INSIGHT INTO
ILLNESS

Fragile capillaries: A significant finding

A test result is considered *positive* when many petechiae (tiny red spots caused by bleeding under the skin) show up below the blood pressure cuff. Both the size and number of petechiae are used to determine abnormalities.

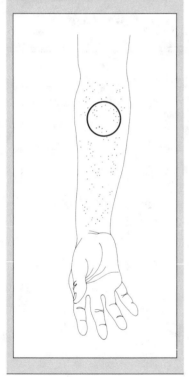

TOURNIQUET TEST

Also called the *capillary fragility test,* this test helps evaluate bleeding tendencies. It measures the ability of the capillaries, the body's smallest blood vessels, to remain intact under pressure, which is controlled by a blood pressure cuff placed around the upper arm.

Why is this test done?

The tourniquet test may be performed for the following reasons:
- To identify abnormal bleeding tendencies
- To assess the fragility of capillary walls
- To identify a low platelet count.

What should you know before the test?

- You don't need to change your diet before this test.
- The test requires use of a blood pressure cuff. You may feel slight discomfort from the pressure of the cuff on your arm.

What happens during the test?

- A nurse or medical technician checks your skin temperature and the room temperature. Normal temperatures help to ensure accurate results.
- A small space on your forearm is selected and marked. Ideally, the site is free of petechiae, which are minute, round purplish red spots caused by bleeding under the skin. If petechiae are present on the site before starting the test, they are counted and the number is recorded for future reference.
- A blood pressure cuff is fastened around your arm and inflated. This pressure is maintained for 5 minutes; then the cuff is released.
- The nurse or medical technician counts the number of petechiae that appear in the marked space.

What happens after the test?

You'll open and close your hand a few times to help blood return to your forearm.

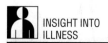

INSIGHT INTO
ILLNESS

How your doctor looks at bruises

Your doctor may use the following terms to identify what you commonly call a rash or a bruise. Types of purpuric lesions —purplish spots from blood seeping into the skin — include petechiae, ecchymoses, and hematomas.

Petechiae

These red or brown lesions are painless, round, and as tiny as pinpoints. Petechiae result from a leakage of red blood cells into skin tissue, and they usually appear and fade in groups.

Ecchymoses

These lesions are another form of blood leakage and are larger than petechiae. Ecchymoses are purple, blue, or yellow-green bruises that vary in size and shape. They can occur anywhere on the body as a result of traumatic injury. In people with bleeding disorders, ecchymoses usually appear on the arms and legs.

Hematomas

A noticeable bruise that's painful and swollen is a hematoma. Hematomas are usually the result of traumatic injury. Superficial hematomas are red, whereas deep hematomas are blue. Although their size varies widely, hematomas typically exceed 1 centimeter in diameter.

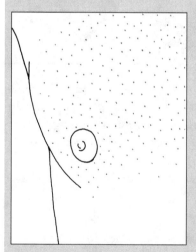

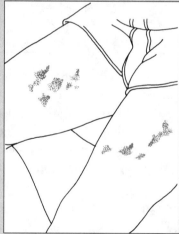

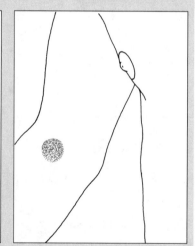

Does the test have risks?

- This test should not be repeated on the same arm within 1 week.
- This test is not recommended if you have disseminated intravascular coagulation or other bleeding disorders or if many petechiae are already present.

What are the normal results?

A few petechiae may normally be present before the test. Less than 10 petechiae on the forearm, 5 minutes after the test, is considered normal, or negative. More than 10 petechiae is considered a positive result.

What do abnormal results mean?

More than 10 petechiae can indicate a platelet defect or a weakness of the capillary walls, called *vascular purpura*. (See *Fragile capillaries: A significant finding,* page 312.) It may occur in a long list of bleeding disorders.

Conditions that are not related to bleeding defects, such as scarlet fever, measles, flu, chronic kidney disease, high blood pressure, and diabetes with vascular disease, may also increase capillary fragility. An abnormal number of petechiae sometimes appear before menstruation or other times in healthy people, especially women over age 40. (See *How your doctor looks at bruises,* page 313.)

PLATELET CLOTTING

Platelets are the crucial element in forming blood clots. The platelet aggregation test measures how well they are doing their job.

After injury to a blood vessel, the clot-forming elements in the blood, called *platelets*, gather at the injury site. Here the platelets clump together to form an aggregate (clot), that helps stop bleeding and promote healing. A test called the *platelet aggregation test* is used to measure how quickly the platelets in a blood sample clump together after an aggregating agent is added to the test tube.

Why is this test done?

The platelet aggregation test may be performed for the following reasons:
- To determine if blood clots properly
- To detect bleeding disorders.

What should you know before the test?

- You will be asked to fast or to maintain a nonfat diet for 8 hours before the test.

- This test requires a blood sample, which takes less than 3 minutes to collect.
- You may feel slight discomfort from the needle puncture and tourniquet pressure.
- Aspirin and aspirin compounds are withheld for 14 days before the test. Azolid, Anturan, phenothiazines, antihistamines, anti-inflammatory drugs, and tricyclic antidepressants are withheld for 48 hours before the test.
- Because many medications may alter the results of this test, you should be as drug free as possible before the test. If you've taken aspirin within the past 14 days and the test cannot be postponed, the lab is asked to verify the presence of aspirin in the sample. If test results are abnormal for this sample, you must stop taking aspirin and the test is repeated in 2 weeks. (See *Aspirin's effect on blood clotting.*)

What happens during the test?

A nurse or medical technician inserts a needle into a vein, usually in your forearm. A blood sample is collected in a tube, which is then sent to a lab for testing.

What happens after the test?

- Pressure is applied to the needle puncture site for 5 minutes or until bleeding stops.
- You may resume your usual diet and medications.
- If swelling develops at the needle puncture site, warm soaks are applied to the area to ease discomfort.

What are the normal results?

Normal aggregation occurs in 3 to 5 minutes, but findings depend on temperature and vary with the lab. Aggregation curves that are obtained by using special compounds in the blood sample help to distinguish various platelet defects.

What do abnormal results mean?

Abnormal findings may indicate von Willebrand's disease, Bernard-Soulier syndrome, storage pool disease, Glanzmann's thrombasthenia, or polycythemia vera.

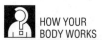 HOW YOUR BODY WORKS

Aspirin's effect on blood clotting

Aspirin inhibits platelet aggregation — the ability of platelets to move together and form a mass at the site of injury. Platelet aggregation is an important stage of blood clotting. Taking aspirin may cause bleeding time to double in healthy people. In children or in people with bleeding disorders such as hemophilia, bleeding time may be even more prolonged.

Beneficial effects
On the other hand, aspirin's action on blood vessels may cause vasodilation (widening of the blood vessels). Low aspirin dosage — 80 milligrams daily or 325 milligrams every other day — may prevent thrombosis (blood clot formation) in an artery or vein that hinders the flow of blood.

ACTIVATED PARTIAL THROMBOPLASTIN TIME

The activated partial thromboplastin time test evaluates all the clotting factors of blood except platelets. This test measures the time it takes for a fibrin clot to form after special compounds called reagents are added to a blood sample. An activator, which is used to shorten clotting time, may also be added to the sample.

Why is this test done?

The activated partial thromboplastin time test may be performed for the following reasons:
- To determine if your blood clots normally
- To help check your bleeding tendencies before surgery
- To screen for clotting factor deficiencies that are present at birth
- To monitor heparin therapy.

What should you know before the test?

- You don't need to change your diet before this test.
- The test requires a blood sample, which takes less than 3 minutes to collect.
- You may feel slight discomfort from the needle puncture and tourniquet pressure.

What happens during the test?

A nurse or medical technician inserts a needle into a vein, usually in your forearm. A blood sample is collected in a tube, which is then sent to a lab for testing.

What happens after the test?

- If swelling develops at the needle puncture site, warm soaks are applied to the area to ease discomfort.
- If you're receiving heparin therapy, this test may be repeated at regular intervals to measure your response to treatment.

What are the normal results?

Normally, a fibrin clot forms 25 to 36 seconds after adding reagents to the sample. If you're on anticoagulant therapy, the doctor specifies the normal test results, adjusted for the therapy you're receiving.

What do abnormal results mean?

Prolonged activated partial thromboplastin time may indicate a deficiency of certain clotting factors or the presence of heparin, fibrin split products, fibrinolysins, or circulating anticoagulants.

PROTHROMBIN TIME

Fibrin is a type of protein that's essential to the clotting of blood. The prothrombin time test measures how long it takes for a fibrin clot to form in a specially treated blood sample.

Why is this test done?

The prothrombin time test may be performed for the following reasons:
- To see if your blood clots normally
- To provide an overall evaluation of certain clotting factors in the blood
- To monitor response to anticoagulants (drugs that are given to thin the blood).

What should you know before the test?

- You don't need to change your diet before the test.
- This test requires a blood sample, which takes less than 3 minutes to collect.
- You may feel slight discomfort from the needle puncture and tourniquet pressure.
- The nurse or medical technician checks your history for the use of medications that may affect test results.
- If this test is used to monitor the effects of blood-thinning drugs, it's performed daily when therapy begins and is repeated at longer intervals when medication levels stabilize.

If you are receiving drugs that cause your blood to become thinner, your doctor may want to measure your prothrombin time.

What happens during the test?

A nurse or medical technician inserts a needle into a vein, usually in your forearm. A blood sample is collected in a tube, which is then sent to a lab for testing.

What happens after the test?

If swelling develops at the needle puncture site, warm soaks are applied to the area to ease discomfort.

What are the normal results?

Normally, prothrombin times range from 10 to 14 seconds. The times vary, however, depending on the source of the clotting factor and the type of sensing devices that are used to measure clot formation. In a person who's receiving blood-thinning drugs, prothrombin time is usually between one and a half and two times the normal time.

What do abnormal results mean?

Prolonged prothrombin time may indicate deficiencies in several specific clotting factors. It may also be due to liver disease or therapy with blood-thinning drugs. Prolonged prothrombin time that exceeds two and a half times the control time is commonly associated with abnormal bleeding.

Prolonged prothrombin time also can be caused by a long list of drugs, thyroid hormones, vitamin A, or overuse of alcohol.

Prolonged or shortened prothrombin time can follow the use of antibiotics, barbiturates, pain relievers, or mineral oil.

CLOTTING FACTORS II, V, VII, AND X

Blood contains a number of elements, called *factors*, that help cause clotting. This test detects a deficiency of four specific factors. (See *Testing for factor XIII deficiency*.)

Why is this test done?

This test may be performed for the following reasons:
- To check blood clotting
- To identify a specific factor deficiency

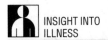
INSIGHT INTO
ILLNESS

Testing for factor XIII deficiency

When a person experiences poor wound healing and other symptoms of a bleeding disorder — despite normal results of coagulation screening tests — a factor XIII assay is recommended.

What is factor XIII?
Factor XIII is responsible for stabilizing the fibrin clot, the final step in the clotting process. If the clot is unstable, it breaks loose, resulting in scarring and poor wound healing. Deficiency of this factor is usually transmitted genetically but may result from liver disease or from tumors.

What happens in this test?
A plasma sample is incubated in a special solution after normal clotting takes place. The clot is observed for 24 hours. If the clot dissolves, a severe factor XI!I deficiency exists.

What are the effects of factor XIII deficiency?
The effects of factor XIII deficiency include the following:
- umbilical bleeding in newborns
- recurrent bleeding under the skin, bruising or clotting in an organ or tissue, and poor wound healing
- bleeding in a joint cavity
- miscarriage (rarely)
- bleeding within the ovaries
- prolonged bleeding after injury (bleeding may begin immediately or may be delayed as long as 12 to 36 hours).

How is it treated?
Treatment with intravenous infusions of plasma or cryoprecipitate may improve the prognosis; some people even live normal lives.

- To study blood-clotting defects
- To monitor the effects of blood component therapy in a factor-deficient person.

What should you know before the test?
- You don't need to change your diet before this test.
- Oral anticoagulants are usually withheld before the test.
- This test requires a blood sample, which takes less than 3 minutes to collect.
- You may feel slight discomfort from the needle puncture and tourniquet pressure.
- If you're factor deficient and receiving blood component therapy, you may need a series of tests.

What happens during the test?

A nurse or medical technician inserts a needle into a vein, usually in your forearm. A blood sample is collected in a tube, which is then sent to a lab for testing.

What happens after the test?

- If swelling develops at the needle puncture site, warm soaks are applied to the area to ease discomfort.
- If you have a bleeding disorder, a pressure bandage may be applied to stop bleeding at the needle puncture site.

Does the test have risks?

If you have a suspected clotting problem, special care is taken to avoid excessive probing during the test, the tourniquet is removed promptly from your arm to avoid bruising, and pressure is applied to the puncture site for 5 minutes, or until the bleeding stops.

What are the normal results?

Clotting time should be between 50% and 150% of the norm.

What do abnormal results mean?

If the clotting time is prolonged, the person may be deficient in the factor being tested. Deficiency of factor II, factor VII, or factor X may indicate liver disease or vitamin K deficiency. Deficiency of factor X may also indicate scattered intravascular coagulation. Factor V deficiency suggests severe liver disease, disseminated intravascular coagulation, or fibrinogenolysis. Deficiencies of all four factors may be present at birth; absence of factor II is lethal.

CLOTTING FACTORS VIII, IX, XI, AND XII

Blood contains a number of elements, called *factors*, that help cause clotting. This test detects a deficiency of four specific factors.

Why is this test done?

This test may be performed for the following reasons:
- To check blood clotting
- To identify a specific factor deficiency
- To study blood-clotting defects
- To monitor the effects of blood component therapy in a factor-deficient person.

What should you know before the test?

- You don't need to change your diet before this test.
- The test requires a blood sample, which takes less than 3 minutes to collect.
- You may feel slight discomfort from the needle puncture and tourniquet pressure.
- Oral anticoagulants are usually withheld before the test.
- If you're factor deficient and receiving blood component therapy, a series of tests may be needed to monitor therapeutic progress.

What happens during the test?

A nurse or medical technician inserts a needle into a vein, usually in your forearm. A blood sample is collected in a tube, which is then sent to a lab for testing.

What happens after the test?

- If swelling develops at the needle puncture site, warm soaks are applied to the area to ease discomfort.
- If you have a bleeding disorder, you may need a pressure bandage to stop bleeding at the needle puncture site.
- You may resume taking any medications that were discontinued before the test.

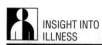

INSIGHT INTO
ILLNESS

Distinguishing between hemophilia A and hemophilia B

When blood studies confirm a hemophilia diagnosis, you're typically told you have either type A or type B hemophilia.

 Hemophilia A, or classic hemophilia, occurs with deficient levels of factor VIII, and *hemophilia B*, or Christmas disease (named for a patient), results from deficient levels of factor IX.

Both types of hemophilia cause the same symptoms, but treatment differs. Knowing which type of hemophilia you have helps the doctor prescribe the most effective treatment.

Hemophilia A

If you have hemophilia A, your factor VIII assay value may be 0% to 30% of normal. Test findings reflect a prolonged activated partial thromboplastin time. However, you'll have a normal platelet count and function and normal bleeding and prothrombin times.

Hemophilia B

If you have hemophilia B, your test findings will show that your blood lacks factor IX. What's more, you'll have baseline coagulation values similar to those for hemophilia A but with normal amounts of factor VIII.

Does the test have risks?

If you're suspected of having a blood-clotting problem, excessive probing is avoided during the test, the tourniquet is removed promptly to avoid bruising, and pressure is applied to the puncture site for 5 minutes, or until the bleeding stops.

What are the normal results?

Clotting time should be between 50% and 150% of the norm.

What do abnormal results mean?

If the clotting time is prolonged, the person may be deficient in the factor being tested. Factor VIII deficiency may indicate hemophilia A, von Willebrand's disease, or factor VIII inhibitor. An acquired deficiency of factor VIII may be caused by disseminated intravascular coagulation or fibrinolysis.

Factor IX deficiency may suggest the presence of hemophilia B, liver disease, factor IX inhibitor, vitamin K deficiency, or therapy with the drug warfarin. Factor VIII and IX inhibitors occur after transfusions in people who are deficient in either factor. (See *Distinguishing between hemophilia A and hemophilia B*.)

Factor XI deficiency may appear after trauma or surgery, or briefly in newborns. Factor XII deficiency may be inherited or acquired and may also appear briefly in newborns.

THROMBIN TIME

This test is also called the *thrombin clotting time test*. In it, thrombin, an enzyme that promotes clotting, is added to a person's blood sample. Thrombin is also added to a normal, or control, sample in the lab. The clotting time for each sample is compared and recorded. This test provides a quick, but imprecise, estimate of how much fibrinogen, a clot-promoting protein, is in the blood.

Why is this test done?

The thrombin time test may be performed for the following reasons:

- To determine if your blood clots normally
- To detect fibrinogen deficiency or defect

- To help the doctor diagnose disseminated intravascular coagulation and liver disease
- To monitor the effectiveness of treatment with heparin or thrombolytic agents.

What should you know before the test?

- This test requires a blood sample, which takes less than 3 minutes to collect.
- You may feel slight discomfort from the needle puncture and tourniquet pressure.
- You don't need to change your diet before the test.
- If possible, heparin therapy is withheld before the test.

What happens during the test?

A nurse or medical technician inserts a needle into a vein, usually in your forearm. A blood sample is collected in a tube, which is then sent to a lab for testing.

What happens after the test?

If swelling develops at the needle puncture site, warm soaks are applied to the area to ease discomfort.

What are the normal results?

Normal thrombin times range from 10 to 15 seconds.

What do abnormal results mean?

A prolonged thrombin time may indicate the presence of heparin therapy, liver disease, disseminated intravascular coagulation, or hypofibrinogenemia. People with prolonged thrombin time may require measurement of fibrinogen levels. If the doctor suspects disseminated intravascular coagulation, the test for fibrin split products is also necessary.

FIBRINOGEN

Also called *factor I,* fibrinogen is a clot-promoting element in blood. Fibrinogen deficiency can produce mild to severe bleeding. This test is used to determine the amount of fibrinogen in a blood sample.

Why is this test done?

This test may be performed for the following reasons:

- To see if your blood clots normally
- To help the doctor diagnose suspected clotting or bleeding disorders caused by fibrinogen abnormalities.

Fibrinogen is an element in the blood that promotes clotting; absence of this element may cause severe bleeding.

What should you know before the test?

- You don't need to change your diet before the test.
- This test requires a blood sample, which takes less than 3 minutes to collect.
- You may feel slight discomfort from the needle puncture and tourniquet pressure.
- The nurse or medical technician will check your drug history for the use of any medications that may affect test results. Usually these drugs are withheld before the test.

What happens during the test?

A nurse or medical technician inserts a needle into a vein, usually in your forearm. A blood sample is collected in a tube, which is then sent to a lab for testing.

What happens after the test?

If swelling develops at the needle puncture site, warm soaks are applied to the area to ease discomfort.

Does the test have risks?

If you are actively bleeding, have an infection or illness, or have received a blood transfusion within 4 weeks, this test is not recommended.

What are the normal results?

Fibrinogen levels normally range from 195 to 365 milligrams per deciliter of blood.

What do abnormal results mean?

Depressed fibrinogen levels may indicate inherited blood disorders; severe liver disease; cancer of the prostate, pancreas, or lung; or bone marrow lesions. Complications or injury in childbirth may cause low fibrinogen levels.

Elevated fibrinogen levels may indicate inflammatory disorders or cancer of the stomach, breast, or kidney.

FIBRIN SPLIT PRODUCTS

After a fibrin clot forms in response to an injury, the clot is eventually broken down by plasmin, a fibrin-dissolving enzyme. The resulting fragments are known as *fibrin split products*, or *fibrinogen degradation products*. In this test, fibrin split products are detected in the diluted serum that's left in a blood sample after clotting.

Why is this test done?

A fibrin split products test may be performed for the following reasons:

- To see if your blood clots normally
- To detect fibrin split products in the circulation
- To help assess fibrin-related problems such as disseminated intra-vascular coagulation. (See *Causes of disseminated intravascular coagulation*, page 326.)

What should you know before the test?

- You don't need to change your diet before the test.
- This test requires a blood sample, which takes less than 3 minutes to collect.
- You may feel slight discomfort from the needle puncture and tourniquet pressure.

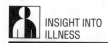

INSIGHT INTO
ILLNESS

Causes of disseminated intravascular coagulation

Disseminated intravascular coagulation is a condition that is marked by widespread clogging of blood vessels and abnormal bleeding. Many disorders can lead to disseminated intravascular coagulation. Below are some of the most well-known causes.

Obstetric
Amniotic fluid embolism, eclampsia, retained dead fetus, retained placenta, abruptio placentae, and toxemia

Cancerous
Sarcoma, spreading carcinoma, acute leukemia, prostatic cancer, and giant hemangioma

Infectious
Acute bacteremia, septicemia, rickettsemia, and infection from viruses, fungi, or protozoa

Necrotic
Injury, destruction of brain tissue, extensive burns, heatstroke, rejection of transplant, and liver necrosis

Cardiovascular
Fat embolism, acute venous thrombosis, cardiopulmonary bypass surgery, hypovolemic shock, heart attack, and high blood pressure

Other
Snakebite, cirrhosis, transfusion of incompatible blood, purpura, and glomerulonephritis

▪ A nurse or medical technician checks your history for the use of heparin or other medications that may interfere with test results. If you're using such medications, the lab must be notified.

What happens during the test?
A nurse or medical technician inserts a needle into a vein, usually in your forearm. A blood sample is collected in a specially treated tube, which is then immediately sent to a lab for testing.

What happens after the test?
If swelling develops at the needle puncture site, warm soaks are applied to the area to ease discomfort.

What are the normal results?
Blood normally contains less than 10 micrograms of fibrin split products per milliliter. A quantitative assay shows less than 3 micrograms per milliliter of blood.

What do abnormal results mean?

Fibrin split products increase due to a long list of disorders, including alcoholic cirrhosis, disseminated intravascular coagulation and subsequent fibrinolysis, congenital heart disease, sunstroke, burns, intrauterine death, a torn placenta, pulmonary blood clot, deep-vein thrombosis, and heart attack. Fibrin split products levels usually exceed 100 micrograms per milliliter in active kidney disease or kidney transplant rejection.

PLASMINOGEN

During the healing process, an enzyme called *plasmin* dissolves clots to prevent excessive clotting and reduced blood flow. Plasmin does not circulate through the body in its active form, however, so it cannot be directly measured. This test is used to measure its circulating precursor, called *plasminogen*.

Why is this test done?

The plasminogen test may be performed for the following reasons:
- To see how well your blood clots normally
- To detect clotting disorders.

What should you know before the test?

- You don't need to change your diet before the test.
- This test requires a blood sample, which takes less than 3 minutes to collect.
- You may feel slight discomfort from the needle puncture and tourniquet pressure.
- The nurse or medical technician will check your drug history for the use of any medications that may affect test results. Usually these drugs are withheld before the test.

What happens during the test?

A nurse or medical technician inserts a needle into a vein, usually in your forearm. A blood sample is collected in a tube, which is then sent to a lab for testing.

What happens after the test?

- If swelling develops at the needle puncture site, warm soaks are applied to the area to ease discomfort.
- You may resume any medications that were withheld before the test.

What are the normal results?

Normal plasminogen levels are 10 to 20 milligrams per deciliter of blood by immunologic methods and 80 to 120 international units per deciliter of blood by functional methods.

What do abnormal results mean?

Diminished plasminogen levels can be caused by disseminated intravascular coagulation (a condition marked by widespread clogging of blood vessels and abnormal bleeding), tumors, and some liver diseases.

11

BLOOD ELEMENT TESTS:
Surveying for Disease

BLOOD GASES & ELECTROLYTES

ARTERIAL BLOOD GAS ANALYSIS

In this test, a sample of blood is collected from an artery, which is a vessel that carries blood from the heart to other parts of the body. Arterial blood gas analysis is used to measure the partial pressures of oxygen and carbon dioxide in blood. Partial pressure is the pressure that an individual gas exerts on the walls of the arteries. Blood pH (or acidity), oxygen content, oxygen saturation, and bicarbonate content are also measured.

Why is this test done?

Arterial blood gas analysis may be performed for the following reasons:
- To evaluate how well the lungs are delivering oxygen to the blood and eliminating carbon dioxide
- To provide information about acid-base disorders
- To monitor respiratory therapy.

What should you know before the test?

- This test requires a blood sample that's collected from the radial, brachial, or femoral artery. These arteries are in the forearm, upper arm, and thigh, respectively.
- You don't need to restrict food or fluids before the test.

What happens during the test?

- Breathe normally while the test is being conducted. Your respiratory rate and rectal temperature are measured and recorded.
- A blood sample is collected from an arterial line that's already in place or by arterial puncture. You may experience a brief cramping or throbbing at the puncture site.

What happens after the test?

- After the sample is collected, pressure is applied to the puncture site for 3 to 5 minutes. Then a gauze pad is taped firmly over the area, without restricting your circulation.
- If you're receiving anticoagulants (blood-thinning drugs) or have a coagulation disorder, pressure is applied to the puncture site for longer than 5 minutes, if necessary.
- Your vital signs are monitored and you're observed for signs of circulatory impairment, such as swelling, discoloration, pain, numbness, or tingling in the bandaged arm or leg.
- You're watched for bleeding from the puncture site.

Does the test have risks?

The nurse or medical technician must wait at least 15 minutes before drawing arterial blood if you're beginning or ending oxygen therapy or if a change is being made in prescribed oxygen therapy.

What are the normal results?

Normal arterial blood gas levels fall within the following ranges:
- Partial pressure of oxygen: 75 to 100 millimeters of mercury
- Partial pressure of carbon dioxide: 35 to 45 millimeters of mercury
- pH: 7.35 to 7.42
- Oxygen content: 15% to 23%
- Oxygen saturation: 94% to 100%
- Bicarbonate: 22 to 26 milliequivalents per liter.

Blood-gas analysis shows the doctor how well your lungs deliver oxygen and eliminate carbon dioxide.

What do abnormal results mean?

Low partial pressure of oxygen, oxygen content, and oxygen saturation levels, with a high partial pressure of carbon dioxide value, may be caused by respiratory muscle weakness or paralysis, head injury, brain tumor, or drug abuse. It can also be caused by airway obstruction, possibly from mucus plugs or a tumor.

Low readings may also be caused by asthma or emphysema, by partially blocked alveoli or pulmonary capillaries, or by alveoli that are damaged or filled with fluid because of disease, hemorrhage, or near-drowning.

Low oxygen content — when respiratory functions are normal — may be caused by severe anemia, decreased blood volume, or reduced oxygen-carrying capacity.

CARBON DIOXIDE CONTENT

When the pressure of carbon dioxide in red blood cells is excessive, carbon dioxide spills out of the cells and dissolves in the plasma, which is fluid that contains blood cells. There, the carbon dioxide combines with water or dissolves to form other compounds.

This test is used to measure the concentration of all forms of carbon dioxide in blood samples. It's commonly ordered for people who have problems with respiration and is usually included in any assessment of electrolyte status. Test results are considered with pH and arterial blood gas levels.

Why is this test done?

Total carbon dioxide content may be measured for the following reasons:

- To determine the amount of carbon dioxide in the blood
- To help evaluate the acid-base balance of the blood.

What should you know before the test?

- This test requires a blood sample, which takes less than 3 minutes to collect.
- You may experience slight discomfort from the needle puncture and tourniquet pressure.
- You don't need to change your diet before the test.
- A nurse or medical technician checks your medication history for any drugs that may affect the test results, including adrenocorticotropic hormone, cortisone, thiazide diuretics, salicylates, paraldehyde, methicillin, dimercaprol, ammonium chloride, or acetazolamide. These drugs may be discontinued. Excessive ingestion of alkaline substances or licorice or accidental ingestion of ethylene glycol or methyl alcohol can also affect test results.

Eating too much licorice or accidentally drinking methyl alcohol could affect the accuracy of this test.

What happens during the test?

A nurse or medical technician inserts a needle into a vein, usually in your forearm. A blood sample is collected in a tube, which is then sent to a lab for testing.

What happens after the test?

If swelling develops at the needle puncture site, warm soaks are applied to the area to ease discomfort.

What are the normal results?

Normal total carbon dioxide levels range from 22 to 34 milliequivalents per liter of blood.

What do abnormal results mean?

High carbon dioxide levels may occur in acid-base disorders, primary aldosteronism, and Cushing's syndrome. Carbon dioxide levels may increase after excessive loss of acids, as in severe vomiting and continuous gastric drainage.

Decreased carbon dioxide levels are common in metabolic acidosis. Levels may also decrease in respiratory alkalosis.

CALCIUM

This test is used to measure the level of calcium in a blood sample. Calcium is an electrolyte, a substance that has an electric charge when it's dissolved in the blood.

Calcium in the blood helps regulate the body's nerve, muscle, and enzyme activity. More than 98% of the body's calcium is in the bones and teeth, however. So, when blood calcium levels fall below normal, calcium moves out of the bones and teeth and dissolves in the blood to restore the blood's calcium balance.

Because calcium is excreted daily, eating calcium-rich foods regularly is necessary to maintain a normal calcium balance. Regular sun exposure also plays a part in calcium metabolism. (See *How sunshine helps you absorb calcium*, page 336.)

Why is this test done?

Calcium levels may be measured for the following reasons:
- To determine blood calcium levels
- To help the doctor diagnose neuromuscular, skeletal, and endocrine disorders; irregular heart rhythms; blood-clotting deficiencies; and acid-base imbalance.

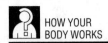

HOW YOUR
BODY WORKS

How sunshine helps you absorb calcium

Most forms of calcium from foods are poorly absorbed from the intestinal tract because they can't be dissolved. But vitamin D — particularly vitamin D_3, which forms when you're exposed to sunshine — and parathyroid hormone play important roles in helping the intestine absorb calcium.

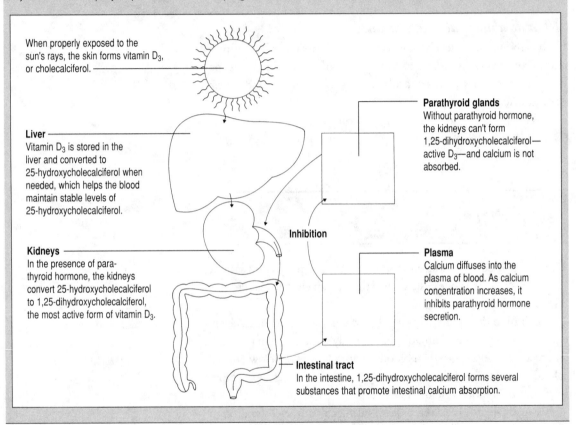

When properly exposed to the sun's rays, the skin forms vitamin D_3, or cholecalciferol.

Liver
Vitamin D_3 is stored in the liver and converted to 25-hydroxycholecalciferol when needed, which helps the blood maintain stable levels of 25-hydroxycholecalciferol.

Kidneys
In the presence of parathyroid hormone, the kidneys convert 25-hydroxycholecalciferol to 1,25-dihydroxycholecalciferol, the most active form of vitamin D_3.

Parathyroid glands
Without parathyroid hormone, the kidneys can't form 1,25-dihydroxycholecalciferol— active D_3—and calcium is not absorbed.

Inhibition

Plasma
Calcium diffuses into the plasma of blood. As calcium concentration increases, it inhibits parathyroid hormone secretion.

Intestinal tract
In the intestine, 1,25-dihydroxycholecalciferol forms several substances that promote intestinal calcium absorption.

What should you know before the test?

- This test requires a blood sample, which takes less than 3 minutes to collect.
- You may experience slight discomfort from the needle puncture.
- You don't need to change your diet before the test.

What happens during the test?

A nurse or medical technician inserts a needle into a vein, usually in your forearm. A blood sample is collected in a tube, which is then sent to a lab for testing.

What happens after the test?

If swelling develops at the needle puncture site, warm soaks are applied to the area to ease discomfort.

What are the normal results?

Normal calcium levels range from 8.9 to 10.1 milligrams per deciliter, or from 4.5 to 5.5 milliequivalents per liter of blood serum (the clear, fluid portion of blood). In children, calcium levels are higher than in adults. Calcium levels can be as high as 12 milligrams per deciliter or 6 milliequivalents per liter during phases of rapid bone growth.

What do abnormal results mean?

Abnormally high serum calcium levels, which is called *hypercalcemia*, may occur with thyroid disorders, Paget's disease of the bone, some cancers, multiple fractures, or prolonged immobilization. High levels may also be caused by low calcium excretion, excessive calcium ingestion, or from overuse of calcium-based antacids.

Hypercalcemia can lead to deep bone pain, flank pain, and muscle weakness. Hypercalcemic crisis begins with nausea, vomiting, and dehydration, leading to stupor, coma, and cardiac arrest.

Low calcium levels, or *hypocalcemia*, may be caused by hypoparathyroidism, total parathyroid removal, or poor calcium absorption. Decreased calcium levels may also occur with Cushing's syndrome, kidney failure, acute pancreatitis, and peritonitis.

Hypocalcemia can lead to numbness and tingling or spasms of the face, arms, and legs; muscle twitching or cramping; tetany; seizures; and irregular heartbeats.

CHLORIDE

This test measures levels of chloride in blood. Chloride is an electrolyte, a substance that has an electric charge when it's dissolved in the blood. (See *Understanding body fluids.*)

Chloride helps regulate blood volume and blood pressure in the arteries. It also affects the body's acid-base balance. Chloride is absorbed through the intestines and is excreted through the kidneys.

Why is this test done?

Chloride levels may be measured for the following reasons:
- To evaluate the chloride content of blood
- To detect acidosis or alkalosis (acid-base imbalance) and electrolyte imbalances
- To help evaluate a person's fluid status.

What should you know before the test?

- This test requires a blood sample, which takes less than 3 minutes to collect.
- You may experience slight discomfort from the needle puncture and tourniquet pressure.
- You don't need to change your diet before the test.
- Your medication history is checked for the use of drugs that may affect test results. Drugs that elevate chloride levels include ammonium chloride, cholestyramine, boric acid, oxyphenbutazone, phenylbutazone, or excessive intravenous sodium chloride. Chloride levels are decreased by thiazides, furosemide, ethacrynic acid, bicarbonates, or prolonged intravenous infusion of dextrose in water.

What happens during the test?

A nurse or medical technician inserts a needle into a vein, usually in your forearm. A blood sample is collected in a tube, which is then sent to a lab for testing.

What happens after the test?

If swelling develops at the needle puncture site, warm soaks are applied to the area to ease discomfort.

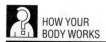
HOW YOUR
BODY WORKS

Understanding body fluids

Fluids, mainly water, account for 60% of an adult's total body weight. The body contains substances that conduct a weak electric current when they are dissolved in fluids. These are called *electrolytes*. Electrolytes with a positive charge are called *cations;* those carrying a negative charge are *anions*. A cation-anion balance results in electric neutrality.

Fluid compartments

Two main compartments house the body's fluids. Within its 100 trillion cells, the intracellular compartment accounts for 40% of the total body weight, which is about 25 liters (or quarts) of fluid.

In the spaces between the cells, the extracellular compartment comprises 15% of the total body weight, or approximately 15 liters of fluid. Intravascular fluid, or plasma in the blood, accounts for the final 5%. A change in the amount or composition of these compartments can be fatal.

Electrolytes

Electrolytes play a crucial role in the body's water distribution, osmolality (proportion of dissolved substances to liquid in a solution), acid-base balance, and neuromuscular (nerve and muscle-based) irritability.

Potassium is the principal cation (positively charged electrolyte), and phosphate is the dominant anion (negatively charged electrolyte) in the intracellular compartment. Like plasma, the interstitial fluids — which surround the cells of most tissues — contains high concentrations of sodium and chloride. Together, fluids and electrolytes nourish and maintain the body.

What are the normal results?

Normal chloride levels range from 100 to 108 milliequivalents per liter of blood serum (the clear, fluid portion of blood).

What do abnormal results mean?

High serum chloride levels, called *hyperchloremia,* may be caused by severe dehydration, kidney failure, head injury with hyperventilation, and primary aldosteronism. Hyperchloremia may cause stupor, rapid deep breathing, and weakness that may lead to coma. Excess chloride, which is acidic, may cause metabolic acidosis.

Low chloride levels, called *hypochloremia,* usually accompany low sodium and potassium levels. Underlying causes include prolonged vomiting, gastric suctioning, intestinal fistula, chronic kidney failure, congestive heart failure or edema with fluid retention, and Addison's disease. Hypochloremia can lead to severe muscle tension, tetany, and depressed breathing. Excessive loss of chloride may cause hypochloremic metabolic alkalosis.

MAGNESIUM

This test measures blood levels of magnesium. Magnesium is an electrolyte, a substance that has an electric charge when it's dissolved in the blood. Magnesium is vital to nerve and muscle functioning. Most is found in the bones and blood cells. A small amount occurs in the fluid around blood cells. Magnesium is absorbed through the small intestine and is excreted in urine and feces.

Why is this test done?

Magnesium levels may be measured for the following reasons:
- To determine the magnesium content in the blood
- To evaluate electrolyte status
- To check nerve and muscle functions
- To assess kidney function.

What should you know before the test?

- Don't use magnesium salts, such as milk of magnesia or Epsom salts, for at least 3 days before the test. You don't need to restrict food or fluids, however.
- This test requires a blood sample, which takes less than 3 minutes to collect.
- You may experience slight discomfort from the needle puncture and tourniquet pressure.

What happens during the test?

A nurse or medical technician inserts a needle into a vein, usually in your forearm. A blood sample is collected in a tube, which is then sent to a lab for testing.

What happens after the test?

If swelling develops at the needle puncture site, warm soaks are applied to the area to ease discomfort.

What are the normal results?

Normal magnesium levels range from 1.7 to 2.1 milligrams per deciliter or from 1.5 to 2.5 milliequivalents per liter of blood serum, which is the clear, fluid portion of blood.

What do abnormal results mean?

Elevated magnesium levels, or *hypermagnesemia,* occur most commonly in kidney failure or when the kidneys excrete inadequate amounts of magnesium. Adrenal insufficiency, or Addison's disease, can also elevate serum magnesium.

Hypermagnesemia can cause lethargy; flushing; sweating; decreased blood pressure; slow, weak pulse; diminished deep-tendon reflexes; muscle weakness; and slow, shallow breathing.

Low magnesium levels, or *hypomagnesemia,* are most commonly caused by chronic alcoholism. Other causes include malabsorption syndrome, diarrhea, faulty absorption after bowel surgery, prolonged bowel or gastric aspiration, acute pancreatitis, primary aldosteronism, severe burns, excessive calcium, and some diuretic therapies.

Hypomagnesemia can lead to leg and foot cramps, hyperactive deep-tendon reflexes, irregular heartbeats, muscle weakness, seizures, twitching, tetany, and tremors.

*P*HOSPHATES

This test measures phosphate levels in the blood. Phosphates are electrolytes, substances that carry electric charges when they're dissolved in the blood. Phosphates affect metabolism, help maintain acid-base balance, and regulate calcium levels. Phosphates are also vital to bone formation; about 85% of the body's phosphates are in the bones.

Most phosphates are absorbed from foods, through the intestines. The kidneys excrete phosphates and regulate blood phosphate levels.

Why is this test done?

Phosphates may be tested for the following reasons:
- To determine phosphate levels in your blood
- To aid diagnosis of kidney disorders and acid-base imbalance
- To detect endocrine, skeletal, and calcium disorders.

What should you know before the test?

- This test requires a blood sample, which takes less than 3 minutes to collect.
- You may experience slight discomfort from the needle puncture and tourniquet pressure.

- You don't need to change your diet before the test.
- Your medication history is checked for drugs that alter phosphate levels, such as vitamin D, anabolic steroids, androgens, phosphate-binding antacids, acetazolamide, insulin, and epinephrine.

What happens during the test?

A nurse or medical technician inserts a needle into a vein, usually in your forearm. A blood sample is collected in a tube, which is then sent to a lab for testing.

What happens after the test?

If swelling develops at the needle puncture site, warm soaks are applied to the area to ease discomfort.

What are the normal results?

Normal phosphate levels range from 2.5 to 4.5 milligrams per deciliter. Children have phosphate levels as high as 7 milligrams per deciliter during periods of increased bone growth.

What do abnormal results mean?

Serum calcium and phosphate levels have an inverse relationship; if one is elevated, the other is lowered. Phosphate levels alone are of limited diagnostic use, so they are interpreted with calcium results. (See "Calcium" pages 335 to 337.)

Low phosphate levels, called *hypophosphatemia*, may be caused by malnutrition, malabsorption, hyperparathyroidism, kidney tubular acidosis, or treatment of diabetic acidosis. In children, hypophosphatemia can suppress normal growth.

High phosphate levels, or *hyperphosphatemia*, may be caused by skeletal disease, healing fractures, thyroid problems, acromegaly, diabetic acidosis, high intestinal obstruction, or kidney failure. Hyperphosphatemia is rarely a medical problem, but it can alter bone metabolism in prolonged cases.

This test measures levels of phosphates, which affect metabolism, help maintain acid-base balance, and regulate calcium levels (vital to bone formation). The kidneys excrete phosphates and regulate blood phosphate levels.

POTASSIUM

This test measures potassium levels in the blood. Potassium helps to maintain the balance among fluid solutions in cells and to regulate muscle activity, enzyme activity, and acid-base balance. Potassium also affects kidney function. It's an electrolyte, a substance that has an electric charge when it's dissolved in the blood.

The body has no efficient method to conserve potassium. The kidneys excrete nearly all that is taken in, even when the body's supply is low. Potassium deficiency can develop rapidly and is quite common. Therefore, it's essential to replenish potassium through the diet. (See *Shopping for potassium,* pages 344 and 345.)

Why is this test done?

Potassium levels may be measured for the following reasons:
- To determine the potassium content of the blood
- To evaluate excess potassium, which is called *hyperkalemia,* or potassium depletion, which is called *hypokalemia*
- To monitor kidney function, acid-base balance, and glucose metabolism
- To evaluate neuromuscular and hormone disorders
- To detect the origin of irregular heartbeats.

What should you know before the test?

- This test requires a blood sample, which takes less than 3 minutes to collect.
- You may experience slight discomfort from the needle puncture and tourniquet pressure.
- You don't need to change your diet before the test.
- Your medication history is checked for the use of drugs that may influence test results. Such medications include diuretics, penicillin G potassium, amphotericin B, methicillin, tetracycline, insulin, or glucose. When possible, these medications are discontinued for the test.

What happens during the test?

A nurse or medical technician inserts a needle into a vein, usually in your forearm. A blood sample is collected in a tube, which is then sent to a lab for testing.

SELF-HELP

Shopping for potassium

Here's a list of foods that can help you maintain your dietary intake of potassium.

FOOD	SERVING SIZE	MILLIEQUIVALENTS OF POTASSIUM
Meats		
Beef	4 ounces (112 grams)	11.2
Chicken	4 ounces (112 grams)	12.0
Scallops	5 large	30.0
Veal	4 ounces (112 grams)	15.2
Vegetables		
Artichokes	1 large bud	7.7
Asparagus (frozen, cooked)	½ cup	5.5
Asparagus, raw	6 spears	7.7
Beans (dried, cooked)	½ cup	10.0
Beans, lima	½ cup	9.5
Broccoli, cooked	½ cup	7.0
Carrots, cooked	½ cup	5.7
Carrots, raw	1 large	8.8
Mushrooms, raw	4 large	10.6
Potato, baked	1 small	15.4
Spinach, fresh, cooked	½ cup	8.5
Squash, winter, baked	½ cup	12.0
Tomato, raw	1 medium	10.4
Fruits		
Apricots, dried	4 halves	5.0
Apricots, fresh	3 small	8.0
Banana	1 medium	12.8
Cantaloupe	½ small	13.0

SELF-HELP

Shopping for potassium *(continued)*

FOOD	SERVING SIZE	MILLIEQUIVALENTS OF POTASSIUM
Fruits *(continued)*		
Figs, dried	7 small	17.5
Peach, fresh	1 medium	6.2
Pear, fresh	1 medium	6.2
Beverages		
Apricot nectar	1 cup (240 milliliters)	9.0
Grapefruit juice	1 cup	8.2
Orange juice	1 cup	11.4
Pineapple juice	1 cup	9.0
Prune juice	1 cup	14.4
Tomato juice	1 cup	11.6

What happens after the test?

If swelling develops at the needle puncture site, warm soaks are applied to the area to ease discomfort.

What are the normal results?

Normal potassium levels range from 3.5 to 5.0 milliequivalents per liter of blood serum (the clear, fluid portion of blood).

What do abnormal results mean?

Hyperkalemia occurs when excessive potassium enters the blood because of burns, crushing injuries, diabetic ketoacidosis, or heart attack. Hyperkalemia may also indicate reduced sodium excretion, possibly due to kidney failure or Addison's disease.

Hyperkalemia can lead to weakness, general discomfort, nausea, diarrhea, colicky pain, muscle irritability progressing to flaccid paralysis, oliguria, and a slow or irregular heartbeat.

Hypokalemia often is caused by aldosteronism or Cushing's syndrome, loss of body fluids, or eating too much licorice.

What you should know about sodium

Americans consume about 20 times more sodium than their bodies need. Consider the following.

Loaded foods

- About three-fourths of the salt you consume is already in the foods you eat and drink.
- Canned, prepared, and "fast" foods are loaded with sodium; so are condiments, such as ketchup. Some foods that don't taste salty are nevertheless high in sodium, such as carbonated beverages, nondairy creamers, cookies, and cakes.
- Other high-sodium food items include baking powder, baking soda, barbecue sauce, bouillon cubes, chili sauce, cooking wine, garlic salt, softened water, and soy sauce.
- Many medicines and other nonfood items, such as alkalizers for indigestion, laxatives, aspirin, cough medicine, mouthwash, and toothpaste, contain sodium.

Reducing the load

- One teaspoon of salt contains 2 grams of sodium — the recommended daily intake. You can maintain this level by not salting your food.
- Even a moderate reduction in salt can lower blood pressure by 10 to 15 points.

Hypokalemia can lead to decreased reflexes; rapid, weak, irregular pulse; mental confusion; hypotension; anorexia; muscle weakness; and paresthesia. In severe cases, ventricular fibrillation, respiratory paralysis, and cardiac arrest can develop.

SODIUM

This test measures sodium levels in serum, which is the clear, fluid portion of blood. Sodium is an electrolyte, a substance that carries an electric charge when it's dissolved in the blood. It affects body water distribution, maintains pressure balance in the fluids that surround cells, and helps nerve and muscle functions. It also affects acid-base balance and influences chloride and potassium levels. Sodium is obtained largely through salt in the diet.

Why is this test done?

Sodium levels may be measured for the following reasons:
- To determine the sodium content of the blood
- To evaluate neuromuscular, kidney, and adrenal functions.

What should you know before the test?

- This test requires a blood sample, which takes less than 3 minutes to collect.
- You may experience slight discomfort from the needle puncture and tourniquet pressure.
- You don't need to change your diet before the test.
- Your medication history is checked for use of drugs that affect sodium levels. Such drugs include most diuretics, corticosteroids, lithium, chlorpropamide, vasopressin, and antihypertensives. When it's possible, medications are discontinued.

What happens during the test?

A nurse or medical technician inserts a needle into a vein, usually in your forearm. A blood sample is collected in a tube, which is then sent to a lab for testing.

What happens after the test?

If swelling develops at the needle puncture site, warm soaks are applied to ease discomfort.

What are the normal results?

Normal sodium levels are 135 to 145 milliequivalents per liter of blood serum, which is the clear, fluid portion of blood.

What do abnormal results mean?

Sodium imbalance can be caused by a loss or gain of sodium or from a change in the body's fluid status.

A high sodium level, which is called *hypernatremia*, may be due to eating too much salt (see *What you should know about sodium*) or drinking too little water. Other causes are water loss due to diabetes insipidus, impaired kidney function, prolonged hyperventilation, sodium retention as in aldosteronism, or severe vomiting or diarrhea.

An abnormally low sodium level, which is called *hyponatremia*, may be caused by eating too little salt or profuse sweating, gastrointestinal suctioning, diuretic therapy, diarrhea, vomiting, adrenal insufficiency, burns, or chronic poor kidney function.

ENZYMES

CREATINE KINASE

Creatine kinase is a type of protein that's known as an enzyme. This enzyme plays a role in the metabolism, or energy production, of muscle cells. Creatine kinase levels reflect normal tissue destruction. A high creatine kinase level in a blood sample indicates injury to cells, as occurs in a heart attack.

Total creatine kinase and levels of three distinct types of creatine kinase, called *isoenzymes*, are usually measured. These are CK-BB (CK$_1$), CK-MB (CK$_2$), and CK-MM (CK$_3$). The initials "M" and "B" denote muscle and brain, respectively, indicating where the isoenzymes occur. CK-BB is found mostly in brain tissue. CK-MM and CK-MB are found primarily in skeletal and heart muscles.

Isoenzyme measurements are used to determine the precise site of tissue destruction in acute heart attack. To obtain more precise information, subunits of CK-MM and CK-MB, called *isoforms*, are measured.

Why is this test done?

Creatine kinase levels may be measured for the following reasons:

- To check your heart and skeletal muscle function
- To detect and diagnose acute heart attack and recurrent heart attack
- To evaluate possible causes of chest pain
- To monitor reduced blood flow to the heart after heart surgery or other treatments that affect heart muscle
- To detect skeletal muscle disorders that do not originate in the nerves.

What should you know before the test?

- You don't need to change your diet before the test but you should avoid drinking alcoholic beverages.
- Use of aminocaproic acid or lithium may interfere with test results. When possible, these drugs are discontinued.
- If you're being evaluated for skeletal muscle disorders, avoid exercising for 24 hours before the test.
- This test requires a blood sample, which takes less than 3 minutes to collect. Multiple blood samples may be needed to detect fluctuations in creatine kinase levels.
- You may experience slight discomfort from the needle puncture and tourniquet pressure.

What happens during the test?

- A nurse or medical technician inserts a needle into a vein, usually in your forearm. A blood sample is collected in a tube, which is then sent to a lab for testing.
- The sample is collected before or within 1 hour of giving intramuscular injections because muscle injury increases the total creatine kinase level.

This enzyme tells the doctor about heart and skeletal muscle function, including the causes of chest pain.

What happens after the test?

▪ If swelling develops at the needle puncture site, warm soaks are applied to the area to ease discomfort.

▪ You may resume taking any medications that were withheld before the test.

What are the normal results?

Total creatine kinase levels range from 25 to 130 international units per liter for men, and from 10 to 150 international units per liter for women. Levels may be significantly higher in very muscular people. Infants up to age 1 have levels two to four times higher than adult levels, possibly reflecting birth trauma and muscle development. Normal ranges for isoenzyme levels are as follows: CK-BB, undetectable; CK-MB, undetectable to 7 international units per liter; CK-MM, 5 to 70 international units per liter (CK-MM makes up 99% of total creatine kinase normally present in blood).

Normal levels of this type of protein may be significantly higher in very muscular people.

What do abnormal results mean?

Detectable CK-BB isoenzyme may indicate possible brain tissue injury, widespread malignant tumors, severe shock, or kidney failure.

CK-MB isoenzyme greater than 5% of total creatine kinase indicates heart attack. In an acute heart attack or following heart surgery, CK-MB rises, peaks in 12 to 24 hours, and usually returns to normal in 24 to 48 hours. Total creatine kinase follows roughly the same pattern.

CK-MB levels may not increase in congestive heart failure or during angina pectoris not accompanied by heart tissue cell death. Serious skeletal muscle injury caused by some muscular dystrophies and other conditions may produce mild CK-MB elevation.

Increasing CK-MM levels follow skeletal muscle damage from injury, such as surgery and intramuscular injections, or from some diseases. A moderate rise in CK-MM levels develops in people with hypothyroidism. Sharp elevations occur with muscular activity caused by agitation, such as in an acute psychotic episode.

Total creatine kinase levels may be elevated in people with severe hypokalemia, carbon monoxide poisoning, malignant hyperthermia, or alcoholic cardiomyopathy. They may also be elevated following seizures and, occasionally, following lung or brain damage.

CREATINE KINASE COMPONENTS

Creatine kinase, an enzyme found in muscle tissue, has three components, which are called *isoenzymes*. These are CK-BB (CK_1), CK-MB (CK_2), and CK-MM (CK_3). The initials "M" and "B" denote muscle and brain, respectively, indicating where the isoenzymes occur; CK-BB is most prevalent in brain tissue; CK-MM and CK-MB are found primarily in skeletal and heart muscle.

Damage to the heart releases CK-MM, CK-MB, and another isoenzyme, called *lactate dehydrogenase*, into the blood. Subcomponents of CK-MM and CK-MB are called $CK-MM_1$, $CK-MM_2$, $CK-MB_1$, and $CK-MB_2$.

Why is this test done?

Creatine kinase isoforms may be measured for the following reasons:
- To confirm or rule out heart attack
- To evaluate skeletal muscle injury.

What should you know before the test?

- This test requires several blood samples, which are drawn at timed intervals. Each takes less than 3 minutes to collect.
- You may experience slight discomfort from the needle puncture and tourniquet pressure.
- You don't need to change your diet before the test.

What happens during the test?

- A nurse or medical technician inserts a needle into a vein, usually in your forearm. A blood sample is collected in a tube, which is then sent to a lab for testing.
- A blood sample is collected every 2 hours as needed.

What happens after the test?

If swelling develops at the needle puncture site, warm soaks are applied to the area to ease discomfort.

What are the normal results?

$CK-MB_2$ concentrations are less than 1.0. The $CK-MB_2$ to $CK-MB_1$ ratio is less than 1.5.

What do abnormal results mean?

An increase in CK-MB indicates heart attack. In more than half of the people who have a heart attack, the ratio of CK-MB$_2$ to CK-MB$_1$ is greater than 1.5 within 2 to 4 hours. By 6 hours after the heart attack, more than 90% of people have a ratio of 1.5 or greater.

*L*ACTATE DEHYDROGENASE

Lactate dehydrogenase is a type of protein that's called an *isoenzyme*. It's involved in the body's metabolic, or energy-producing, process. When cells are damaged, levels of lactate dehydrogenase in the blood become elevated. Measuring total lactate dehydrogenase is of limited diagnostic use, however, because lactate dehydrogenase is present in almost all body tissues. Five tissue-specific forms of lactate dehydrogenase are measured in this test. These are identified by the initials "LD" and a numeral: LD$_1$ and LD$_2$ appear primarily in the heart, red blood cells, and kidneys; LD$_3$ is primarily in the lungs; and LD$_4$ and LD$_5$ are in the liver and the skeletal muscles.

*T*he test helps doctors diagnose heart attack, lung damage, anemias, and liver disease.

Why is this test done?

Lactate dehydrogenase levels may be measured for the following reasons:
- To detect tissue damage
- To aid the diagnosis of heart attack, lung damage, anemias, and liver disease
- To support creatine kinase isoenzyme test results
- To monitor a person's response to some types of chemotherapy.

What should you know before the test?

- You don't need to change your diet before this test.
- A blood sample is required, which takes less than 3 minutes to collect.
- You may experience slight discomfort from the needle puncture and tourniquet pressure.
- If heart attack is suspected, the test is repeated on the next two mornings to monitor changes.

What happens during the test?

A nurse or medical technician inserts a needle into a vein, usually in your forearm. A blood sample is collected in a tube, which is then sent to a lab for testing.

What happens after the test?

If swelling develops at the needle puncture site, warm soaks are applied to the area to ease discomfort.

What are the normal results?

Total lactate dehydrogenase levels normally range from 45 to 90 international units per liter. Normal distribution is as follows:

- LD_1: 14% to 26% of total
- LD_2: 29% to 39% of total
- LD_3: 20% to 26% of total
- LD_4: 8% to 16% of total
- LD_5: 6% to 16% of total.

What do abnormal results mean?

Because many common diseases cause elevations in total lactate dehydrogenase levels, further testing is usually necessary for a diagnosis. In some disorders, total lactate dehydrogenase may be within normal limits, but abnormal proportions of each enzyme indicate specific organ tissue damage.

ASPARTATE AMINOTRANSFERASE

Aspartate aminotransferase is a type of protein called an *enzyme* that's essential to energy production in cells of the body. Aspartate aminotransferase is found in the liver, heart, skeletal muscle, kidneys, pancreas, and red blood cells. It's released into the bloodstream in proportion to the amount of cell damage due to heart or liver problems. The change in aspartate aminotransferase levels over time is a reliable monitoring mechanism.

Why is this test done?

Aspartate aminotransferase levels may be measured for the following reasons:

- To check heart and liver function
- To aid detection and differential diagnosis of acute liver disease
- To monitor a person's progress and prognosis in heart and liver diseases
- To help the doctor diagnose heart attack in correlation with creatine kinase and lactate dehydrogenase levels.

What should you know before the test?

- You don't need to change your diet before the test.
- The test usually requires three blood samples, collected on 3 consecutive days. Each sample takes less than 3 minutes to collect.
- You may experience slight discomfort from the needle puncture and tourniquet pressure.
- Drugs that may interfere with results are usually withheld before the test.

What happens during the test?

A nurse or medical technician inserts a needle into a vein, usually in your forearm. Each blood sample is collected in a tube, which is then sent to a lab for testing.

What happens after the test?

- If swelling develops at the needle puncture site, warm soaks are applied to the area to ease discomfort.
- You may resume taking medications that were withheld before the test.

What are the normal results?

Aspartate aminotransferase levels range from 8 to 20 international units per liter. Normal levels for infants are up to four times higher than those of adults.

What do abnormal results mean?

Aspartate aminotransferase levels fluctuate, reflecting the extent of cell damage. Levels are minimally elevated early in the disease process and extremely elevated during the most acute phase. Depending on when the initial sample is drawn, aspartate aminotransferase levels may increase, indicating increasing disease severity and tissue damage, or decrease, indicating disease resolution and tissue repair.

ALANINE AMINOTRANSFERASE

Alanine aminotransferase is an enzyme — or specialized protein — that's necessary for tissue energy production. Alanine aminotransferase primarily appears in the liver, with lesser amounts in the kidneys, heart, and skeletal muscle. This test is used to measure the levels of alanine aminotransferase that are released to the bloodstream after acute liver cell damage.

Why is this test done?
Alanine aminotransferase may be measured for the following reasons:
- To check liver function
- To detect and evaluate treatment of acute liver disease, especially hepatitis or cirrhosis without jaundice
- To distinguish between heart and liver tissue damage when considered with aspartate aminotransferase levels
- To assess the adverse effects that some drugs may have on the liver.

The test for this enzyme helps the doctor check for bad effects that some drugs may have on the liver.

What should you know before the test?
- This test requires a blood sample, which takes less than 3 minutes to collect.
- You may experience slight discomfort from the needle puncture and tourniquet pressure.
- You don't need to change your diet before the test.
- Drugs that may affect test results are usually withheld.

What happens during the test?
A nurse or medical technician inserts a needle into a vein, usually in your forearm. A blood sample is collected in a tube, which is then sent to a lab for testing.

What happens after the test?

- If swelling develops at the needle puncture site, warm soaks are applied to the area to ease discomfort.
- You may resume taking medications that were withheld before the test.

What are the normal results?

Alanine aminotransferase levels range from 8 to 20 international units per liter.

What do abnormal results mean?

Extremely high alanine aminotransferase levels — up to 50 times normal — suggest viral or severe drug-induced hepatitis or other liver disease with extensive cell damage. Moderate-to-high levels may indicate infectious mononucleosis, chronic hepatitis, intrahepatic cholestasis or cholecystitis, early or improving acute viral hepatitis or severe liver congestion due to heart failure. Slight-to-moderate elevations of alanine aminotransferase may appear in any condition that produces acute liver injury, such as active cirrhosis and drug-induced or alcoholic hepatitis. Marginal elevations occasionally occur in acute heart attack, reflecting secondary liver congestion or the release of small amounts of alanine aminotransferase from heart tissue.

*A*LKALINE PHOSPHATASE

Alkaline phosphatase is an enzyme, or specialized protein, that's involved in bone calcification. (See *Why enzymes cause chemical reactions,* page 356.) It also helps transport the products of metabolism and lipids, or fats, through the body.

This test is used to measure alkaline phosphatase levels in the blood. Alkaline phosphatase measurements reflect the combined activity of several alkaline phosphatase isoenzymes, or subforms, that are found in the liver, bones, kidneys, intestinal lining, and placenta. Bone and liver alkaline phosphatase are always present in the blood of adults, with liver alkaline phosphatase most prominent except during the last 3 months of pregnancy. Intestinal alkaline phosphatase can be a normal finding or it can be an abnormal finding associated with liver disease.

Why enzymes cause chemical reactions

According to current theory, enzymes promote chemical reactions in the body because of their surface activity. Each reactant has its own unique three-dimensional surface, just like a puzzle piece.

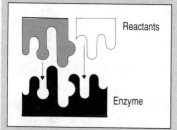

Reactants

Enzyme

An enzyme combines with reactants whose surfaces fit its own.

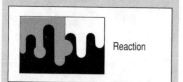

Reaction

To start a reaction, the reactants and an enzyme that's specific— or custom-fitted — to them combine briefly.

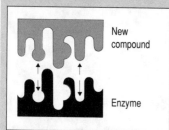

New compound

Enzyme

At the end of the reaction, the two parts separate, leaving the enzyme unchanged.

Why is this test done?

Alkaline phosphatase levels may be measured for the following reasons:

- To check your liver or bone function
- To detect and identify skeletal disease
- To detect liver lesions that cause biliary obstruction, such as tumors or abscesses
- To assess response to vitamin D in the treatment of rickets
- To supplement information from other liver function studies and gastrointestinal enzyme tests.

What should you know before the test?

- You must fast for at least 8 hours before the test because fat intake stimulates intestinal alkaline phosphatase secretion.
- This test requires a blood sample, which takes less than 3 minutes to collect.
- You may experience slight discomfort from the needle puncture and tourniquet pressure.

What happens during the test?

A nurse or medical technician inserts a needle into a vein, usually in your forearm. A blood sample is collected in a tube, which is then sent to a lab for testing.

What happens after the test?

- If swelling develops at the needle puncture site, warm soaks are applied to the area to ease discomfort.
- You may resume your regular diet.

What are the normal results?

Total alkaline phosphatase levels for men range from 90 to 239 international units per liter. For women under age 45, total alkaline phosphatase levels range from 76 to 196 international units per liter. For women over age 45, the range widens to 87 to 250 international units per liter.

What do abnormal results mean?

Although significant alkaline phosphatase elevations are possible with diseases that affect many organs, they are most likely to indicate skeletal disease or bile duct obstruction. Many acute liver diseases cause alkaline phosphatase elevations.

GAMMA GLUTAMYL TRANSFERASE

Gamma glutamyl transferase is an enzyme, or specialized protein, that's involved in the transfer of amino acids across cell membranes and possibly in other aspects of metabolism (energy production). Highest concentrations of gamma glutamyl transferase exist in the kidney tubules, but it also appears in the liver, biliary tract epithelium, pancreas, lymphocytes, brain, and testicles. This test is used to measure gamma glutamyl transferase levels in blood.

Why is this test done?

Gamma glutamyl transferase levels may be measured for the following reasons:
- To evaluate liver function
- To provide information about liver diseases, to assess liver function, and to detect alcohol ingestion
- To distinguish between skeletal disease and liver disease when alkaline phosphatase levels are elevated.

What should you know before the test?

- This test requires a blood sample, which takes less than 3 minutes to collect.
- You may experience slight discomfort from the needle puncture and tourniquet pressure.
- You don't need to change your diet before the test.

What happens during the test?

A nurse or medical technician inserts a needle into a vein, usually in your forearm. A blood sample is collected in a tube, which is then sent to a lab for testing.

What happens after the test?

If swelling develops at the needle puncture site, warm soaks are applied to the area to ease discomfort.

What are the normal results?

Usually, normal levels in women range from 5 to 24 international units per liter. In men, levels range from 8 to 37 international units per liter.

What do abnormal results mean?

Serum gamma glutamyl transferase levels are increased in any acute liver disease. Moderate increases occur in acute pancreatitis, in kidney disease, in prostatic metastases, after surgery, and sometimes with epilepsy or brain tumors. Levels also increase after alcohol ingestion. The sharpest elevations occur with obstructive jaundice and liver metastatic infiltrations. Gamma glutamyl transferase may increase 5 to 10 days after an acute heart attack.

AMYLASE

Amylase is an enzyme, or specialized protein, that's formed primarily in the pancreas and the salivary glands. It helps digest starch and glycogen in the mouth, stomach, and intestine. (See *Turning starch into sugar.*) In suspected acute pancreatic disease, measurement of amylase in the blood or the urine is the most important lab test.

Amylase helps digest starch and glycogen in the mouth, stomach, and intestine.

Why is this test done?

Amylase levels may be measured for the following reasons:
- To check pancreatic function and to diagnose acute pancreatitis
- To distinguish between acute pancreatitis and other causes of abdominal pain that require immediate surgery
- To evaluate possible pancreatic injury caused by abdominal injury or surgery.

What should you know before the test?

- This test requires a blood sample, which takes less than 3 minutes to collect.
- You may experience slight discomfort from the needle puncture and tourniquet pressure.
- You don't need to change your diet before the test, but you must abstain from alcohol.
- Drugs that may elevate amylase levels are withheld before the test.

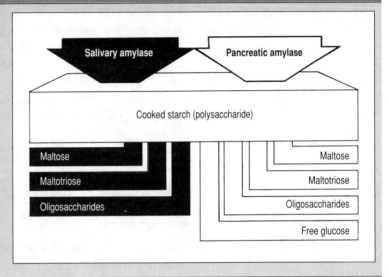

HOW YOUR
BODY WORKS

Turning starch into sugar

Starch is a polysaccharide, meaning it's composed of long chains of simple sugars. It can be digested only after it has been cooked.

Amylase takes over
Within 15 to 30 minutes after starchy foods are eaten, amylase — which is produced by the salivary glands and the pancreas — converts 70% of starch polysaccharides to disaccharides, which include simple sugars such as maltose, glucose, and oligosaccharides.

What happens during the test?

A nurse or medical technician inserts a needle into a vein, usually in your forearm. A blood sample is collected in a tube, which is then sent to a lab for testing.

What happens after the test?

- If swelling develops at the needle puncture site, warm soaks are applied to the area to ease discomfort.
- You may resume taking medications that were withheld before the test.

What are the normal results?

Serum levels range from 30 to 220 international units per liter. A general average is less than 300 international units per liter. More than 20 methods of measuring serum amylase exist, with different ranges of normal levels. Test levels cannot always be converted to a standard measurement.

What do abnormal results mean?

After the onset of acute pancreatitis, amylase levels begin to rise in 2 hours, peak at 12 to 48 hours, and return to normal in 3 to 4 days. Determination of urine levels should follow blood amylase results to rule out pancreatitis. Moderate elevations in blood amylase may accompany obstruction of the bile duct, the pancreatic duct, or at the juncture of these ducts. Other causes are pancreatic injury from perforated peptic ulcer; pancreatic cancer; and acute salivary gland disease. Impaired kidney function may increase amylase levels in blood.

Depressed levels may indicate chronic pancreatitis, pancreatic cancer, cirrhosis, hepatitis, or toxemia of pregnancy.

LIPASE

Lipase is an enzyme, or specialized protein, that's produced in the pancreas and is secreted into the duodenum, where it converts triglycerides and other fats into fatty acids and glycerol.

Destruction of pancreatic cells, which occurs in acute pancreatitis, releases large amounts of lipase into the blood. This test is used to measure blood lipase levels. It is most useful when performed with a serum or urine amylase test.

Why is this test done?

Lipase levels may be measured for the following reasons:
- To evaluate pancreas function
- To help the doctor diagnose acute pancreatitis.

What should you know before the test?

- You must fast overnight before the test.
- Cholinergics, codeine, meperidine, and morphine are usually withheld before the test.
- This test requires a blood sample, which takes less than 3 minutes to collect.
- You may experience slight discomfort from the needle puncture and tourniquet pressure.

INSIGHT INTO
ILLNESS

Blocking the enzyme path

The pancreas secretes lipase, amylase, and other enzymes. These pass through the pancreatic duct into the duodenum, which is the upper portion of the intestine. In pancreatitis — inflammation of the pancreas — and obstruction of the pancreatic duct by a tumor or calculus, these enzymes can't reach their destination. Instead, they're diverted into the bloodstream.

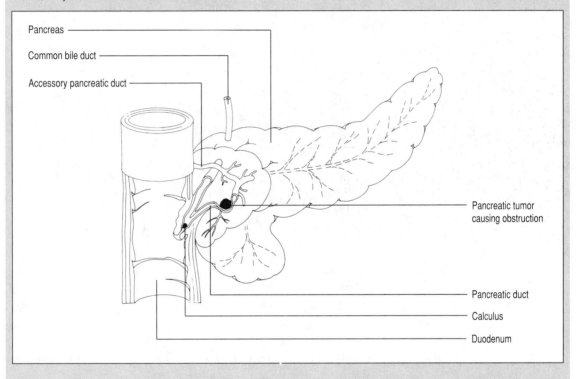

Pancreas

Common bile duct

Accessory pancreatic duct

Pancreatic tumor causing obstruction

Pancreatic duct

Calculus

Duodenum

What happens during the test?

A nurse or medical technician inserts a needle into a vein, usually in your forearm. A blood sample is collected in a tube, which is then sent to a lab for testing.

What happens after the test?

- If swelling develops at the needle puncture site, warm soaks are applied to the area to ease discomfort.
- You may resume taking medications that were withheld before the test.

What are the normal results?

Normal lipase levels are generally less than 300 international units per liter.

What do abnormal results mean?

High lipase levels suggest acute pancreatitis or pancreatic duct obstruction. (See *Blocking the enzyme path,* page 361.) After an acute attack, levels remain elevated up to 14 days. Lipase levels may also increase in other pancreatic injuries, such as perforated peptic ulcer, and with high intestinal obstruction, pancreatic cancer, or kidney disease with impaired excretion.

ACID PHOSPHATASE

Acid phosphatase is a group of enzymes, or specialized proteins, that are found primarily in the prostate gland and semen and, to a lesser extent, in the liver, spleen, red blood cells, bone marrow, and platelets. This test measures total acid phosphatase and the prostatic fraction in a blood sample.

Why is this test done?

Acid phosphatase levels may be measured for the following reasons:
- To check prostate function
- To detect prostate cancer
- To monitor response to therapy for prostate cancer (successful treatment decreases acid phosphatase levels).

What should you know before the test?

- This test requires a blood sample, which takes less than 3 minutes to collect.
- You may experience slight discomfort from the needle puncture and tourniquet pressure.
- You don't need to change your diet before this test.
- You must not use fluorides, phosphates, and clofibrate before the test.

What happens during the test?

A nurse or medical technician inserts a needle into a vein, usually in your forearm. A blood sample is collected in a tube, which is then sent to a lab for testing.

What happens after the test?

- If swelling develops at the needle puncture site, warm soaks are applied to the area to ease discomfort.
- You may resume taking medications that were withheld before the test.

What are the normal results?

Normal levels for total acid phosphatase range from approximately 0.5 to 1.9 international units per liter.

What do abnormal results mean?

High acid phosphatase levels may indicate a prostate tumor that has spread. If the tumor has spread to the bones, high acid phosphatase levels are accompanied by high alkaline phosphatase levels.

Acid phosphatase levels increase moderately in prostatic tissue damage, Paget's disease, Gaucher's disease, and occasionally in other conditions, such as multiple myeloma.

*P*ROSTATE-SPECIFIC ANTIGEN

Antigens are any substances — such as dissolved toxins or bacteria— that evoke responses from a person's immune system. Prostate-specific antigen occurs in normal and benign prostatic tissue, as well as with prostate cancer. This test is used to measure prostate-specific antigen levels in the blood. The results are used to monitor the spread or recurrence of prostate cancer and to evaluate treatment for this disease.

Why is this test done?

Prostate-specific antigen may be measured for the following reasons:
- To monitor the course of prostate cancer
- To monitor and evaluate a person's response to treatment.

What should you know before the test?
- You don't need to change your diet before this test.
- The test requires a blood sample, which takes less than 3 minutes to collect. The sample is collected in the morning, if possible.
- You may experience slight discomfort from the needle puncture and tourniquet pressure.

What happens during the test?
A nurse or medical technician inserts a needle into a vein, usually in your forearm. A blood sample is collected in a tube, which is then sent to a lab for testing.

What happens after the test?
If swelling develops at the needle puncture site, warm soaks are applied to the area to ease discomfort.

What are the normal results?
Normal levels for prostate-specific antigen should not exceed 2.7 nanograms per milliliter of blood serum in men under age 40 or 4 nanograms per milliliter in men age 40 or older.

What do abnormal results mean?
About 80% of men with prostate cancer have prostate-specific antigen levels greater than 4 nanograms per milliliter. Prostate-specific antigen results alone do not confirm a diagnosis of prostate cancer, however; about 20% of men with benign prostatic tissue growth also have levels greater than 4 nanograms per milliliter. Further assessment and testing, including tissue biopsy, are needed to confirm cancer.

The results of this test are used to monitor the spread or recurrence of prostate cancer and to evaluate its treatment.

PLASMA RENIN ACTIVITY

Renin is an enzyme, or specialized protein, that's produced in the kidneys. Renin secretion from the kidneys is the first stage of a cycle that controls the body's sodium-potassium balance, fluid volume, and blood pressure. Renin is released into the renal veins — which are in the abdomen, near the kidneys — in response to sodium depletion and blood loss.

This test is a screening procedure for renovascular hypertension, or high blood pressure, but it doesn't confirm this diagnosis.

Why is this test done?

Plasma renin activity may be measured for the following reasons:
- To determine the cause of high blood pressure
- To screen for high blood pressure of kidney-related origin (renovascular hypertension)
- To help plan treatment of essential hypertension, a genetic disease that's often aggravated by excessive sodium intake
- To help identify primary aldosteronism (a disorder caused by excessive secretion of the hormone aldosterone)
- To confirm primary aldosteronism (for this, the *sodium-depleted plasma renin* test is used)
- To help identify high blood pressure linked to renovascular disease that affects one or both sides of the body (for this, *renal vein catheterization* is used).

What should you know before the test?

- A nurse or technician checks your history for the use of any substances that may affect the test results, including diuretics, antihypertensives, vasodilators, oral contraceptives, and licorice. Discontinue use of these and maintain a normal-sodium diet for 2 to 4 weeks before the test.
- For the sodium-depleted renin test, you'll receive furosemide. If you have angina or cerebrovascular insufficiency, you'll receive chlorthiazide and follow a low-salt diet for 3 days. (See *Preparing for renin testing: Pass up the salt,* page 367.)
- You'll be asked to collect your urine for 24 hours before the test.
- For several days before the test, you won't receive radiation treatments.
- The test requires a blood sample, which takes less than 3 minutes to collect. The sample is collected in the morning, if possible.
- You may experience slight discomfort from the needle puncture and tourniquet pressure.
- If a recumbent sample is ordered, you must remain in bed for at least 2 hours before the sample is obtained because posture influences renin secretion. If an upright sample is ordered, you must stand or sit upright for 2 hours before the test is performed.
- If renal vein catheterization is ordered, you'll be asked to sign an informed consent form. This procedure is done in the X-ray department. Before the test, you'll receive a local anesthetic.

Because posture influences renin secretion, one version of the test requires a blood sample after you spend 2 hours in bed.

What happens during the test?

During peripheral vein sample collection:

- A nurse or medical technician inserts a needle into a vein, usually in your forearm. A blood sample is collected in a tube, which is then sent to a lab for testing.
- The lab is notified if you're fasting and whether you're upright or supine during specimen collection.

During renal vein catheterization:

- A flexible tube, called a *catheter*, is advanced to the kidneys through the large vein in your thigh. Samples are taken from both of your renal veins and from the major vein to your heart.

What happens after the test?

After peripheral vein sample collection:

- If swelling develops at the needle puncture site, warm soaks are applied to the area to ease discomfort.
- You may resume your usual diet.
- You may resume taking medications that were discontinued before the test.

After renal vein catheterization:

- Pressure is applied to the catheterization site for 10 to 20 minutes to prevent bleeding.
- Your vital signs are monitored, and the catheterization site is checked every half hour for 2 hours, then every hour for 4 hours, to ensure that the bleeding has stopped.
- You may resume your usual diet.
- You may resume taking medications that were discontinued before the test.

Does the test have risks?

After renal vein catheterization, you're checked for blue skin coloration, loss of pulse, or skin coolness, which are signs of clot formation and clogged arteries.

What are the normal results?

Levels of plasma renin activity and of aldosterone decrease with advancing age. Results vary with the type of test.

Sodium-depleted, upright, peripheral vein: For ages 18 to 39, the range is from 2.9 to 24 nanograms per milliliter per hour; the average is 10.8 nanograms per milliliter per hour. For age 40 and over, the

SELF-HELP

Preparing for renin testing: Pass up the salt

Before undergoing renin testing, you must severely restrict your intake of sodium for 3 days. This restriction is important to the accuracy of the test. If you are following this diet at home, observe these precautions.

- Eat only the foods included in the meal plan provided by the doctor. You may delete foods from the diet, but you may not add foods.
- Measure all portions, using standard measuring cups and spoons.
- Use 4 ounces (112 grams) *unsalted* beefsteak or ground beef for lunch and 4 ounces *unsalted* chicken for dinner. (Amount refers to weight before cooking.)
- You may eat the following *unsalted* (fresh or frozen) vegetables: asparagus, green or wax beans, cabbage, cauliflower, lettuce, and tomatoes.
- Use only the specified amount of coffee.
- If you are thirsty between meals, drink distilled water, but *no other* food or beverages.
- Prepare all foods without salt; don't use salt at the table.

Breakfast
1 egg, poached or boiled, or fried in *unsalted* fat
2 slices *unsalted* toast
1 shredded wheat biscuit or ⅔ cup *unsalted* cooked cereal
4 ounces (120 milliliters) half-and-half or milk
8 ounces (240 milliliters) coffee
1 cup orange juice
Sugar, jam or jelly, and *unsalted* butter, as desired

Lunch
4 ounces *unsalted* tomato juice
4 ounces *unsalted* beefsteak or ground beef; may be broiled, or fried in unsalted fat
½ cup *unsalted* potato
½ cup *unsalted* green beans or other allowed vegetable
1 serving fruit
8 ounces coffee
1 slice *unsalted* bread
Sugar, jam or jelly, and *unsalted* butter, as desired

Dinner
4 ounces *unsalted* chicken; may be baked or broiled, or fried in *unsalted* fat
½ cup *unsalted* potato
1 slice *unsalted* bread
Lettuce salad (vinegar and oil dressing)
½ cup unsalted green beans or other allowed vegetable
1 serving fruit
8 ounces coffee
Sugar, jam or jelly, and *unsalted* butter, as desired

range is from 2.9 to 10.8 nanograms per milliliter per hour; the average is 5.9 nanograms per milliliter per hour.

Sodium-replete, upright, peripheral vein: For ages 18 to 39, the range is from 0.6 to 4.3 nanograms per milliliter per hour; the average is 1.9 nanograms per milliliter per hour. For age 40 and over, the range is from 1.0 to 3.0 nanograms per milliliter per hour; the average is 1.0 nanograms per milliliter per hour.

Renal vein catheterization: The ratio of the renin level in the renal vein to the level in the inferior vena cava is less than 1.5 to 1.0.

What do abnormal results mean?

Elevated renin levels may occasionally occur in high blood pressure of several types, cirrhosis, hypokalemia (potassium depletion), and hypovolemia (depletion of body fluid) caused by bleeding. Other causes are renin-producing kidney tumors and hypofunction of the adrenal gland (Addison's disease). High renin levels may also be found in chronic kidney failure with parenchymal disease, end-stage kidney disease, and transplant rejection.

Decreased renin levels may indicate hypervolemia due to a high-sodium diet, salt-retaining steroids, primary aldosteronism, Cushing's syndrome, licorice ingestion syndrome, or essential high blood pressure with low renin levels.

High serum and urine aldosterone levels, with low plasma renin activity, help identify primary aldosteronism. In the sodium-depleted renin test, low plasma renin confirms primary aldosteronism.

CHOLINESTERASE

The cholinesterase test measures the amounts of two similar enzymes, or specialized proteins: acetylcholinesterase and pseudocholinesterase. Acetylcholinesterase is present in nerve tissue, red cells of the spleen, and the gray matter of the brain. Pseudocholinesterase is produced primarily in the liver and appears in small amounts in the pancreas, intestine, heart, and white matter of the brain. (See *Sending an impulse from nerves to muscles.*)

When poisoning by an organophosphate (which is in nerve gases and many insecticides) is suspected, either cholinesterase may be measured. In suspected poisoning by muscle relaxant, the person lacks adequate pseudocholinesterase, which normally inactivates the muscle relaxant. In this case, measurement of pseudocholinesterase is required.

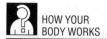

HOW YOUR BODY WORKS

Sending an impulse from nerves to muscles

Each time a nerve impulse arrives at the junction between a nerve fiber and a skeletal muscle fiber, the nerve terminals release about 300 vesicles, or bubbles, of the enzyme acetylcholine into the synaptic clefts, as seen in the diagram.

An important pause

The action of the enzyme acetylcholinesterase allows the muscle fiber to recover, or relax. Without acetylcholinesterase, muscle excitation would be continuous.

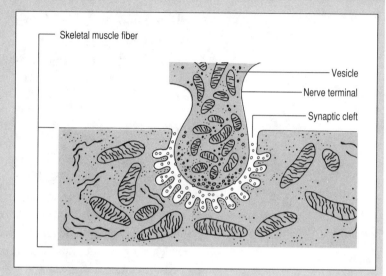

Skeletal muscle fiber

Vesicle

Nerve terminal

Synaptic cleft

Why is this test done?

Cholinesterase levels may be measured for the following reasons:

- To check muscle function or the extent of poisoning
- To evaluate a person's potential response to cholinesterase-related substances before surgery or electroconvulsive therapy
- To determine a person's possible side effects from muscle relaxants
- To check overexposure to insecticides containing organophosphate compounds
- To check liver function and (rarely) aid diagnosis of liver disease.

What should you know before the test?

- This test requires a blood sample, which takes less than 3 minutes to collect.
- You may experience slight discomfort from the needle puncture and tourniquet pressure.
- When possible, medications that affect serum cholinesterase levels are withheld before the test.

What happens during the test?

A nurse or medical technician inserts a needle into a vein, usually in your forearm. A blood sample is collected in a tube, which is then sent to a lab for testing.

What happens after the test?

- If swelling develops at the needle puncture site, warm soaks are applied to the area to ease discomfort.
- You may resume taking medications that were withheld before the test.

What are the normal results?

Pseudocholinesterase levels range from 8 to 18 international units per milliliter of blood serum.

What do abnormal results mean?

Severely lowered pseudocholinesterase levels suggest an inherited deficiency or organophosphate insecticide poisoning. Levels near zero require emergency treatment.

Pseudocholinesterase levels are usually normal in early liver obstruction and are decreased with liver damage, such as hepatitis or cirrhosis. Levels also decline because of acute infections, chronic malnutrition, anemia, heart attack, obstructive jaundice, and cancer.

Glucose-6-phosphate Dehydrogenase

Glucose-6-phosphate dehydrogenase is an enzyme, or specialized protein, that's found in most cells of the body. It's involved in metabolizing glucose, a form of sugar that the body uses for energy. This test can detect glucose-6-phosphate dehydrogenase deficiency, which is a hereditary condition that allows destruction of red blood cells.

About 10% of all African American men in the United States inherit mild glucose-6-phosphate dehydrogenase deficiency. Some people of Mediterranean descent inherit a severe deficiency. In some whites, fava beans may produce episodes of red blood cell destruction. Although deficiency of glucose-6-phosphate dehydrogenase provides partial immunity to one type of malaria, it causes a bad reaction to antimalarial drugs.

Why is this test done?

Glucose-6-phosphate dehydrogenase levels may be measured for the following reasons:

- To detect an inherited enzyme deficiency that affects red blood cells
- To diagnose hemolytic anemia caused by glucose-6-phosphate dehydrogenase deficiency.

What should you know before the test?

- This test requires a blood sample, which takes less than 3 minutes to collect.
- You may experience slight discomfort from the needle puncture and tourniquet pressure.
- You don't need to change your diet before the test.
- A nurse or medical technician checks your history for recent blood transfusion or ingestion of aspirin, sulfonamides, phenacetin, nitrofurantoin, vitamin K derivatives, antimalarials, or fava beans. These substances cause red blood cell destruction in people who are glucose-6-phosphate dehydrogenase–deficient.

The test may identify a specific anemia or an inherited enzyme deficiency that affects red blood cells.

What happens during the test?

A nurse or medical technician inserts a needle into a vein, usually in your forearm. A blood sample is collected in a tube, which is then sent to a lab for testing.

What happens after the test?

If swelling develops at the needle puncture site, warm soaks are applied to the area to ease discomfort.

What are the normal results?

Serum levels of glucose-6-phosphate dehydrogenase vary with the measurement method used. Results are reported as normal or abnormal.

What do abnormal results mean?

If the results of initial tests are positive, a quantitative assay for glucose-6-phosphate dehydrogenase may be performed. People with some types of genetically linked anemia exhibit symptoms only when they experience stress, illness, or exposure to drugs or agents that set off episodes of red blood cell destruction.

Tay-Sachs Screening

This test measures levels of hexosaminidase in blood serum or amniotic fluid. Hexosaminidase is an enzyme, or specialized protein that's found primarily in brain tissue. Deficiency of hexosaminidase A, an isoenzyme, indicates Tay-Sachs disease, a fatal disorder that affects people of Ashkenazic Jewish ancestry about 100 times more often than the general population. Both parents must carry the defective gene to transmit Tay-Sachs disease to their children.

Both parents must carry the defective gene to transmit Tay-Sachs disease to their children.

Why is this test done?
Hexosaminidase A may be measured for the following reasons:
- To identify carriers of Tay-Sachs disease
- To confirm or rule out Tay-Sachs disease in newborns
- To establish prenatal diagnosis of hexosaminidase A deficiency.

What should you know before the test?
- This test requires a blood sample, which takes less than 3 minutes to collect.
- You may experience slight discomfort from the needle puncture and tourniquet pressure.
- You don't need to change your diet before the test.
- When the test is performed prenatally, you're instructed on preparations for amniocentesis.

What happens during the test?
- A nurse or medical technician inserts a needle into a vein, usually in your forearm. A blood sample is collected in a tube, which is then sent to a lab for testing.
- When testing a newborn, blood is drawn from the baby's arm, neck, or umbilical cord. The procedure is safe and quickly performed.

What happens after the test?

- If swelling develops at the needle puncture site, warm soaks are applied to the area to ease discomfort.
- After testing a newborn, a small bandage is placed on the site of the needle puncture.
- If both you and your partner are carriers of Tay-Sachs disease, you'll be referred for genetic counseling. If either partner's blood test result is negative, the child won't get Tay-Sachs disease.

What are the normal results?

Total blood serum levels of hexosaminidase range from 5 to 12.9 international units per liter; hexosaminidase A accounts for 55% to 76% of the total.

What do abnormal results mean?

Absence of hexosaminidase A indicates Tay-Sachs disease, even though total hexosaminidase levels may be normal.

GALACTOSEMIA SCREENING

This test involves measuring levels of galactose-1-phosphate uridyl transferase. This enzyme, or specialized protein, is involved in the metabolism of lactose, a type of sugar that comes from milk. Deficiency of this enzyme may lead to galactosemia, which is a hereditary disorder. Galactosemia can impair eye, brain, and liver development, causing irreversible cataracts, mental retardation, and cirrhosis, unless it's detected and treated soon after birth.

A simple screening test for galactose-1-phosphate uridyl transferase deficiency is required in some hospitals for all newborns. Prenatal testing of amniotic fluid can also detect transferase deficiency, but this is rarely performed.

Why is this test done?

Galactose-1-phosphate uridyl transferase may be tested for the following reasons:

- To screen newborns for galactosemia
- To detect carriers of galactosemia who may transmit the disorder to their children.

What should you know before the test?

- When testing an adult, the test requires a blood sample, which takes less than 3 minutes to collect.
- You may experience slight discomfort from the needle puncture and tourniquet pressure.
- You don't need to change your diet before the test.
- Your medical history is checked for a recent exchange transfusion. If you've had a transfusion, the lab is notified or the test is postponed.

To screen for galactosemia in an infant, a small amount of umbilical cord blood or blood from a heel stick is collected.

What happens during the test?

- For a *qualitative*, or screening, test on a newborn, a small amount of umbilical cord blood or blood from a heel puncture is collected on special paper, which is then sent to a lab for testing.
- For a *quantitative* test on an adult, a nurse or medical technician inserts a needle into a vein, usually in the forearm. A blood sample is collected in a tube, which is then sent to a lab for testing.

What happens after the test?

- If swelling develops at the needle puncture site, warm soaks are applied to the area to ease discomfort.
- If test results indicate galactosemia, you're referred for nutrition counseling and provided with a galactose- and lactose-free diet for your newborn. A soybean or meat-based formula may be substituted for milk.

What are the normal results?

Normally, the qualitative test is negative. The normal range for the quantitative test is 18.5 to 28.5 international units of transferase per gram of hemoglobin.

What do abnormal results mean?

A positive qualitative test may indicate a transferase deficiency. A follow-up quantitative test is performed as soon as possible. Quantitative test results of less than 5 international units per gram of hemoglobin indicate galactosemia. Levels between 5 and 18.5 international units per gram of hemoglobin may indicate a carrier state.

ANGIOTENSIN-CONVERTING ENZYME

This test measures serum levels of angiotensin-converting enzyme, which is found in lung capillaries and, in lesser concentrations, in blood vessels and kidney tissue. Its primary function is to help regulate blood pressure in arteries. However, measurement of angiotensin-converting enzyme is of little use in diagnosing high blood pressure.

Why is this test done?
Angiotensin-converting enzyme may be measured for the following reasons:
- To diagnose sarcoidosis, Gaucher's disease, or leprosy
- To monitor a person's response to therapy for sarcoidosis.

What should you know before the test?
- You must fast for 12 hours before this test.
- The test requires a blood sample, which takes less than 3 minutes to collect.
- You may experience slight discomfort from the needle puncture and tourniquet pressure.
- Because young people have variable angiotensin-converting enzyme levels, the test may be postponed if you're under age 20.

What happens during the test?
A nurse or medical technician inserts a needle into a vein, usually in your forearm. A blood sample is collected in a tube, which is then sent to a lab for testing.

What happens after the test?
If swelling develops at the needle puncture site, warm soaks are applied to the area to ease discomfort.

What are the normal results?
Normal levels are 6.1 to 21.1 international units of angiotensin-converting enzyme per liter of blood serum.

What do abnormal results mean?

Elevated serum angiotensin-converting enzyme levels may indicate sarcoidosis, Gaucher's disease, or leprosy, but results must be correlated with the person's clinical condition. In some people, elevated angiotensin-converting enzyme levels may be caused by liver diseases, hyperthyroidism, or diabetic retinopathy.

Serum angiotensin-converting enzyme levels decline as the person responds to steroid or prednisone therapy for sarcoidosis.

FATS & LIPOPROTEINS

TRIGLYCERIDES

Triglycerides are the main storage form of fats in the body. They constitute about 95% of fatty tissue. Results of this test are used in the quantitative analysis of triglycerides in the blood. This test is not diagnostic, but it permits early detection of hyperlipemia (excessive lipids in the blood), which increases the risk of heart disease.

Why is this test done?

Triglycerides may be measured for the following reasons:
- To detect disorders of fat metabolism
- To screen for hyperlipemia
- To help identify nephrotic syndrome, which is marked by massive fluid retention and other symptoms
- To determine the risk of heart disease.

What should you know before the test?

- This test requires a blood sample, which takes less than 3 minutes to collect.
- You may experience slight discomfort from the needle puncture and tourniquet pressure.
- Abstain from food for 10 to 14 hours before the test and abstain from alcohol for 24 hours. You can have water.

- Medications that may interfere with the accuracy of test results are withheld.

What happens during the test?
A nurse or medical technician inserts a needle into a vein, usually in your forearm. A blood sample is collected in a tube, which is then sent to a lab for testing.

What happens after the test?
- If swelling develops at the needle puncture site, warm soaks are applied to the area to ease discomfort.
- You may resume taking medications that were withheld before the test.
- You may resume your regular diet.

What are the normal results?
Triglyceride levels are age- and sex-related. There's some controversy about normal ranges, although levels of 40 to 160 milligrams per deciliter of blood for men and 35 to 135 milligrams per deciliter for women are widely accepted.

What do abnormal results mean?
Increased or decreased triglyceride levels in the blood suggest an abnormality. Additional tests are required for a definitive diagnosis.

A mild-to-moderate increase in triglyceride levels indicates bile duct obstruction, diabetes, nephrotic syndrome, glandular diseases, or alcohol abuse. Markedly increased levels, without an identifiable cause, reflect hyperlipoproteinemia that's present at birth. More tests are needed to confirm this diagnosis.

Decreased serum levels are rare, mainly caused by malnutrition or a condition called *abetalipoproteinemia.*

Normal triglyceride levels are age- and sex-related, and there's some controversy about normal ranges.

CHOLESTEROL

Cholesterol is a component of cell membranes and certain structures in the blood. It's taken into the body in foods and metabolized in the liver and other body tissues. This test measures total cholesterol levels in the blood. High levels may increase a person's risk of heart disease. (See *Getting cholesterol under control.*) Further testing is needed, though, to determine the ratios of different cholesterol types, which affect the risk level.

Why is this test done?

Cholesterol may be measured for the following reasons:

- To check the body's fat metabolism
- To measure the risk of heart disease
- To aid diagnosis of nephrotic syndrome, pancreatitis, liver disease, hypothyroidism, and hyperthyroidism.

What should you know before the test?

- This test requires a blood sample, which takes less than 3 minutes to collect.
- You may experience slight discomfort from the needle puncture and tourniquet pressure.
- Don't to eat or drink for 12 hours before the test.
- Drugs that influence cholesterol levels will be withheld before the test.

What happens during the test?

A nurse or medical technician inserts a needle into a vein, usually in your forearm. A blood sample is collected in a tube, which is then sent to a lab for testing.

What happens after the test?

- If swelling develops at the needle puncture site, warm soaks are applied to the area to ease discomfort.
- You may resume taking medications that were withheld before the test.
- You may resume your usual diet.

What are the normal results?

Total cholesterol levels vary with age and sex. The normal range is 170 to 200 milligrams per deciliter of blood serum. Levels of 280 to 320 milligrams per deciliter are considered elevated.

SELF-HELP

Getting cholesterol under control

Changing your diet helps reduce your cholesterol level. You'll need to reduce the amount of saturated fats you eat. This means cutting down drastically on eggs, dairy products, and fatty meats. Rely instead on poultry, fish, fruits, vegetables, and high-fiber breads. Use this list as a starting point for your new diet.

FOOD	ELIMINATE	SUBSTITUTE
Bread and cereals	Breads with whole eggs listed as a major ingredient	Oatmeal, multigrain, and bran cereals; whole-grain breads; rye bread
	Egg noodles	Pasta, rice
	Pies, cakes, doughnuts, biscuits, high-fat crackers and cookies	Angel food cake; low-fat cookies, crackers, home-baked goods
Eggs and dairy products	Whole milk, 2% milk, imitation milk	Skim milk, 1% milk, buttermilk
	Cream, half-and-half, most nondairy creamers, whipped toppings	None
	Whole milk yogurt and cottage cheese	Nonfat or low-fat yogurt, low-fat (1% or 2%) cottage cheese
	Cheese, cream cheese, sour cream, light cream cheese, light sour cream	None
	Egg yolks	Egg whites
	Ice cream	Sherbet, frozen tofu
Fats and oils	Coconut, palm, and palm kernel oils	Unsaturated vegetable oils (corn, olive, canola, safflower, sesame, soybean, and sunflower)
	Butter, lard, bacon fat	Unsaturated margarine and shortening, diet margarine
	Dressings made with egg yolks	Mayonnaise, unsaturated or low-fat salad dressings
	Chocolate	Baking cocoa
Meat, fish, and poultry	Fatty cuts of beef, lamb, or pork	Lean cuts of beef, lamb, or pork
	Organ meats, spare ribs, cold cuts, sausage, hot dogs, bacon	Poultry
	Sardines, roe	Sole, salmon, mackerel

What do abnormal results mean?

Elevated serum cholesterol, which is called *hypercholesterolemia*, may indicate risk of heart disease, as well as hepatitis, lipid disorders, bile duct blockage, nephrotic syndrome, obstructive jaundice, pancreatitis, and hypothyroidism.

Low serum cholesterol, called *hypocholesterolemia*, is commonly associated with malnutrition, liver damage, and hyperthyroidism. Abnormal cholesterol levels frequently require further testing to pinpoint the cause.

PHOSPHOLIPIDS

This test measures phospholipid levels in your blood. Phospholipids are forms of fat in the body that contain phosphorus. They're a major component of cell membranes and are involved in cell permeability and in controlling enzyme activity in the membrane. They help carry fats through the intestines and from the liver and other fat deposits to other body tissues. Phospholipids are also essential for gas exchange in the lungs.

Why is this test done?

Phospholipids may be measured for the following reasons:
- To determine how the body metabolizes fats
- To aid in the evaluation of fat metabolism
- To aid diagnosis of an underactive thyroid, diabetes, nephrotic syndrome, chronic pancreatitis, obstructive jaundice, and hypolipoproteinemia.

What should you know before the test?

- This test requires a blood sample, which takes less than 3 minutes to collect.
- You may experience slight discomfort from the needle puncture and tourniquet pressure.
- Abstain from drinking alcohol for 24 hours before the test and from food and fluids after midnight the night before the test.

What happens during the test?

A nurse or medical technician inserts a needle into a vein, usually in your forearm. A blood sample is collected in a tube, which is then sent to a lab for testing.

What happens after the test?

- If swelling develops at the needle puncture site, warm soaks are applied to the area to ease discomfort.
- You may resume your usual diet.

What are the normal results?

Normal phospholipid levels range from 180 to 320 milligrams per deciliter of blood. Although men usually have higher levels than women, levels in pregnant women exceed those of men.

What do abnormal results mean?

Elevated phospholipid levels may indicate hypothyroidism, diabetes, nephrotic syndrome, chronic pancreatitis, or obstructive jaundice.

Decreased levels may indicate primary hypolipoproteinemia.

Although men usually have higher normal phospholipid levels than women, levels in pregnant women are even higher.

LIPOPROTEIN-CHOLESTEROL FRACTIONS: HDL AND LDL

When a person's total cholesterol levels are found to be elevated, this test can isolate and measure the two primary types of cholesterol fractions in the blood. These are known as *high-density lipoproteins (HDLs),* popularly known as "good" cholesterol, and *low-density lipoproteins (LDLs),* or "bad" cholesterol. The relative levels of these cholesterol types have opposite effects on the incidence of heart disease. In other words, a high level of "good" high-density lipoproteins reduces the risk of heart disease. Conversely, a high level of "bad" low-density lipoproteins increases the risk of heart disease.

Why is this test done?

A lipoprotein-cholesterol test is performed to check a person's risk of heart disease.

What should you know before the test?

- This test requires a blood sample, which takes less than 3 minutes to collect.
- You may experience slight discomfort from the needle puncture and tourniquet pressure.
- Maintain your normal diet for 2 weeks before the test, but abstain from alcohol for 24 hours before the test. Fast and avoid exercise for 12 to 14 hours before the test.
- Medications that may influence test results are withheld before the test.

What happens during the test?

A nurse or medical technician inserts a needle into a vein, usually in your forearm. A blood sample is collected in a tube, which is then sent to a lab for testing.

What happens after the test?

- If swelling develops at the needle puncture site, warm soaks are applied to the area to ease discomfort.
- You may resume taking medications that were withheld before the test.
- You may resume your usual diet.

What are the normal results?

Normal cholesterol levels vary according to age, sex, geographic region, and ethnic group. Normal HDL levels range from 29 to 77 milligrams per deciliter of blood. Normal LDL levels range from 62 to 185 milligrams per deciliter.

What do abnormal results mean?

High LDL levels increase the risk of heart disease. Elevated HDL levels generally reflect a healthy state but can also indicate chronic hepatitis, early-stage primary biliary cirrhosis, or alcohol consumption. Rarely, a sharp increase to as high as 100 milligrams per deciliter in one type of HDL called *alpha$_2$-high-density lipoprotein* may indicate heart disease.

LIPOPROTEIN PHENOTYPING

Lipoproteins are the forms in which fats are transported in the blood. Lipoprotein phenotyping is used to determine levels of the four major lipoproteins: *chylomicrons, very low-density lipoproteins, low-density lipoproteins,* and *high-density lipoproteins*. Detecting altered lipoprotein patterns is the key to identifying metabolic disorders known as *hyperlipoproteinemia* or *hypolipoproteinemia*.

Why is this test done?

Lipoprotein phenotyping is performed for the following reasons:
- To evaluate how the body metabolizes fats
- To classify hyperlipoproteinemia or hypolipoproteinemia.

What should you know before the test?

- This test requires a blood sample, which takes less than 3 minutes to collect.
- You may experience slight discomfort from the needle puncture and tourniquet pressure.
- Abstain from alcohol for 24 hours before the test and fast after midnight before the test. Eat a low-fat meal the night before the test.
- A nurse or medical technician checks your drug history for the use of heparin, which may affect test results.
- You mustn't take antilipemics such as cholestyramine for about 2 weeks before the test.
- If you're hospitalized for any condition that might significantly alter lipoprotein metabolism, such as diabetes, nephrosis, or an underactive thyroid, the lab is notified.

Preparing for the test means no alcohol for 24 hours and no exercise or food for 14 hours.

What happens during the test?

A nurse or medical technician inserts a needle into a vein, usually in your forearm. A blood sample is collected in a tube, which is then sent to a lab for testing.

What happens after the test?

- If swelling develops at the needle puncture site, warm soaks are applied to the area to ease discomfort.
- You may resume taking medications that were withheld before the test.

- You may resume your regular diet.

What are the normal results?

Several types of lipoproteins normally exist in the body. The lab reports characteristic patterns among the various lipoproteins.

What do abnormal results mean?

Lipoprotein disorders are identified by characteristic patterns among a person's lipoproteins. The disorders are classified as either hyperlipoproteinemias or hypolipoproteinemias. There are six types of hyperlipoproteinemias: I, IIa, IIb, III, IV, and V. Types IIa, IIb, and IV are relatively common. All hypolipoproteinemias are rare.

PROTEINS & PIGMENTS

PROTEIN COMPONENTS

The two major proteins in blood are called *albumin* and *globulins*. This test is used to measure the levels of these proteins in blood serum, the clear fluid portion of blood. The proteins are measured and classified as five distinct fractions: albumin and $alpha_1$, $alpha_2$, beta, and gamma globulins.

Why is this test done?

Protein components are tested for the following reasons:
- To determine the protein content of blood
- To aid diagnosis of liver disease, protein deficiency, kidney disorders, and gastrointestinal and tumor-causing diseases.

What should you know before the test?

- This test requires a blood sample, which takes less than 3 minutes to collect.
- You may experience slight discomfort from the needle puncture and tourniquet pressure.
- You don't need to change your diet before the test.

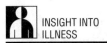

INSIGHT INTO
ILLNESS

How illness can affect blood protein levels

Abnormal levels of the two major proteins in the blood, albumin or the globulins, may occur in many different disorders.

Increased levels

Total proteins
- Dehydration
- Vomiting, diarrhea
- Diabetic acidosis
- Fulminating and chronic infections
- Multiple myeloma
- Monocytic leukemia
- Chronic inflammatory disease, such as rheumatoid arthritis or early-stage Laënnec's cirrhosis

Albumin
Multiple myeloma

Globulins
- Chronic syphilis
- Tuberculosis
- Subacute bacterial endocarditis
- Multiple myeloma
- Collagen diseases
- Systemic lupus erythematosus
- Rheumatoid arthritis
- Diabetes mellitus
- Hodgkin's disease

Decreased levels

Total proteins
- Malnutrition
- Gastrointestinal disease
- Blood dyscrasias
- Essential hypertension
- Hodgkin's disease
- Uncontrolled diabetes mellitus
- Malabsorption
- Hepatic dysfunction
- Toxemia of pregnancy
- Nephroses
- Surgical and traumatic shock
- Severe burns
- Hemorrhage
- Hyperthyroidism
- Benzene and carbon tetrachloride poisoning
- Congestive heart failure

Albumin
- Malnutrition
- Nephritis/nephrosis
- Diarrhea
- Plasma loss from burns
- Hepatic disease
- Hodgkin's disease
- Hypogamma-globulinemia
- Peptic ulcer
- Acute cholecystitis
- Sarcoidosis
- Collagen diseases
- Systemic lupus erythematosus
- Rheumatoid arthritis
- Essential hypertension
- Metastatic cancer
- Hyperthyroidism

Globulins
Levels vary in neoplastic and kidney diseases, liver dysfunction, and some blood disorders.

- Your medication history is checked for drugs that may influence protein levels. When possible, use of such medications is discontinued.

What happens during the test?
A nurse or medical technician inserts a needle into a vein, usually in your forearm. A blood sample is collected in a tube, which is then sent to a lab for testing.

What happens after the test?
If swelling develops at the needle puncture site, warm soaks are applied to the area to ease discomfort.

What are the normal results?
Normal total protein levels are 6.6 to 7.9 grams per deciliter of serum. The albumin fraction ranges from 3.3 to 4.5 grams per deciliter. The $alpha_1$-globulin fraction ranges from 0.1 to 0.4 gram per deciliter; $alpha_2$-globulin ranges from 0.5 to 1 gram per deciliter. Beta globulin ranges from 0.7 to 1.2 grams per deciliter; gamma globulin ranges from 0.5 to 1.6 grams per deciliter.

What do abnormal results mean?
For common findings, see *How illness can affect blood protein levels,* page 385.

HAPTOGLOBIN

This test measures the levels of haptoglobin, which is a type of protein that's produced in the liver. When many red blood cells are destroyed, the haptoglobin level decreases rapidly and may remain low for 5 to 7 days, until the liver produces more of it.

Why is this test done?
Haptoglobin may be measured for the following reasons:
- To determine the condition of red blood cells and the rate of their destruction
- To distinguish between types of protein in the blood

- To investigate transfusion reactions that lead to red blood cell destruction
- To establish proof of paternity.

What should you know before the test?

- This test requires a blood sample, which takes less than 3 minutes to collect.
- You may experience slight discomfort from the needle puncture and tourniquet pressure.
- You don't need to change your diet before the test.
- Your medication history is checked for drugs that may influence haptoglobin levels, including steroids and androgens.

What happens during the test?

A nurse or medical technician inserts a needle into a vein, usually in your forearm. A blood sample is collected in a tube, which is then sent to a lab for testing.

What happens after the test?

If swelling develops at the needle puncture site, warm soaks are applied to the area to ease discomfort.

What are the normal results?

Normal haptoglobin levels are 38 to 270 milligrams per deciliter of blood serum.

Haptoglobin is absent in 90% of newborns, but levels usually increase to normal by 4 months of age.

What do abnormal results mean?

Extremely low haptoglobin levels may occur in acute and chronic red blood cell destruction, severe hepatocellular disease, infectious mononucleosis, and transfusion reactions. Liver disease inhibits haptoglobin production. If your serum haptoglobin levels are very low, you must be monitored for symptoms of red blood cell destruction: chills, fever, back pain, flushing, distended neck veins, irregular heartbeat and breathing, and low blood pressure.

In about 1% of the population — including 4% of blacks — haptoglobin is permanently absent; this disorder is known as *congenital ahaptoglobinemia.*

Haptoglobin is absent in 90% of newborns, but their levels usually increase to normal by 4 months of age.

Strikingly elevated serum haptoglobin levels occur in diseases that are marked by chronic inflammatory reactions or tissue destruction, such as rheumatoid arthritis and malignant tumors.

TRANSFERRIN

Transferrin is a type of protein that's formed in the liver. It's also called *siderophilin*. Iron in the body comes from iron-rich foods or from the breakdown of red blood cells. Transferrin transports iron from the blood to the liver, spleen, and bone marrow, where it's used or stored. This test provides a quantitative analysis of transferrin levels in the blood. Results are used to evaluate iron metabolism. Iron level is usually measured at the same time.

Why is this test done?
Transferrin may be measured for the following reasons:
- To determine the cause of anemia and to evaluate iron metabolism in iron deficiency anemia
- To determine the iron-transporting capacity of the blood.

What should you know before the test?
- This test requires a blood sample, which takes less than 3 minutes to collect.
- You may experience slight discomfort from the needle puncture and tourniquet pressure.
- You don't need to change your diet before the test.
- Your medication history is checked for the use of drugs that may influence transferrin levels.

Iron in the body comes from iron-rich foods or from the breakdown of red blood cells.

What happens during the test?
A nurse or medical technician inserts a needle into a vein, usually in your forearm. A blood sample is collected in a tube, which is then sent to a lab for testing.

What happens after the test?
If swelling develops at the needle puncture site, warm soaks are applied to the area to ease discomfort.

What are the normal results?

Normal transferrin levels range from 220 to 400 micrograms of transferrin per deciliter of blood serum; 65 to 170 micrograms per deciliter are usually bound to iron.

What do abnormal results mean?

Inadequate transferrin levels may lead to impaired hemoglobin production and, possibly, anemia. Depressed serum levels may indicate inadequate production of transferrin due to liver damage or excessive protein loss from kidney disease. Decreased transferrin levels may also be caused by acute or chronic infection or cancer.

Elevated serum transferrin levels may be a sign of a severe iron deficiency.

AMINO ACID SCREENING

This test checks infants for errors of amino acid metabolism. Amino acids are the chief component of all proteins. The body contains at least 20 amino acids — 10 of these aren't formed in the body and must be acquired through the diet. Certain inborn enzyme deficiencies interfere with normal metabolism of amino acids and cause accumulation or deficiency of them. (See *Amino acids: No sooner collected than spent,* page 390.)

Why is this test done?

Amino acid screening may be performed for the following reasons:
- To determine how well an infant's body produces and uses amino acids
- To screen for inborn errors of amino acid metabolism.

What should you know before the test?

- The infant must not be given food or liquids for 4 hours before the test.
- A small amount of blood is taken from the infant's heel. Collecting the sample takes only a few minutes.

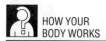

HOW YOUR
BODY WORKS

Amino acids: No sooner collected than spent

Unlike carbohydrates or fats, protein is not stored by the body. Instead, the body breaks down proteins and forms an amino acid pool. From this pool, amino acids react with products of carbohydrate and fat metabolism through such processes as oxidative deamination, transamination, and ammonia transport. These reactions create new proteins as well as hormones, enzymes, or nonprotein nitrogen compounds such as creatine.

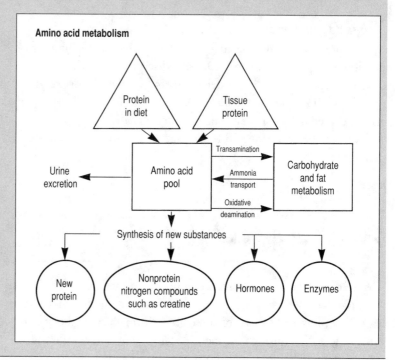

Amino acid metabolism

What happens during the test?

A nurse or medical technician makes a shallow skin puncture and collects a few drops of blood in a narrow tube.

What happens after the test?

- If a hematoma develops at the puncture site, warm soaks are applied to ease the infant's discomfort.
- You may resume your child's usual diet.

What are the normal results?

The test result shows a normal amino acid pattern in the blood.

What do abnormal results mean?

Excessive amino acids typically produce conditions called *overflow aminoacidurias*. Inborn abnormalities of the amino acid transport system in the kidneys produce disorders that are called *renal aminoac-idurias*. Comparing blood and urine test results helps the doctor distinguish between the two types of aminoacidurias. The amino acid patterns are normal in renal aminoacidurias and abnormal in over-flow aminoacidurias.

PHENYLALANINE SCREENING

This test is also called the *Guthrie screening test*. It's used to screen infants for high levels of phenylalanine in the blood. It's a required test in many states.

Phenylalanine is a naturally occurring amino acid that's essential to growth and nitrogen balance. Accumulation of phenylalanine in the blood may indicate a serious enzyme deficiency. This result may indicate a condition that's called *phenylketonuria* or *PKU*. To ensure accurate results, the test must be performed after 3 to 4 full days of milk or formula feeding. (See *How PKU is inherited*, page 392.)

Why is this test done?
Phenylalanine screening is performed to screen infants for possible phenylketonuria.

What should you know before the test?
This test requires a blood sample. A small amount of blood is drawn from the infant's heel.

What happens during the test?
A nurse or medical technician performs a heel puncture and collects three drops of blood on a filter paper.

What happens after the test?
If swelling develops at the puncture site, warm soaks are applied to ease the infant's discomfort.

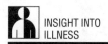

INSIGHT INTO
ILLNESS

How PKU is inherited

Phenylketonuria, also called *PKU*, is an inherited disorder that, if untreated, can cause mental retardation and other problems. In PKU, an accumulation of phenylalanine and other substances hinders normal nervous system development.

Hereditary risk

Being a heterozygous carrier of a trait means that, although there are no outward signs of the trait, it may be passed on to one's children. When *both* parents carry a recessive (hidden) trait for PKU, there's a 25% chance that their child will inherit both recessive genes. If so, the child will require a restricted diet to avoid retardation.

Diet therapy

Avoiding dietary phenylalanine prevents accumulation of toxic compounds and thereby prevents mental retardation. As the child matures, the body develops alternative ways to process phenylalanine.

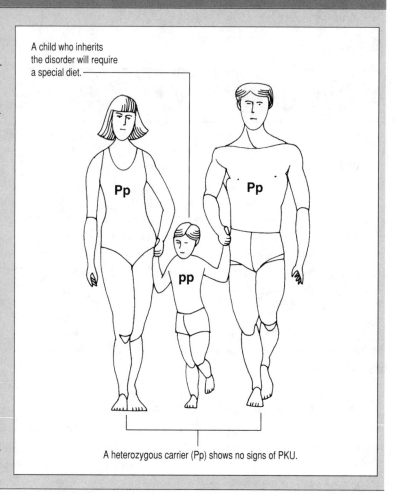

A child who inherits the disorder will require a special diet.

Pp

Pp

pp

A heterozygous carrier (Pp) shows no signs of PKU.

What are the normal results?

A negative test indicates normal phenylalanine levels of less than 2 milligrams of phenylalanine per deciliter of blood. This indicates no appreciable danger of phenylketonuria.

What do abnormal results mean?

At birth, an infant with phenylketonuria usually has normal phenylalanine levels, but after milk or formula feeding begins, levels gradually increase. A positive test result suggests the *possibility* of phenyl-ketonuria.

Diagnosis requires exact serum phenylalanine measurement and urine testing. A positive test may also be caused by liver disease, galactosemia, or delayed development of certain enzyme systems. Although this disease is a common cause of mental deficiency, early detection and continuous treatment with a low-phenylalanine diet can prevent permanent mental retardation.

AMMONIA

A form of nitrogen, ammonia helps maintain the acid-base balance in the body. This test measures levels of ammonia in the blood plasma (the clear fluid of the blood that contains suspended cells and dissolved proteins.)

Normally, ammonia passes through the liver before it's excreted in urine. In diseases such as cirrhosis of the liver, ammonia can bypass the liver and accumulate in the blood. Plasma ammonia levels may help indicate the severity of liver damage.

Why is this test done?
Ammonia may be measured for the following reasons:
- To check liver function
- To help monitor severe liver disease and the effectiveness of therapy
- To recognize impending or established liver-related coma.

What should you know before the test?
- You're asked to fast overnight before the test.
- This test requires a blood sample, which takes less than 3 minutes to collect.
- You may experience slight discomfort from the needle puncture and tourniquet pressure.
- Certain medications influence ammonia levels in the blood plasma and will be discontinued, if possible.

In diseases such as cirrhosis of the liver, ammonia can bypass the damaged liver and accumulate in the blood.

What happens during the test?

A nurse or medical technician inserts a needle into a vein, usually in your forearm. A blood sample is collected in a tube, which is then sent to a lab for testing.

What happens after the test?

- If swelling develops at the needle puncture site, warm soaks are applied to the area to ease discomfort.
- When plasma ammonia levels are high, you're watched for signs of liver related coma.

What are the normal results?

Normal ammonia levels are less than 50 micrograms of ammonia per deciliter of blood plasma.

What do abnormal results mean?

Elevated plasma ammonia levels commonly occur in severe liver disease — such as cirrhosis and acute liver necrosis — and may lead to liver-related coma. Elevated ammonia levels are also possible in Reye's syndrome, severe congestive heart failure, gastrointestinal hemorrhage, and erythroblastosis fetalis.

BLOOD UREA NITROGEN

This test measures the nitrogen found in urea, which is the chief end product of protein metabolism in the body. Urea is formed in the liver from ammonia and is excreted by the kidneys. The blood urea nitrogen level reflects protein intake and kidney function.

Why is this test done?

Blood urea nitrogen may be measured for the following reasons:
- To evaluate your kidney function and check for kidney disease
- To aid assessment of fluid use and balance in the body.

What should you know before the test?

- You don't need to restrict food or fluids before the test, but you should avoid a diet high in meat.

- This test requires a blood sample, which takes less than 3 minutes to collect.
- You may experience slight discomfort from the needle puncture and tourniquet pressure.
- Your medication history is checked for use of drugs that influence blood urea nitrogen levels, and they may be discontinued.

What happens during the test?

A nurse or medical technician inserts a needle into a vein, usually in your forearm. A blood sample is collected in a tube, which is then sent to a lab for testing.

What happens after the test?

If swelling develops at the needle puncture site, warm soaks are applied to the area to ease discomfort.

What are the normal results?

Blood urea nitrogen levels normally range from 8 to 20 milligrams of nitrogen per deciliter of blood, with slightly higher levels in elderly people.

What do abnormal results mean?

Elevated blood urea nitrogen levels occur in kidney disease, reduced blood flow to the kidneys possibly caused by dehydration, urinary tract obstruction, and in conditions that cause protein breakdown, such as burns.

Depressed blood urea nitrogen levels occur in severe liver damage, malnutrition, and overhydration.

Depressed blood urea nitrogen levels show up in people with severe liver damage, malnutrition, and excessive liquid intake.

CREATININE

Creatinine occurs in the blood in amounts proportional to the body's muscle mass. Analysis of creatinine levels in the blood provides a more sensitive measure of kidney damage than blood urea nitrogen levels.

Why is this test done?

Creatinine levels may be measured for the following reasons:

- To check kidney function
- To screen for kidney damage.

What should you know before the test?

- This test requires a blood sample, which takes less than 3 minutes to collect.
- You may experience slight discomfort from the needle puncture and tourniquet pressure.
- You're asked to restrict food and fluids for about 8 hours before the test.
- Your history is checked for the use of drugs that may influence test results.

What happens during the test?

A nurse or medical technician inserts a needle into a vein, usually in your forearm. A blood sample is collected in a tube, which is then sent to a lab for testing.

What happens after the test?

If swelling develops at the needle puncture site, warm soaks are applied to the area to ease discomfort.

What are the normal results?

Normal creatinine concentrations in men are from 0.8 to 1.2 milligrams of creatinine per deciliter of blood; in women, from 0.6 to 0.9 milligrams per deciliter.

What do abnormal results mean?

Elevated creatinine levels generally indicate kidney disease that has seriously damaged 50% or more of the tissue. Elevated levels may also be associated with gigantism and acromegaly.

URIC ACID

Uric acid, a component of urine, normally appears in the bloodstream before being excreted. Excessive uric acid in the blood is a primary sign of gout, which is a hereditary form of arthritis. This test measures the levels of uric acid in a blood sample. Disorders of metabolism and impaired kidney excretion characteristically raise the levels of uric acid in the blood.

Why is this test done?

Uric acid levels are measured to detect gout or kidney dysfunction.

What should you know before the test?

- This test requires a blood sample, which takes less than 3 minutes to collect.
- You may experience slight discomfort from the needle puncture and tourniquet pressure.
- You must fast for 8 hours before the test.
- Your medication history is checked for use of drugs that may influence test results. They may be discontinued before the test.

Excessive uric acid in the blood is a primary sign of gout, which is a hereditary form of arthritis.

What happens during the test?

A nurse or medical technician inserts a needle into a vein, usually in your forearm. A blood sample is collected in a tube, which is then sent to a lab for testing.

What happens after the test?

If swelling develops at the needle puncture site, warm soaks are applied to the area to ease discomfort.

What are the normal results?

Uric acid concentrations in men normally range from 4.3 to 8.0 milligrams of uric acid per deciliter of blood; in women, from 2.3 to 6.0 milligrams per deciliter.

What do abnormal results mean?

Increased uric acid levels may indicate gout or impaired kidney function. Levels may also increase with congestive heart failure, glycogen storage disease, infections, hemolytic or sickle cell anemia, polycythemia, tumors, and psoriasis.

Low uric acid levels may indicate poor kidney tubular absorption, as in Fanconi's syndrome, or acute liver atrophy.

Bilirubin

Bilirubin is a clear yellow or orange fluid found in bile. It's produced by the breakdown of red blood cells. This test is used to measure the levels of bilirubin in the blood. After leaving the bloodstream, bilirubin is normally excreted with bile, which aids in food digestion. Proper bilirubin excretion is especially important in newborns because excessive bilirubin can accumulate in the brain, causing irreparable damage.

Adults must fast at least 4 hours before the test. Fasting isn't necessary for newborns.

Why is this test done?
Bilirubin may be measured for the following reasons:
- To evaluate liver function and to help diagnose obstructions in the bile system
- To evaluate the condition of red blood cells and to help diagnose anemia due to red blood cell destruction
- To aid the diagnosis of jaundice and to monitor its progress
- To determine a newborn's possible need for a transfusion or phototherapy to control excessive bilirubin.

What should you know before the test?
- This test requires a blood sample, which takes less than 3 minutes to collect.
- You (or your newborn) may experience slight discomfort from the needle puncture and tourniquet pressure.
- You don't need to restrict fluids but should fast for at least 4 hours before the test. Fasting is not necessary for newborns.
- Your medication history is checked for the use of drugs that interfere with bilirubin levels. They may be discontinued before the test.

What happens during the test?
- A nurse or medical technician inserts a needle into a vein, usually in your forearm. A blood sample is collected in a tube, which is then sent to a lab for testing.

- When a newborn is tested, a heel puncture is performed, and a small tube is filled to the designated level with blood.

What happens after the test?

If swelling develops at the needle puncture site, warm soaks are applied to the area to ease discomfort.

What are the normal results?

When measured by the *indirect serum bilirubin* method, normal adult levels are 1.1 milligrams of bilirubin per deciliter of blood serum or less; normal adult levels, when measured by the *direct serum bilirubin* method, are less than 0.5 milligrams of bilirubin per deciliter of blood serum. Total bilirubin in the newborn ranges from 1.0 to 12.0 milligrams per deciliter.

What do abnormal results mean?

Elevated indirect serum bilirubin levels often indicate liver damage and can reveal severe red blood cell destruction that causes hemolytic anemia. If cell destruction continues, both direct and indirect bilirubin results may increase. Other causes of elevated indirect levels include inborn enzyme deficiencies, such as Gilbert's disease.

Elevated direct serum bilirubin levels usually indicate bile system obstruction.

In newborns, levels of 18.0 milligrams of bilirubin or more per deciliter of blood indicate the need for blood exchange transfusion.

CARBOHYDRATES

FASTING BLOOD SUGAR

This test is also called the *fasting plasma glucose test*. Glucose is a form of sugar that's found in fruits and other foods. It's also an important component of blood and is the body's chief source of energy. This test is used to measure blood sugar levels following a 12- to 14-hour fast. Normally, increases in blood sugar levels are kept in check by the secretion of insulin. This test is commonly used to screen for diabetes, in which the absence or deficiency of insulin allows persistently high sugar levels.

Why is this test done?

The fasting blood sugar test is performed for the following reasons:
- To detect disorders of glucose metabolism
- To screen for diabetes
- To monitor drug or diet therapy in people with diabetes.

What should you know before the test?

- This test requires a blood sample, which takes less than 3 minutes to collect.
- You may experience slight discomfort from the needle puncture and tourniquet pressure.
- You must fast for 12 to 14 hours before the test.
- Before the test, you're asked to suspend the use of drugs that may affect test results. If you have diabetes, you may take your medication after the test.
- Watch for feelings of weakness, restlessness, nervousness, hunger, and sweating. Report these symptoms of hypoglycemia, or low blood sugar, immediately.

What happens during the test?

A nurse or medical technician inserts a needle into a vein, usually in your forearm. A blood sample is collected in a tube, which is then sent to a lab for testing.

What happens after the test?

- If swelling develops at the needle puncture site, warm soaks are applied to the area to ease discomfort.
- Eat a balanced meal or a snack after the test, and resume taking medications that were withheld before the test.

What are the normal results?

Generally, normal levels, after a 12- to 14-hour fast, are 70 to 100 milligrams of true glucose for each deciliter of blood.

What do abnormal results mean?

Confirmation of diabetes requires fasting blood sugar levels of 140 milligrams per deciliter or more, obtained on two or more occasions.

While you're fasting to prepare for the test, watch for feelings of weakness, restlessness, nervousness, hunger, and sweating.

When borderline or briefly elevated levels are reported, a 2-hour postprandial blood sugar test or the oral glucose tolerance test may be performed to confirm the diagnosis.

Increased fasting blood sugar levels can be caused by pancreatitis, recent acute illness such as heart attack, Cushing's syndrome, acromegaly, and pheochromocytoma. High blood sugar (hyperglycemia) may also stem from hyperlipoproteinemia, chronic liver disease, nephrotic syndrome, brain tumor, sepsis, or gastrectomy with dumping syndrome, and is typical in eclampsia, anoxia, and seizure disorder.

Depressed blood sugar levels can be caused by hyperinsulinism, insulinoma, von Gierke's disease, functional or reactive hypoglycemia, myxedema, adrenal insufficiency, congenital adrenal hyperplasia, hypopituitarism, malabsorption syndrome, and some liver disorders.

TWO-HOUR POSTPRANDIAL BLOOD SUGAR

This test is a valuable tool for detecting diabetes, a condition that causes persistently high blood sugar levels. It's used when someone has symptoms of diabetes, such as extreme thirst and excessive urination, or when results of the fasting plasma blood sugar test suggest diabetes.

Why is this test done?
The two-hour postprandial blood sugar test is performed for the following reasons:
- To evaluate sugar metabolism
- To aid diagnosis of diabetes
- To monitor drug or diet therapy in people with diabetes.

What should you know before the test?
- This test requires a blood sample, which takes less than 3 minutes to collect.
- You may experience slight discomfort from the needle puncture and tourniquet pressure.

How blood sugar levels vary with age

After age 50, normal blood sugar levels increase markedly and steadily, sometimes reaching 160 milligrams or more of glucose per deciliter of blood. In a younger person, a glucose concentration greater than 145 milligrams per deciliter suggests incipient diabetes and requires further evaluation.

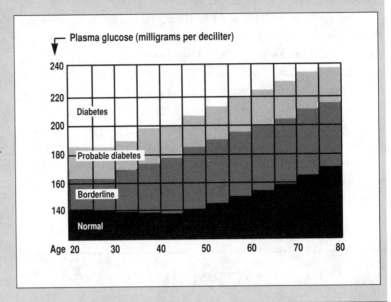

- Eat a balanced meal or one containing 100 grams of carbohydrate before the test and then fast for 2 hours. Avoid smoking and strenuous exercise after the meal.

What happens during the test?

A nurse or medical technician inserts a needle into a vein, usually in your forearm. A blood sample is collected in a tube, which is then sent to a lab for testing.

What happens after the test?

- If swelling develops at the needle puncture site, warm soaks are applied to the area to ease discomfort.
- You may resume your usual diet and normal activity.

What are the normal results?

In a person who doesn't have diabetes, the postprandial blood sugar level is less than 145 milligrams of sugar per deciliter of blood; levels are slightly elevated in people who are over age 87. (See *How blood sugar levels vary with age*.)

What do abnormal results mean?

Two 2-hour postprandial blood sugar levels of 200 milligrams per deciliter or more indicate diabetes mellitus. High levels may also occur with pancreatitis, Cushing's syndrome, acromegaly, and pheochromocytoma. High levels may also be caused by hyperlipoproteinemia, chronic liver disease, nephrotic syndrome, brain tumor, sepsis, gastrectomy with dumping syndrome, eclampsia, anoxia, or seizure disorders.

Low sugar levels occur in hyperinsulinism, insulinoma, von Gierke's disease, myxedema, adrenal insufficiency, congenital adrenal hyperplasia, hypopituitarism, malabsorption syndrome, and some cases of liver insufficiency.

ORAL GLUCOSE TOLERANCE TEST

This test checks your body's ability to process glucose, a form of sugar that's your chief source of energy. During this test, sugar levels in the blood and urine are monitored for 3 hours after drinking a large dose of sugar solution. This is the most sensitive way to evaluate borderline cases of diabetes, a disorder that causes high sugar levels in the blood.

Why is this test done?

The oral glucose tolerance test is performed for the following reasons:
- To evaluate sugar metabolism
- To confirm diabetes
- To aid diagnosis of abnormally low blood sugar levels (called *hypoglycemia*) and malabsorption syndrome.

What should you know before the test?

- You're asked to eat a high-carbohydrate diet for 3 days and then to fast for 10 to 16 hours before the test. (See *Following a high-carbohydrate diet*, page 404.)
- Don't smoke, drink coffee or alcohol, or exercise strenuously for 8 hours before or during the test.
- This test requires five blood samples and usually five urine specimens. You may experience slight discomfort from the needle punctures and the pressure of the tourniquet.

SELF-HELP

Following a high carbohydrate diet

To prepare for the oral glucose tolerance test and to ensure accurate results, follow a high-carbohydrate diet like the one below for at least 3 days before the test. If you find the diet too restrictive, follow your regular diet but eat 12 extra slices of bread each day.

BREAKFAST
1 serving fruit
Eggs, as desired
5 bread exchanges*
1 cup milk
Butter or margarine
Coffee or tea, if desired

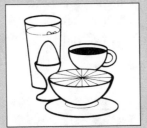

LUNCH AND DINNER
Meat, as desired
5 bread exchanges*
2 vegetables
1 serving fruit
1 cup milk
Butter or margarine
Coffee or tea, if desired

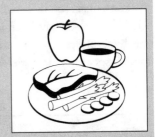

*One of the following equals one bread exchange

1 slice bread, white or whole wheat
1½-inch cube of cornbread
½ hamburger or hot dog roll
½ cup dry cereal (avoid sugar-coated
  varieties)
½ cup cooked cereal
½ cup noodles, spaghetti, or macaroni
½ cup cooked dried beans or peas
⅓ cup corn or ½ small ear of corn
1 biscuit

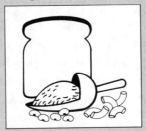

½ corn muffin
1 roll
5 saltine crackers
2 graham crackers
½ cup grits or rice
1 small white potato
½ cup mashed potato
¼ cup sweet potato
¼ cup baked beans
¼ cup pork and beans

- Bring a book or other quiet diversion with you to the test because the procedure usually takes 3 hours and can last as long as 6 hours.
- Your medication history is checked for drugs that may affect test results. Such drugs are usually withheld before the test.
- Watch for and immediately report any feelings of weakness, restlessness, nervousness, hunger, or sweating; these may indicate hypoglycemia.

What happens during the test?

- A nurse or medical technician first obtains a fasting blood sample. A needle is inserted into a vein, usually in your forearm. A blood sample is collected in a tube, which is then sent to a lab for testing.

- A urine specimen is collected immediately following the blood sample.
- After collecting these samples, you're given a dose of dissolved sugar to drink. The time it takes for you to finish it is recorded. You're encouraged to drink the entire solution within 5 minutes.
- Blood samples are drawn 30 minutes, 1 hour, 2 hours, and 3 hours after you drink the sugar solution.
- Urine specimens are collected at the same intervals.
- You may lie down if you feel faint from the needle punctures.
- You're encouraged to drink water throughout the test to promote adequate urination.

What happens after the test?
- If swelling develops at the needle puncture site, warm soaks are applied to the area to ease discomfort.
- You may resume taking medications that were withheld before the test.
- After the test, eat a balanced meal or a snack, and be alert for a hypoglycemic reaction.

Does the test have risks?
- Extended monitoring to detect hypoglycemia should not be performed on a person who is suspected of having a tumor-causing condition called *insulinoma*. Prolonged fasting may lead to fainting and coma.
- If you develop severe hypoglycemia, the test is discontinued and you'll be given orange juice with sugar added to drink. You may receive intravenous sugar to reverse the reaction.

What are the normal results?
Normal sugar levels peak at 160 to 180 milligrams of sugar per deciliter of blood within 30 minutes to 1 hour after consuming the oral sugar test dose. Sugar returns to fasting levels or lower within 2 to 3 hours. Urine sugar tests remain negative throughout.

What do abnormal results mean?
Depressed glucose tolerance, in which levels peak sharply before falling slowly to fasting levels, may confirm diabetes or may be caused by Cushing's disease, hemochromatosis, pheochromocytoma, or central nervous system lesions.

Bring a book or other quiet diversion with you because this test usually takes 3 hours and can last as long as 6 hours.

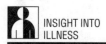

Effects of low blood sugar

Various body organs respond differently to conditions of low blood sugar. The symptoms you're most likely to notice if you have this condition are headache, sweating, and nausea.

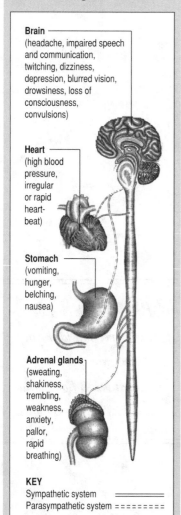

Brain
(headache, impaired speech and communication, twitching, dizziness, depression, blurred vision, drowsiness, loss of consciousness, convulsions)

Heart
(high blood pressure, irregular or rapid heartbeat)

Stomach
(vomiting, hunger, belching, nausea)

Adrenal glands
(sweating, shakiness, trembling, weakness, anxiety, pallor, rapid breathing)

KEY
Sympathetic system ══════
Parasympathetic system ═ ═ ═ ═ ═

Increased glucose tolerance, in which levels may peak at less than normal, may indicate insulinoma, malabsorption syndrome, adrenocortical insufficiency (Addison's disease), or an underactive thyroid or pituitary gland.

BETA-HYDROXYBUTYRATE

This test is used to measure the levels of beta-hydroxybutyric acid in the blood. Beta-hydroxybutyrate is one of three ketone bodies that are products of fatty acid metabolism in the liver. The other two ketone bodies are acetoacetate and acetone. An accumulation of all three ketone bodies is referred to as *ketosis;* excessive formation of ketone bodies in the blood is called *ketonemia.*

Why is this test done?
Beta-hydroxybutyric acid may be measured for the following reasons:
- To evaluate ketones in your blood
- To diagnose carbohydrate deprivation, which may be caused by starvation, digestive disturbances, dietary imbalances, or frequent vomiting
- To aid diagnosis of diabetes resulting from poor carbohydrate utilization
- To aid diagnosis of glycogen storage diseases, specifically von Gierke's disease
- To monitor the effect of insulin therapy during treatment of diabetic ketoacidosis
- To monitor a person's status during emergency management of hypoglycemia, acidosis, excessive alcohol ingestion, or unexplained changes in electrolyte balance. (See *Effects of low blood sugar.*)

What should you know before the test?
- This test requires a blood sample, which takes less than 3 minutes to collect.
- You may experience slight discomfort from the needle puncture and tourniquet pressure.
- You don't need to change your diet before the test.

What happens during the test?

A nurse or medical technician inserts a needle into a vein, usually in your forearm. A blood sample is collected in a tube, which is then sent to a lab for testing.

What happens after the test?

If swelling develops at the needle puncture site, warm soaks are applied to the area to ease discomfort.

What are the normal results?

The normal value for beta-hydroxybutyrate levels is less than 0.4 millimols per liter of blood serum or plasma.

What do abnormal results mean?

Elevated levels may suggest worsening of ketosis. Levels that are greater than 2 millimols per liter require immediate treatment.

GLYCOSYLATED HEMOGLOBIN

The glycosylated hemoglobin test is also called the *total fasting hemoglobin test*. It's used for monitoring diabetes therapy.

Hemoglobin is a pigment in blood cells that assists in oxygen transport. Three minor forms of hemoglobin are measured in this test: hemoglobin A_{1a}, hemoglobin A_{1b}, and hemoglobin A_{1c}.

Measuring glycosylated hemoglobin levels gives the doctor information about the average blood sugar level during the preceding 2 to 3 months. This test requires collection of only one blood sample every 6 to 8 weeks and can therefore be used for evaluating long-term effectiveness of diabetes therapy.

Why is this test done?

The glycosylated hemoglobin test is performed to evaluate diabetes therapy.

What should you know before the test?

■ This test requires a blood sample, which takes less than 3 minutes to collect.

With only one blood sample every 6 to 8 weeks, the test can evaluate long-term diabetes therapy.

- You may experience slight discomfort from the needle puncture and tourniquet pressure.
- You don't need to change your diet or prescribed medication regimen before the test.

What happens during the test?

A nurse or medical technician inserts a needle into a vein, usually in your forearm. A blood sample is collected in a tube, which is then sent to a lab for testing.

What happens after the test?

- If swelling develops at the needle puncture site, warm soaks are applied to the area to ease discomfort.
- You may schedule an appointment in 6 to 8 weeks for appropriate follow-up testing.

What are the normal results?

Normal glycosylated hemoglobin levels are reported as a percentage of the total hemoglobin within a red blood cell.

What do abnormal results mean?

In diabetes, hemoglobins A_{1a} and A_{1b} constitute approximately 2.5% to 3.9% of total hemoglobin; hemoglobin A_{1c} constitutes 8% to 11.9%; and total glycosylated hemoglobin level is 10.9% to 15.5%. As effective therapy brings diabetes under control, levels approach the normal range.

ORAL LACTOSE TOLERANCE TEST

This test measures blood sugar levels after you drink a dose of lactose, which is a form of sugar that's found in milk. The test is used to screen for lactose intolerance. Lactose intolerance may be caused by a deficiency of the intestinal enzyme lactase, which normally splits lactose into simpler sugars. The undigested lactose remains in the intestine, which leads to symptoms such as abdominal cramps and watery diarrhea.

True congenital, or inborn, lactase deficiency is rare. Usually, lactose intolerance is acquired later in life because lactase levels generally decrease with age.

Why is this test done?

The oral lactose tolerance test is performed to determine if a person's symptoms are caused by lactose intolerance.

What should you know before the test?

- You must fast and avoid strenuous activity for 8 hours before the test.
- This test may require a stool sample.
- This test also requires the collection of four blood samples. You may feel slight discomfort from the needle punctures and the pressure of the tourniquet, but collecting each blood sample takes less than 3 minutes. The entire procedure may take as long as 2 hours.
- Your medication history is checked for drugs that may affect plasma glucose levels, and they may be discontinued.

What happens during the test?

- A nurse or medical technician first obtains a fasting blood sample. A needle is inserted into a vein, usually in your forearm. A blood sample is collected in a tube, which is then sent to a lab for testing.
- You're asked to drink the lactose solution, and the time is recorded.
- Blood samples are collected 30, 60, and 120 minutes after you drink the lactose.
- A stool sample is collected 5 hours after you drink the lactose.

What happens after the test?

- If swelling develops at the needle puncture site, warm soaks are applied to the area to ease discomfort.
- You may resume your usual diet, medications, and activities.

Does the test have risks?

You may experience symptoms of lactose intolerance, such as abdominal cramps, nausea, bloating, flatulence, and watery diarrhea. The test administrator will monitor you for these symptoms.

What are the normal results?

Normally, glucose levels in the blood increase more than 20 milligrams of glucose per deciliter over fasting levels within 15 to 60 minutes after you drink the lactose. Stool sample analysis shows normal pH of 7 to 8 and low glucose content.

What do abnormal results mean?

An increase in plasma glucose of less than 20 milligrams per deciliter indicates lactose intolerance, as does stool acidity, or pH of 5.5 or less, and high glucose content. Accompanying signs and symptoms provoked by the test also suggest but do not confirm the diagnosis, as such symptoms may appear in people with normal lactase activity after consuming the lactose. Small-bowel biopsy with lactase assay may confirm the diagnosis.

*L*ACTIC ACID

The test is recommended for all people with symptoms of lactic acidosis, such as rapid, deep breathing.

Lactic acid, which occurs in the blood as lactate, is made primarily in muscle cells and red blood cells. It's produced during carbohydrate metabolism and is normally metabolized, or converted to energy, by the liver. Blood lactate concentration depends on the rates of production and metabolism. Levels may increase significantly during exercise.

Lactate and pyruvate, another product of carbohydrate metabolism, react together in a process that's regulated by oxygen supply. When oxygen is low, pyruvate converts to lactate. When oxygen is adequate, lactate converts to pyruvate. When the liver fails to metabolize lactose sufficiently or when excess pyruvate converts to lactate, severe elevations of lactic acid, called *lactic acidosis,* may result.

Measurement of blood lactate levels is recommended for all people with symptoms of lactic acidosis, such as rapid, deep breathing.

Why is this test done?

Lactic acid levels are measured to help determine the cause of lactic acidosis.

What should you know before the test?

- This test requires a blood sample, which takes less than 3 minutes to collect.
- You may experience slight discomfort from the needle puncture and tourniquet pressure.
- Fast overnight before the test, and rest for at least 1 hour before the test.

What happens during the test?

- A nurse or medical technician inserts a needle into a vein, usually in your forearm. A blood sample is collected in a tube, which is then sent to a lab for testing.
- During blood collection, don't clench your fist because this may raise blood lactate levels.

What happens after the test?

- If swelling develops at the needle puncture site, warm soaks are applied to the area to ease discomfort.
- You may resume your normal diet.

What are the normal results?

Lactate levels range from 0.93 to 1.65 milliequivalents of lactate per liter of blood. Pyruvate levels range from 0.08 to 0.16 milliequivalent per liter. Normally, the lactate to pyruvate ratio is less than 10 to 1.

What do abnormal results mean?

Elevated lactate levels are usually associated with low oxygen levels in tissues and may be caused by strenuous muscle exercise, shock, hemorrhage, septicemia, heart attack, pulmonary embolism, and cardiac arrest.

Increased lactate levels may also be caused by disorders such as diabetes, leukemias and lymphomas, liver disease, or kidney failure, or from enzyme-based defects such as Von Gierke's disease.

Lactic acidosis can occur when large doses of Tylenol (or other acetaminophen-containing drugs) or alcohol are consumed.

VITAMINS

FOLIC ACID

This test is used to measure the amount of folic acid in a blood sample. It's often performed with a test for vitamin B_{12} levels. Like vitamin B_{12}, folic acid influences red blood cell production, overall body growth, and the formation of genes, which carry the genetic information in cells. Folic acid is also called *pteroylglutamic acid, folacin,* or *folate.*

Normally, a person's diet supplies folic acid from liver, kidney, yeast, fruits, leafy vegetables, eggs, and milk. Eating too little of these foods may cause a deficiency, especially during pregnancy. This test is called for when certain blood disorders are suspected.

Foods that contain folic acid include liver, kidney, yeast, fruits, leafy vegetables, eggs, and milk. Eating too little of these foods may cause a deficiency, especially during pregnancy.

Why is this test done?
Folic acid levels may be measured for the following reasons:
- To determine the folic acid level in the blood
- To help diagnose anemia from folic acid or vitamin B_{12} deficiency
- To assess folic acid stores in pregnancy.

What should you know before the test?
- You'll be instructed to fast overnight before this test.
- This test requires a blood sample, which takes less than 3 minutes to collect. You may experience slight discomfort from the needle puncture and tourniquet pressure while the sample is drawn.
- The doctor or nurse will review your medication history to see if you are taking drugs that may affect test results, such as phenytoin or pyrimethamine. When possible, such medications will be withheld. If they can't be withheld, the lab will be notified.

What happens during the test?
A nurse or medical technician inserts a needle into a vein, usually in your forearm. A blood sample is collected in a tube, which is then sent to a lab for testing.

What happens after the test?

▪ If swelling develops at the needle puncture site, warm soaks will be applied to the area to ease discomfort.

▪ You may resume taking medications that were discontinued before the test.

What are the normal results?

Normal levels range from 3 to 16 nanograms of folic acid per milliliter of blood.

What do abnormal results mean?

Levels of folic acid in the blood below 2 nanograms per milliliter may indicate blood-related abnormalities, such as anemia, decreased white blood cell count, and decreased platelet count. Low folic acid levels can also be caused by metabolism problems, inadequate dietary intake, chronic alcoholism, poor absorption, or pregnancy.

Levels greater than 20 nanograms per milliliter may indicate excessive dietary intake of folic acid or folic acid supplements. Even when taken in large doses, this vitamin is nontoxic.

VITAMIN A AND CAROTENE

This test measures the amount of vitamin A — which is also called *retinol* — in the blood. Vitamin A, a fat-soluble vitamin, is derived from carotene, a substance that's found in leafy green vegetables and yellow fruits and vegetables. In a person's diet, vitamin A also is found in eggs, poultry, meat, and fish. Vitamin A is important for reproduction, bone growth, vision — especially night vision — and for forming the *epithelium,* or cells that cover and protect various organs and body parts. (See *Fat-soluble vitamins,* page 414.)

Why is this test done?

Vitamin A and carotene tests may be performed for the following reasons:

▪ To measure the level of vitamin A in the blood and to investigate suspected vitamin A deficiency or toxicity

▪ To diagnose visual disturbances, especially night blindness and a drying condition of the eyes called *xerophthalmia*

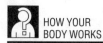

HOW YOUR BODY WORKS

Fat-soluble vitamins

Vitamins are classified as either fat soluble or water soluble. Fat-soluble vitamins — which include vitamins A, D, E, and K — are absorbed with the fats in certain foods.

Vital but toxic too

Although these vitamins are necessary for survival, excessive or prolonged intake of most fat-soluble vitamins — especially in doses that exceed the recommended daily amounts — can have toxic effects. That's because the body stores these vitamins and does not readily excrete them.

Functions unclear

Fat-soluble vitamins have different functions that are only partially understood: Vitamin A helps to maintain night vision and cell health; vitamin D regulates the body's use of calcium and phosphorus, which are important for healthy bones; vitamin E is associated with several production processes in the body; and vitamin K is necessary for proper blood clotting.

- To diagnose some skin diseases
- To screen for poor vitamin absorption.

What should you know before the test?

- You should fast overnight before the test, but you may drink water.
- This test requires a blood sample, which takes less than 3 minutes to collect. You may experience slight discomfort from the needle puncture and tourniquet pressure while the sample is drawn.

What happens during the test?

A nurse or medical technician inserts a needle into a vein, usually in your forearm. A blood sample is collected in a tube, which is then sent to a lab for testing.

What happens after the test?

- If swelling develops at the needle puncture site, warm soaks will be applied to the area to ease discomfort.
- You may resume your usual diet.

What are the normal results?

Normal levels differ according to age and sex. For children, the range of levels is 30 to 80 micrograms of vitamin A per deciliter of blood. For adults, it is 30 to 65 micrograms per deciliter. Levels for men are usually 20% higher.

What do abnormal results mean?

Low levels of vitamin A — a condition called *hypovitaminosis A* — may indicate impaired fat absorption from various conditions such as infectious hepatitis. Low levels are also associated with a form of malnutrition known as *protein-calorie malnutrition*. Similar decreases in vitamin A levels may also be caused by chronic kidney inflammation.

High vitamin A levels — called *hypervitaminosis A* — usually indicate excessive intake of vitamin A supplements or of foods high in vitamin A. Increased levels are also associated with uncontrolled diabetes.

Low carotene levels may indicate impaired fat absorption or, rarely, insufficient carotene in the diet. Carotene levels may also be suppressed during pregnancy. Elevated carotene levels indicate excessive dietary intake of this nutrient.

Vitamin B₂

This test is used to evaluate the amount of vitamin B_2 — or riboflavin — in the blood. Vitamin B_2 is essential for a person's growth and tissue activity. This test is more reliable than a urine vitamin B_2 test. (See *Water-soluble vitamins.*)

Why is this test done?
Vitamin B_2 testing may be performed for the following reasons:
- To evaluate vitamin B_2 levels
- To detect vitamin B_2 deficiency.

What should you know before the test?
- Maintain a normal diet before the test.
- This test requires a blood sample, which takes less than 3 minutes to collect.
- You may experience slight discomfort from the needle puncture and tourniquet pressure.

What happens during the test?
A nurse or medical technician inserts a needle into a vein, usually in your forearm. A blood sample is collected in a tube, which is then sent to a lab for testing.

What happens after the test?
- If swelling develops at the needle puncture site, warm soaks will be applied to the area to ease discomfort.
- If a deficiency is detected, you should know that good dietary sources of vitamin B_2 are milk products, liver and kidneys, fish, green leafy vegetables, and legumes.

What are the normal results?
Normal levels are 3 to 5 micrograms of vitamin B_2 per deciliter of blood.

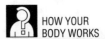
HOW YOUR
BODY WORKS

Water-soluble vitamins

Vitamins are classified as either fat soluble or water soluble. Water-soluble vitamins include vitamin C and the B complex vitamins. Vitamin C is necessary for making some proteins and for maintaining healthy bone and cartilage.

B complex vitamins
- Vitamin B_1, called thiamine, prevents the disease beriberi and plays a role in energy metabolism.
- Vitamin B_2 is essential for growth and tissue function.
- Vitamin B_6, or pyridoxine, is essential to protein metabolism and contributes to cell growth and blood formation.
- Vitamin B_{12} is essential for red blood cell production.

What do abnormal results mean?

Test results below 3 micrograms per deciliter indicate vitamin B_2 deficiency. This can be caused by insufficient dietary intake of vitamin B_2, poor absorption of nutrients, or conditions that increase metabolic demands, such as stress.

VITAMIN B_{12}

This test is used to measure the amount of vitamin B_{12} in the blood. Vitamin B_{12} is also called *cyanocobalamin, antipernicious anemia factor,* or *extrinsic factor.* The test for vitamin B_{12} is often performed with a test for folic acid levels.

Vitamin B_{12} is essential to red blood cell production, nervous system health, and the formation of genes, which carry the genetic information in cells. This vitamin is found almost exclusively in animal products, such as meat, shellfish, milk, and eggs. (See *Vitamin B_{12} absorption.*)

Why is this test done?

Vitamin B_{12} testing may be performed for the following reasons:
- To determine the amount of vitamin B_{12} in the blood
- To help diagnose anemia and determine whether it's due to vitamin B_{12} or folic acid deficiency
- To help diagnose some central nervous system disorders.

What should you know before the test?

- If your folic acid level is also being measured, you'll be instructed to fast overnight before the test.
- This test requires a blood sample, which takes less than 3 minutes to collect. You may experience slight discomfort from the needle puncture and tourniquet pressure.
- Your medication history will be checked for the use of drugs — such as para-aminosalicylic acid, phenytoin, neomycin, and colchicine — that may alter test results. These drugs may be withheld before the test. If they can't be withheld, the lab will be notified.

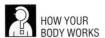

HOW YOUR
BODY WORKS

Vitamin B$_{12}$ absorption

As vitamin B$_{12}$ is metabolized, it's absorbed at many locations in the body where it's used to produce red blood cells and support nervous system function.

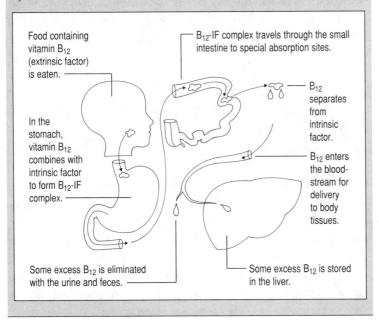

Food containing vitamin B$_{12}$ (extrinsic factor) is eaten.

In the stomach, vitamin B$_{12}$ combines with intrinsic factor to form B$_{12}$-IF complex.

B$_{12}$-IF complex travels through the small intestine to special absorption sites.

B$_{12}$ separates from intrinsic factor.

B$_{12}$ enters the blood-stream for delivery to body tissues.

Some excess B$_{12}$ is eliminated with the urine and feces.

Some excess B$_{12}$ is stored in the liver.

What happens during the test?

A nurse or medical technician inserts a needle into a vein, usually in your forearm. A blood sample is collected in a tube, which is then sent to a lab for testing.

What happens after the test?

▪ If swelling develops at the needle puncture site, warm soaks will be applied to the area to ease discomfort.
▪ You may resume your usual diet.

What are the normal results?

Normal levels range from 100 to 700 picograms of vitamin B$_{12}$ per milliliter of blood.

What do abnormal results mean?

Low levels of this vitamin in the blood may indicate inadequate dietary intake, especially in strict vegetarians. Low levels are also associated with poor absorption of nutrients by the intestine, as occurs with celiac disease, poor absorption of vitamin B_{12} alone, conditions of increased metabolism such as an overactive thyroid, pregnancy, and central nervous system damage.

High levels of vitamin B_{12} may be caused by excessive dietary intake; liver disease, such as cirrhosis or acute or chronic hepatitis; and conditions known as *myeloproliferative disorders,* including some leukemias.

VITAMIN C

This test is used to measure levels of vitamin C, or ascorbic acid, in a blood sample. Vitamin C is needed to maintain healthy cartilage and bone. It also promotes iron absorption, influences folic acid metabolism, and may be necessary for withstanding the stresses of injury and infection.

This vitamin is present in generous amounts in citrus fruits, berries, tomatoes, raw cabbage, green peppers, and green leafy vegetables. Severe vitamin C deficiency, also called *scurvy,* causes fragility of tiny blood vessels, joint abnormalities, and various other symptoms.

Why is this test done?

Vitamin C testing may be performed for the following reasons:
- To detect the amount of vitamin C in the blood
- To aid diagnosis of scurvy, scurvy-like conditions, and disorders such as malnutrition and poor nutrient absorption.

What should you know before the test?

- You'll be instructed to fast overnight before the test.
- This test requires a blood sample, which takes less than 3 minutes to collect.
- You may experience slight discomfort from the needle puncture and tourniquet pressure.

Megadoses of vitamin C: Miracle cure or dangerous myth?

In the early 1970s, Nobel Laureate Linus Pauling sparked interest in vitamin C when he suggested that megadoses of this vitamin may increase a person's resistance to infections and cancer and lower blood cholesterol levels. Pauling recommended daily doses of vitamin C that are two to five times the recommended amount — 60 milligrams daily for adults — and much higher doses during times of stress or illness. He especially advocated very high doses to treat cancer and to relieve common cold symptoms.

Outcome of recent research
To date, research hasn't supported Pauling's theories. In fact, a recent study has shown that high-dose vitamin C is no more effective than a placebo, or fake pill, in the treatment of cancer. Other studies have shown that high-dose vitamin C has little or no effect on the severity of colds. But despite this, many people supplement their diets with high doses of vitamin C. And, in addition to delaying proper treatment, some of them experience severe side effects.

Dangers of vitamin C overload
The most common side effects of excessive vitamin C are diarrhea and vomiting. However, in some people, high-doses of vitamin C may trigger or intensify gout and lead to the formation of kidney stones. Vitamin C also promotes iron absorption, which may lead to iron toxicity. If a person is receiving drug therapy, high doses of vitamin C may also interfere with the way medications work.

What happens during the test?

A nurse or medical technician inserts a needle into a vein, usually in your forearm. A blood sample is collected in a tube, which is then sent to a lab for testing.

What happens after the test?

- If swelling develops at the needle puncture site, warm soaks will be applied to the area to ease discomfort.
- You may resume your usual diet.

What are the normal results?

Normally, 0.3 milligram or more of vitamin C per deciliter of blood is acceptable.

What do abnormal results mean?

People with levels of 0.2 to 0.29 milligram of vitamin C per deciliter are considered "at risk." Levels under 0.2 milligram per deciliter indicate vitamin C deficiency. Vitamin C levels diminish during pregnancy to a low point immediately after giving birth. Depressed levels occur with infection, fever, and anemia. Severe deficiencies result in scurvy.

High levels occur when vitamin C is consumed. Excess vitamin C is normally excreted in the urine, but excessive concentrations can cause urinary problems. (See *Megadoses of vitamin C: Miracle cure or dangerous myth?* page 419.)

VITAMIN D₃

Also called *cholecalciferol*, vitamin D_3 is important for bone growth and overall health. It's produced in the skin by the sun's ultraviolet rays. It also occurs naturally in fish liver oils, egg yolks, liver, and butter.

To become active, vitamin D is converted to a substance called *25-hydroxycholecalciferol*. This test is performed to determine the amount of 25-hydroxycholecalciferol in the blood.

Why is this test done?
Vitamin D_3 tests may be performed for the following reasons:
- To measure vitamin D in the body
- To evaluate skeletal diseases, such as rickets
- To help diagnose a condition called *hypercalcemia*, or excessive calcium in the blood
- To detect vitamin D toxicity
- To monitor therapy with vitamin D_3.

What should you know before the test?
- You don't have to restrict food or fluids before this test.
- The test requires a blood sample, which takes less than 3 minutes to collect. You may experience slight discomfort from the needle puncture and tourniquet pressure while the sample is drawn.
- The doctor or nurse will check your medication history for use of drugs that could alter test results, such as corticosteroids or anticonvulsants. If possible, these drugs are withheld. If they cannot be withheld, the lab will be notified.

Vitamin D deficiency can cause a condition known as rickets, or bone softening.

What happens during the test?
A nurse or medical technician inserts a needle into a vein, usually in your forearm. A blood sample is collected in a tube, which is then sent to a lab for testing.

What happens after the test?

- If swelling develops at the needle puncture site, warm soaks will be applied to the area to ease discomfort.
- You may resume taking medications that were discontinued before the test.

What are the normal results?

In summer, the range for the active form of vitamin D is from 15 to 80 nanograms of 25-hydroxycholecalciferol per milliliter of blood. In winter, it's 14 to 42 nanograms per milliliter.

What do abnormal results mean?

Low or undetectable levels may be caused by vitamin D deficiency, which can cause a condition known as *rickets,* or bone softening. A deficiency may be caused by a poor diet, decreased exposure to the sun, or impaired absorption of vitamin D from liver disease, pancreatitis, celiac disease, cystic fibrosis, or surgery that removes part of the stomach or small bowel.

Levels over 100 nanograms per milliliter may indicate excessive self-medication or prolonged vitamin therapy. Elevated levels with excess calcium in the blood may be due to hypersensitivity to vitamin D.

TRACE ELEMENTS

MANGANESE

This test measures the amount of manganese in a blood sample. Manganese is a trace element, meaning extremely small amounts of it are present in the body. Although its function is only partially understood, manganese is known to activate several substances called *enzymes* that are essential to a person's metabolism. Dietary sources of manganese include unrefined cereals, green leafy vegetables, and nuts.

Manganese toxicity may be caused by inhaling manganese dust or fumes — a hazard in the steel and dry-cell battery industries — or from drinking contaminated water.

Why is this test done?

Manganese tests may be performed for the following reasons:
- To determine the level of manganese in the blood
- To detect manganese toxicity.

What should you know before the test?

- You don't need to restrict your diet before this test.
- The test requires a blood sample, which takes less than 3 minutes to collect. You may experience slight discomfort from the needle puncture and tourniquet pressure as the sample is drawn.
- The doctor or nurse will check your medication history for use of drugs that may influence test results, such as estrogens and glucocorticoids. When possible, such drugs will be withheld before the test. If they cannot be withheld, the lab will be notified.

What happens during the test?

A nurse or medical technician inserts a needle into a vein, usually in your forearm. A blood sample is collected in a tube, which is then sent to a lab for testing.

What happens after the test?

- If swelling develops at the needle puncture site, warm soaks will be applied to the area to ease discomfort.
- You may resume taking medications that were discontinued before the test.

What are the normal results?

Normal levels for this nutrient range from 0.04 to 1.4 micrograms of manganese per deciliter of blood.

What do abnormal results mean?

Extremely high levels indicate manganese toxicity, which requires prompt medical attention to prevent central nervous system deterioration. Low manganese levels may indicate insufficient dietary intake, although deficiency hasn't been linked to disease.

ZINC

This test measures the amount of zinc in the blood. Extremely small amounts of zinc are present in the body, but it plays a critical role in maintaining good health. Zinc deficiency — called *hypozincemia* — can seriously impair a person's metabolism, growth, and development.

Zinc occurs naturally in water and in most foods. High concentrations are found in meat, seafood, dairy products, whole grains, nuts, and legumes.

Why is this test done?

Zinc testing may be performed for the following reasons:
- To determine the concentration of zinc in the blood
- To detect zinc deficiency or toxicity.

What should you know before the test?

- You don't need to change or restrict your diet before this test.
- This test requires a blood sample, which takes less than 3 minutes to collect. You may experience slight discomfort from the needle puncture and tourniquet pressure while the sample is drawn.
- The doctor or nurse will check your drug history for use of medications — such as zinc-chelating agents and corticosteroids — that may interfere with the test results. When possible, such drugs will be withheld before the test. If they cannot be withheld, the lab will be notified.

What happens during the test?

A nurse or medical technician inserts a needle into a vein, usually in your forearm. A blood sample is collected in a tube, which is then sent to a lab for testing.

What happens after the test?

- If swelling develops at the needle puncture site, warm soaks will be applied to the area to ease discomfort.
- You may resume taking medications that were discontinued before the test.

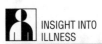

INSIGHT INTO ILLNESS

Toxic zinc exposure: 14 high-risk jobs

Approximately 50,000 industrial workers are at risk for toxic exposure to zinc oxide. Overexposure can be caused by inhaling dust or fumes in the following industries and occupations:
- Alloy manufacturing
- Brass foundry work
- Bronze foundry work
- Electric fuse manufacturing
- Gas welding
- Electroplating
- Galvanizing
- Junk metal refining
- Paint manufacturing
- Metal cutting
- Metal spraying
- Rubber manufacturing
- Roof making

What are the normal results?

Normal levels range from 70 to 150 micrograms of zinc per deciliter of blood.

What do abnormal results mean?

Levels below 70 micrograms per deciliter indicate zinc deficiency. Low levels may be due to insufficient dietary intake, an underlying disease, or a hereditary deficiency. Markedly depressed levels are common in people with leukemia. Low zinc levels are common in persons with alcoholic cirrhosis of the liver, heart attack, ileitis, chronic kidney failure, rheumatoid arthritis, and some anemias.

Elevated and potentially toxic zinc levels may be caused by accidental ingestion or exposure while working at an industrial site. (See *Toxic zinc exposure: 14 high-risk jobs*, page 423.)

12

HORMONE TESTS:
Tracking the Body's Messengers

PITUITARY HORMONES

CORTICOTROPIN

This test measures the amount of corticotropin in a blood sample. Corticotropin is a hormone, a chemical that's secreted by the pituitary gland in the brain. This hormone affects the activity of another gland in the body, the adrenal gland, and causes it to secrete steroid hormones. Corticotropin also may be called *adrenocorticotropic hormone*.

This test may be ordered for people with signs of adrenal insufficiency, which means that their adrenal gland is not functioning adequately. It also may be ordered for a person with signs of Cushing's syndrome, which occurs when the adrenal gland secretes too much of its hormones. (See *Where do hormones come from?* page 428.)

Why is this test done?

Corticotropin levels may be measured for the following reasons:
- To determine if hormonal secretion is normal
- To help diagnose deficient activity by the adrenal gland
- To diagnose Cushing's syndrome.

What should you know before the test?

- A low-carbohydrate diet is generally recommended for 2 days before the test. This requirement may vary, depending on the lab. In addition, you must fast and limit your physical activity for 10 to 12 hours before the test.
- The test requires a blood sample, which takes less than 3 minutes to collect. While the sample is being drawn, you may experience slight discomfort from the needle puncture and tourniquet pressure.
- The lab needs up to 4 days to complete the analysis.
- The doctor or nurse will ask if you take any medications that may affect test results, such as corticosteroids, estrogens, amphetamines, spironolactone, calcium gluconate, or alcohol. Usually, these drugs are withheld for 48 hours or longer before the test.

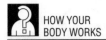

HOW YOUR
BODY WORKS

Where do hormones come from?

Different glands throughout the body store and secrete hormones, allowing these powerful, complex chemicals to circulate through the bloodstream. Hormones both stimulate and inhibit the activity of specific glands or organs. The glands and organs, in turn, also secrete hormones that maintain chemical balance in the body. This illustration shows the body's glands and the hormones they secrete.

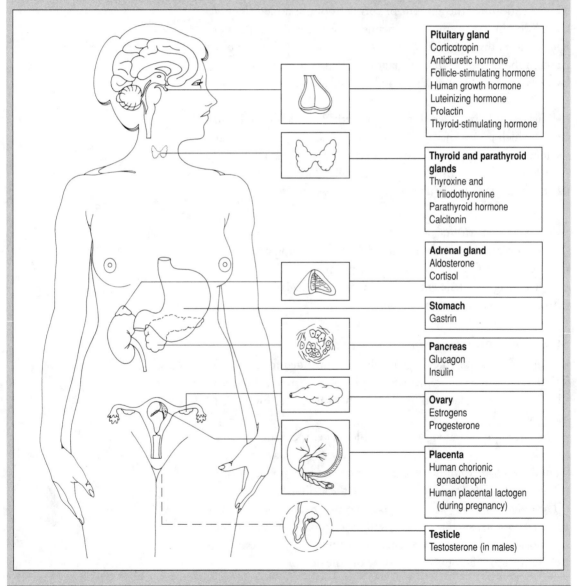

Pituitary gland
Corticotropin
Antidiuretic hormone
Follicle-stimulating hormone
Human growth hormone
Luteinizing hormone
Prolactin
Thyroid-stimulating hormone

Thyroid and parathyroid glands
Thyroxine and
  triiodothyronine
Parathyroid hormone
Calcitonin

Adrenal gland
Aldosterone
Cortisol

Stomach
Gastrin

Pancreas
Glucagon
Insulin

Ovary
Estrogens
Progesterone

Placenta
Human chorionic
  gonadotropin
Human placental lactogen
  (during pregnancy)

Testicle
Testosterone (in males)

What happens during the test?

- If the doctor suspects you're experiencing adrenal hypofunction (inadequate adrenal gland activity), a blood sample is collected between 6 a.m. and 8 a.m.
- If the doctor suspects you're experiencing Cushing's syndrome, a blood sample is collected between 6 p.m. and 11 p.m., which is the time of lowest hormonal secretion.
- A nurse or medical technician inserts a needle into a vein, usually in your forearm. A blood sample is collected in a tube, which is then sent to a lab for testing.

What happens after the test?

- If swelling develops at the needle puncture site, warm soaks are applied to the area to ease discomfort.
- You may resume your usual diet and medications.

What are the normal results?

The Mayo Clinic sets baseline values at less than 60 picograms of corticotropin per milliliter of blood, but these values may vary, depending on the lab.

What do abnormal results mean?

The doctor interprets the test results in light of the person's signs and symptoms.

Suspected adrenal insufficiency

A higher-than-normal corticotropin level may indicate primary adrenal insufficiency, or Addison's disease. A low-normal corticotropin level suggests secondary adrenal insufficiency resulting from pituitary or hypothalamic dysfunction.

Suspected adrenal hyperfunction

An elevated corticotropin level that remains continuously high for several days suggests Cushing's disease. Moderately elevated corticotropin levels suggest pituitary-dependent adrenal hyperplasia or nonadrenal tumors such as oat cell carcinoma of the lungs.

A low-normal corticotropin level implies adrenal hyperfunction (overactivity) caused by an adrenocortical tumor or hyperplasia.

RAPID CORTICOTROPIN TEST

This is the most effective test for evaluating adrenal hypofunction, or inadequate adrenal gland activity. It may also be called the *rapid adrenocorticotropic hormone test* or the *cosyntropin test*.

In this test, baseline levels of cortisol are compared to levels of the hormone after an injection of cosyntropin, a synthetic form of corticotropin. A definitively high morning cortisol level rules out adrenal hypofunction and makes further testing unnecessary.

Why is this test done?

The rapid corticotropin test may be performed for any of the following reasons:
- To determine if your condition is due to a hormonal deficiency
- To determine if a problem with the functioning of the adrenal gland is primary hypofunction (originating from within the gland itself) or secondary hypofunction (originating from elsewhere in the body).

What should you know before the test?

- You may be required to fast for 10 to 12 hours before the test, and you must be relaxed and resting quietly for 30 minutes before the test.
- The test takes at least 1 hour to perform; three blood samples are taken and an injection is given.
- You may experience slight discomfort from the needle punctures and tourniquet pressure when the blood samples are drawn.
- You'll be instructed to refrain from taking corticotropin and all steroid medications before the test. If such drugs must be continued, the lab must be notified.

What happens during the test?

- A nurse or medical technician inserts a needle into a vein, usually in your forearm. A blood sample is collected in a tube, which is then sent to a lab for testing. This is used to determine your preinjection, or baseline, cortisol level.
- Cosyntropin is injected into a vein or muscle.

- Blood samples are collected 30 and 60 minutes after the cosyntropin injection.

What happens after the test?

- If swelling develops at the needle puncture sites, warm soaks are applied to the area to ease discomfort.
- You're observed for signs of a rare allergic reaction to cosyntropin, such as hives and itching, or an irregular heartbeat.
- You may resume your usual diet.
- Resume taking medications that were discontinued before the test.

What are the normal results?

Normally, cortisol levels rise 7 micrograms per deciliter of blood or more above the baseline value, to a peak of 18 micrograms per deciliter or more 60 minutes after the cosyntropin injection. Generally, a doubling of the baseline value indicates a normal response. A normal result means that the person does not have adrenal insufficiency.

What do abnormal results mean?

In people with primary adrenal hypofunction, cortisol levels remain low. However, if test results show below-normal increases in cortisol, further testing may be needed to distinguish between primary and secondary adrenal hypofunction.

GROWTH HORMONE

Human growth hormone is also called *somatotrophic hormone*. A protein secreted by the pituitary gland, it's the primary regulator of human growth. Unlike other pituitary hormones, human growth hormone has no single target gland; it affects many body tissues. Hypersecretion (overabundance) or hyposecretion (inadequacy) of this hormone may cause conditions such as dwarfism or gigantism. Altered human growth hormone levels are common in people with pituitary problems.

Why is this test done?

Human growth hormone levels may be measured for the following reasons:

- To help determine the cause of abnormal growth
- To distinguish dwarfism from other diagnoses; retarded growth in children also can be caused by pituitary or thyroid hypofunction
- To confirm a diagnosis of gigantism (abnormal height) or acromegaly (abnormal enlargement of the hands, feet, nose, and jaw)
- To aid diagnosis of pituitary or hypothalamic tumors
- To help evaluate human growth hormone therapy.

What should you know before the test?

- You'll be instructed to fast and to limit your physical activity for 10 to 12 hours before the test.
- This test requires a blood sample, which takes less than 3 minutes to collect. The lab requires at least 2 days for analysis. You may experience slight discomfort from the needle puncture and tourniquet pressure while the sample is being drawn.
- Another blood sample may have to be drawn the following day for comparison.
- The doctor or nurse will check your medication history for medications that affect human growth hormone levels, such as pituitary-based steroids. Usually, such medications are withheld before the test.
- You should relax and lie down for 30 minutes before the test; stress and physical activity elevate human growth hormone levels.

What happens during the test?

A nurse or medical technician inserts a needle into a vein, usually in your forearm. A blood sample is collected in a tube, which is then sent to a lab for testing.

What happens after the test?

- If swelling develops at the needle puncture site, warm soaks are applied to the area to ease discomfort.
- You may resume your usual diet.
- Resume taking medications that were discontinued before the test.

What are the normal results?

Normal human growth hormone levels for men range from undetectable to 5 nanograms of this hormone per milliliter of blood; for

> *Human growth hormone is the primary regulator of human growth. Unlike other pituitary hormones, it has no single target gland; it affects many body tissues.*

women, from undetectable to 10 nanograms per milliliter. Higher values in women are due to estrogen effects. Children generally have higher human growth hormone levels, ranging from undetectable to 16 nanograms per milliliter.

What do abnormal results mean?

Increased human growth hormone levels may indicate a pituitary or hypothalamic tumor that causes gigantism in children and acromegaly in adults and adolescents. People with diabetes sometimes have elevated human growth hormone levels without acromegaly. Growth hormone suppression testing is necessary to confirm a diagnosis.

Pituitary infarction, tumors, or cancer that has spread from another part of the body may reduce human growth hormone levels. Dwarfism may be due to low human growth hormone levels, although only 15% of all cases of growth failure are related to endocrine dysfunction. Confirmation of the diagnosis requires other lab tests.

GROWTH HORMONE SUPPRESSION TEST

This test is used to evaluate excessive amounts of human growth hormone from the pituitary gland. It may also be called the *glucose loading test*.

Normally, glucose — in the form of a sugary solution you drink during the test — should suppress the hormone's secretion. In a person with excessively high levels, failure of the glucose to suppress the secretion of growth hormone indicates a pituitary problem. This result confirms a diagnosis of acromegaly (abnormal enlargement of the hands, feet, nose, and jaw) or gigantism (abnormal height).

Why is this test done?

The growth hormone suppression test may be performed for any of the following reasons:
- To determine the cause of abnormal growth
- To assess elevated human growth hormone levels
- To confirm a diagnosis of gigantism in children and acromegaly in adults.

What should you know before the test?

▪ This test takes about 1 hour to complete, but the lab requires at least another 2 days to complete its analysis.

▪ You'll be instructed to fast and to limit your physical activity for 10 to 12 hours before the test; you may be asked to relax and lie down for 30 minutes immediately before the test.

▪ A nurse or technician checks your medication history. Usually, all steroids — including estrogens and progestogens — and other pituitary-based hormones are withheld before the test.

▪ When testing begins, you must drink a sugary solution. You may experience some nausea after drinking the solution.

▪ This test also requires two blood samples, each of which takes less than 3 minutes to collect. While the samples are being drawn, you may experience slight discomfort from the needle puncture and tourniquet pressure.

What happens during the test?

▪ A nurse or medical technician inserts a needle into a vein, usually in your forearm. A blood sample is collected in a tube, which is then sent to a lab for testing.

▪ You next take the sugary solution by mouth. To prevent nausea, you may drink the solution slowly.

▪ After about 2 hours, another blood sample is drawn and sent to the lab.

What happens after the test?

▪ If swelling develops at the needle puncture site, warm soaks are applied to the area to ease discomfort.

▪ You may resume your usual diet.

▪ With the doctor's permission, you may resume taking medications that were discontinued before the test.

What are the normal results?

Normally, glucose suppresses human growth hormone to levels ranging from undetectable to 3 nanograms of this hormone per milliliter of blood in 30 minutes to 2 hours. In children, rebound stimulation may occur after 2 to 5 hours.

What do abnormal results mean?

In a person with active acromegaly, baseline levels are elevated — 75 nanograms per milliliter — and aren't suppressed to less than 5 nanograms per milliliter during the test. Unchanged or increasing human growth hormone levels in response to glucose loading indicate excess secretion of human growth hormone and may confirm suspected acromegaly — abnormal enlargement of the hands, feet, nose, and jaw — or gigantism, which is abnormal height. This response may be verified by repeating the test after a 1-day rest.

INSULIN TOLERANCE TEST

This test measures blood levels of human growth hormone and corticotropin, another hormone, after administering insulin.

Insulin-induced hypoglycemia — or low blood sugar — stimulates secretion of human growth hormone and corticotropin. A failure of insulin to stimulate hormone secretion indicates poor functioning of the pituitary or adrenal gland and helps confirm insufficient human growth hormone or corticotropin.

Why is this test done?

The insulin tolerance test may be performed for the following reasons:

- To evaluate hormonal secretion
- To help the doctor diagnose human growth hormone or corticotropin deficiency
- To identify pituitary dysfunction
- To differentiate between primary and secondary adrenal hypofunction.

What should you know before the test?

- You must fast and restrict physical activity for 10 to 12 hours before the test. You may be asked to relax and lie down for 90 minutes before the test.
- The test requires intravenous administration of insulin and the collection of several blood samples.
- You may experience slight discomfort from the needle puncture and tourniquet pressure while the blood samples are drawn.

- You may experience an increased heart rate, perspiration, hunger, and anxiety after receiving the insulin. These symptoms usually pass quickly, but if they become severe, the test will be discontinued.
- The test takes about 2 hours and results are usually available in 2 days.

What happens during the test?

- A nurse or medical technician inserts a needle into a vein, usually in your forearm. Three blood samples are collected in tubes, which are then sent to a lab for testing. These provide baseline values of glucose (sugar), human growth hormone, and corticotropin in your blood.
- Insulin is then infused into your bloodstream for 1 to 2 minutes.
- Additional blood samples are collected 15, 30, 45, 60, 90, and 120 minutes after you're given the insulin. A collection device called an *indwelling venous catheter* is used so you don't have to undergo repeated needle punctures.

What happens after the test?

- If swelling develops at the needle puncture site, warm soaks are applied to the area to ease discomfort.
- You may resume your usual diet and activities.
- Resume taking medications that were discontinued before the test.

Does the test have risks?

- This test isn't recommended for people with cardiovascular or cerebrovascular disorders, epilepsy, or low baseline cortisol levels.
- There's a risk of developing a severe hypoglycemic reaction to insulin. The nurse or technician will have a concentrated sugar solution readily available should this occur.

What are the normal results?

Normally, a person's blood sugar decreases to 50% of the fasting level 20 to 30 minutes after the insulin is given. This stimulates a 10- to 20-nanogram increase over baseline values in both human growth hormone and corticotropin. Peak levels occur 60 to 90 minutes after the insulin is given.

What do abnormal results mean?

Failure of the insulin to stimulate an increase in hormone levels may indicate a problem in the hypothalamus or the pituitary or adrenal gland. An increase in human growth hormone levels of less than 10 nanograms per deciliter may indicate a human growth hormone deficiency. However, a definitive diagnosis of deficiency requires an additional test such as the arginine test. Further testing is needed to find out where the abnormality originates.

An increase in corticotropin levels of less than 10 nanograms per deciliter may indicate insufficient adrenal activity. Further testing is done to confirm and supplement the diagnosis.

ARGININE TEST

Also known as the *human growth hormone stimulation test,* this test measures the level of the hormone after an injection of arginine, a substance that normally stimulates the secretion of this hormone.

The results are used to identify dysfunction of the pituitary gland in infants and children with growth retardation and to confirm human growth hormone deficiency.

Why is this test done?
The arginine test may be performed for the following reasons:
- To identify human growth hormone deficiency
- To aid the diagnosis of pituitary tumors
- To confirm human growth hormone deficiency in infants and children with low baseline levels.

What should you know before the test?
- You must fast and limit physical activity for 10 to 12 hours before the test.
- This test requires intravenous infusion of a drug and collection of several blood samples. It takes at least 2 hours to perform; results will be available in 2 days.
- You may experience slight discomfort from the needle puncture and tourniquet pressure while the blood samples are drawn.
- Before the test, the doctor or nurse will check your medication history. Usually, steroid medications, including pituitary-based hormones, are withheld before the test.

- Because human growth hormone levels might increase after exercise or excitement, you should relax and lie down for at least 90 minutes before the test.

What happens during the test?

- A nurse or medical technician inserts a needle into a vein, usually in your forearm. A blood sample is collected in a tube, which is then sent to a lab for testing.
- Arginine is provided intravenously for 30 minutes. A device called an *indwelling venous catheter* is used to avoid repeated needle punctures; this also minimizes your stress and anxiety.
- After the arginine is given, three more blood samples are collected at 30-minute intervals.

What happens after the test?

- If swelling develops at the needle puncture site, warm soaks are applied to the area to ease discomfort.
- You may resume your usual diet.
- With the doctor's permission, you may resume taking medications that were discontinued before the test.

What are the normal results?

Arginine should raise human growth hormone levels to more than 10 nanograms of hormone per milliliter of blood in men, 15 nanograms per milliliter in women, and 48 nanograms per milliliter in children. Such an increase may appear 30 minutes after arginine infusion is discontinued or in the samples drawn 60 and 90 minutes later.

What do abnormal results mean?

Elevated fasting levels of arginine and increases that occur during sleep help rule out human growth hormone deficiency. Failure of human growth hormone levels to increase after arginine is given indicates a low reserve of pituitary human growth hormone. In children, this deficiency causes dwarfism; in adults, it can indicate panhypopituitarism. When human growth hormone levels fail to reach 10 nanograms per milliliter, retesting is required at the same time of day as the original test.

FOLLICLE-STIMULATING HORMONE

A follicle is a tiny sack that surrounds each egg in a woman's ovary. Follicle-stimulating hormone is produced in the pituitary gland and stimulates the growth and maturation of the follicles. This test measures the amounts of follicle-stimulating hormone in a blood sample. The results indicate how well the gonads (sex glands) are functioning.

This test is vital to infertility studies, and it's performed more often on women than on men. Levels of follicle-stimulating hormone in the blood fluctuate widely in women. Therefore, daily testing may be necessary for 3 to 5 days, or multiple samples may be drawn on the same day.

A test for follicle-stimulating hormone is vital to infertility studies. It's performed more often on women than on men.

Why is this test done?

The follicle-stimulating hormone test may be performed for the following reasons:

- To determine if a woman's hormonal secretion is normal
- To diagnose infertility and menstrual disorders
- To diagnose precocious puberty in girls before age 9 and in boys before age 10
- To diagnose hypogonadism (inadequate sex gland activity).

What should you know before the test?

- Your don't need to fast or limit physical activity before this test.
- This test requires a blood sample, which takes less than 3 minutes to collect. While the sample is being drawn, you may experience slight discomfort from the needle puncture and tourniquet pressure.
- The doctor or nurse will check your medication history. Drugs — including those that contain estrogens or progestogens — are usually withheld for 48 hours before the test because they may interfere with test results.
- You may be asked to relax and lie down for 30 minutes before the test.

What happens during the test?

A nurse or medical technician inserts a needle into a vein, usually in your forearm. A blood sample is collected in a tube, which is then sent to a lab for testing. The lab requires at least 3 days to complete the analysis.

What happens after the test?

- If swelling develops at the needle puncture site, warm soaks are applied to the area to ease discomfort.
- You may resume your usual diet.
- With the doctor's permission, you may resume taking medications that were discontinued before the test.

What are the normal results?

Normal results vary greatly, depending on a person's age, stage of sexual development, and — for a woman — the phase of her menstrual cycle. For women who menstruate, normal results are as follows:

- Early menstrual cycle phase: 5 to 20 micro-international units of the hormone per milliliter of blood
- Midcycle peak: 15 to 30
- Late cycle phase: 5 to 15.

Approximate values for adult men are 5 to 20 micro-international units of the hormone per milliliter of blood; for menopausal women, 50 to 100.

What do abnormal results mean?

Low follicle-stimulating hormone levels may cause male or female infertility. Low levels may be caused by anorexia nervosa, panhypopituitarism, or hypothalamic lesions.

High follicle-stimulating hormone levels in women may indicate ovarian failure associated with Turner's syndrome or Stein-Leventhal syndrome. Elevated levels may occur with precocious puberty and in postmenopausal women. In men, abnormally high follicle-stimulating hormone levels may indicate destruction of the testes from mumps or X-ray exposure, testicular failure, seminoma, or male climacteric. Absence of the gonads at birth and early-stage acromegaly (abnormal enlargement of the hands, feet, nose, and jaw) may cause follicle-stimulating hormone levels to increase in both sexes.

LUTEINIZING HORMONE

This test measures the amount of luteinizing hormone in a blood sample. In women, luteinizing hormone is secreted during the menstrual cycle. This causes ovulation and helps the body prepare for possible conception. In men, continuous luteinizing hormone secretion stimulates the testes to release testosterone, a hormone that affects sperm production.

Why is this test done?

The luteinizing hormone test may be performed for the following reasons:

- To determine if the secretion of female hormones is normal
- To detect ovulation
- To assess male or female infertility
- To evaluate amenorrhea
- To monitor therapy designed to induce ovulation.

What should you know before the test?

- You usually don't need to fast or restrict your activities before the test.
- This test requires a blood sample, which takes less than 3 minutes to collect. While the sample is being drawn, you may experience slight discomfort from the needle puncture and tourniquet pressure.
- The doctor or nurse will check your medication history before the test. Drugs that may interfere with the test results, such as steroids—including estrogens or progesterone—are usually withheld for 48 hours before the test.

What happens during the test?

A nurse or medical technician inserts a needle into a vein, usually in your forearm. A blood sample is collected in a tube, which is then sent to a lab for testing. The lab needs at least 3 days to complete the analysis.

What happens after the test?

- If swelling develops at the needle puncture site, warm soaks are applied to the area to ease discomfort.

- With the doctor's permission, you may resume taking medications that were discontinued before the test.

What are the normal results?

Normal values may have a wide range:
- Adult men: 1 to 10 international units of luteinizing hormone per liter of blood
- Adult women: values depend on the phase of a woman's menstrual cycle: During the early phase, 1 to 20 international units per liter; during ovulation, 25 to 100; after ovulation, 0.2 to 20
- Postmenopausal women: 20 to 100
- Boys before puberty: less than 0.5
- Girls before puberty: less than 0.2.

What do abnormal results mean?

In women, absence of a midcycle peak in luteinizing hormone secretion may indicate failure to ovulate. Decreased or low-normal levels may indicate poor gonadal activity; these findings are commonly associated with faulty menstruation. High luteinizing hormone levels may indicate an inborn absence of ovaries or ovarian failure associated with Stein-Leventhal syndrome, Turner's syndrome, menopause, or early-stage acromegaly (abnormal enlargement of the hands, feet, nose, and jaw).

In men, low values may indicate gonadal dysfunction of hypothalamic or pituitary origin. High values may indicate testicular failure or damaged or absent testes.

PROLACTIN

The hormone prolactin is also known as *lactogenic hormone* or *lactogen*. It's essential for the development of the mammary glands during pregnancy and for stimulating and maintaining milk production after giving birth. Prolactin is secreted in men and nonpregnant women, but its function in them is unknown. Prolactin levels increase in response to sleep and to physical or emotional stress.

In this test, the amount of prolactin in a blood sample is measured. Prolactin levels normally increase ten- to twentyfold during

The secrets of milk production during pregnancy

During pregnancy, certain hormones help prepare the breasts for lactation (milk production). Estrogen causes the breasts to grow by increasing their fat content; progesterone causes fat globule growth and alveolar duct development.

After childbirth, the mother's pituitary gland secretes prolactin, a hormone that causes the release of colostrum, a liquid nutrient that precedes the flow of milk from the breasts. Usually, within 3 days, the breasts secrete large amounts of milk rather than colostrum.

The infant's sucking stimulates nerve endings at the nipple, which allows the expression of milk from the mother's breasts. Sucking also stimulates the release of another hormone, which causes milk to flow into the alveolar ducts and the lactiferous channels.

From here, the milk is available to the infant. Because the infant's sucking stimulates both milk production and milk expression, the more the infant breast-feeds, the more milk the breast produces.

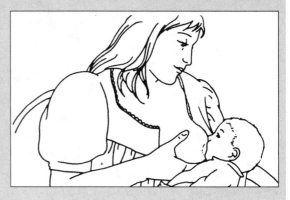

pregnancy. After delivery, prolactin secretion decreases to original levels in mothers who don't breast-feed; secretion increases during breast-feeding. This test is used when pituitary tumors are suspected. (See *The secrets of milk production during pregnancy*.)

Why is this test done?

Prolactin levels may be measured for the following reasons:
- To evaluate hormonal secretion
- To diagnose pituitary dysfunction
- To diagnose hypothalamic dysfunction regardless of cause
- To evaluate amenorrhea (failure to menstruate) and galactorrhea (excessive milk production).

What should you know before the test?

- You don't need to restrict food, fluids, or physical activities before this test; however, you may be asked to relax for about 30 minutes before the test.
- The doctor or nurse will check your medication history. Any drugs that may interfere with test results, such as alcohol, morphine, Al-

domet, estrogens, apomorphine, ergot alkaloids, and levodopa, will usually be withheld before the test.

- This test requires a blood sample, which takes less than 3 minutes to collect. While the sample is being drawn, you may experience slight discomfort from the needle puncture and tourniquet pressure.

What happens during the test?

A nurse or medical technician inserts a needle into a vein, usually in your forearm. A blood sample is collected in a tube, which is then sent to a lab for testing. The lab requires at least 4 days to complete the analysis.

What happens after the test?

- If swelling develops at the needle puncture site, warm soaks are applied to the area to ease discomfort.
- With the doctor's permission, you may resume taking medications that were discontinued before the test.

What are the normal results?

Normal values range from undetectable to 23 nanograms of prolactin per deciliter of blood in non-breast-feeding women.

What do abnormal results mean?

Abnormally high prolactin levels — 100 to 300 nanograms per milliliter — suggest Forbes-Albright syndrome. Rarely, high levels may be caused by severe endocrine disorders, such as an underactive thyroid, or some types of infertility. Additional measurements on two other occasions may be needed to diagnose slight elevations.

Decreased prolactin levels in a breast-feeding woman cause failure of milk production and may be associated with Sheehan's syndrome. Abnormally low prolactin levels have also been found occasionally with empty-sella syndrome, in which the pituitary gland is flattened and appears empty.

THYROID-STIMULATING HORMONE

Thyroid-stimulating hormone, or thyrotropin, helps increase the size, number, and activity of thyroid cells. It also stimulates the release of hormones that affect a person's metabolism and that are essential for normal growth and development.

In this test, the amount of thyroid-stimulating hormone in a blood sample is measured. The test is used to detect hypothyroidism (deficient thyroid gland activity).

Why is this test done?

Thyroid-stimulating hormone levels may be measured for the following reasons:
- To assess thyroid gland activity
- To diagnose hypothyroidism
- To help determine the cause of hypothyroidism
- To monitor drug therapy for hypothyroidism.

What should you know before the test?

- This test requires a blood sample, which takes less than 3 minutes to collect. While the sample is being drawn, you may experience slight discomfort from the needle puncture and tourniquet pressure.
- The doctor or nurse will check your drug history. Steroids, thyroid hormones, aspirin, and other drugs that may influence test results are usually discontinued before the test.
- You may be asked to relax and lie down for 30 minutes before the test.

What happens during the test?

A nurse or medical technician inserts a needle into a vein, usually in your forearm. A blood sample is collected in a tube, which is then sent to a lab for testing. The lab requires up to 2 days to complete the analysis.

What happens after the test?

- If swelling develops at the needle puncture site, warm soaks are applied to the area to ease discomfort.
- With the doctor's permission, you may resume taking medications that were discontinued before the test.

What are the normal results?

Normal results for adults and children range from undetectable to 15 micro-international units of thyroid-stimulating hormone per milliliter.

What do abnormal results mean?

Thyroid-stimulating hormone levels that exceed 20 micro-international units per milliliter of blood suggest hypothyroidism or, possibly, a goiter due to an iodine deficiency. Thyroid-stimulating hormone levels may be slightly elevated in a person with thyroid cancer whose thyroid gland functions normally.

Low or undetectable thyroid-stimulating hormone levels may be normal, but occasionally indicate hypothyroidism. Low thyroid-stimulating hormone levels also are caused by thyroiditis, and from an overactive thyroid or Graves' disease. Further testing is necessary to confirm a diagnosis.

THYROID & PARATHYROID HORMONES

THYROXINE

Thyroxine is a hormone that is secreted by the thyroid gland. Only a minute fraction of this thyroxine circulates freely in the blood. It's enough, though, to influence many functions in the body, such as metabolism, reproduction, growth, and development. (See *Step by step: The formation of thyroid hormones,* opposite, and *The thyroid gland: Creator of crucial hormones,* page 448.)

The thyroxine test is one of the most common diagnostic tools for evaluating the thyroid. It's used to measure the total circulating thyroxine level when thyroxine-binding globulin is normal. An alternative test is the Murphy-Pattee test.

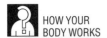

HOW YOUR BODY WORKS

Step by step: The formation of thyroid hormones

You need to eat foods containing iodine to enable your thyroid gland to manufacture its important hormones. The thyroid requires approximately 1 milligram of dietary iodine every week. These diagrams show how iodine gets the job done.

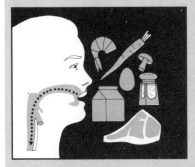

1 You ingest iodine when you eat seafoods, vegetables, eggs and dairy products, meat, and iodized salt.

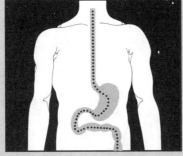

2 After digestion, the iodine contained in these foods is absorbed into the blood from the small bowel.

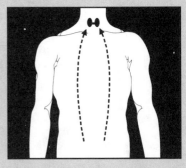

3 Iodine travels through the bloodstream and accumulates in the thyroid gland.

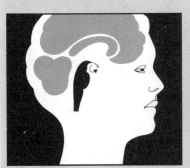

4 Meanwhile, the hypothalamus synthesizes thyrotropin-releasing hormone, which travels to the pituitary gland.

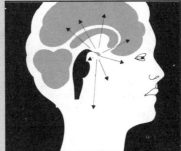

5 In the pituitary, thyrotropin-releasing hormone stimulates the production and release of thyroid-stimulating hormone.

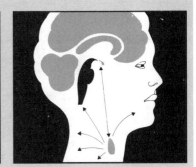

6 Thyroid-stimulating hormone then travels to the thyroid gland, where it stimulates the production of thyroxine and triiodothyronine from iodine, and triggers their release.

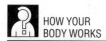

The thyroid gland: Creator of crucial hormones

The thyroid gland straddles the upper windpipe. Its three hormones — thyroxine, triiodothyronine, and calcitonin — are synthesized in colloid follicles (see inset), where the surrounding epithelial cells prepare the hormones for release into the bloodstream.

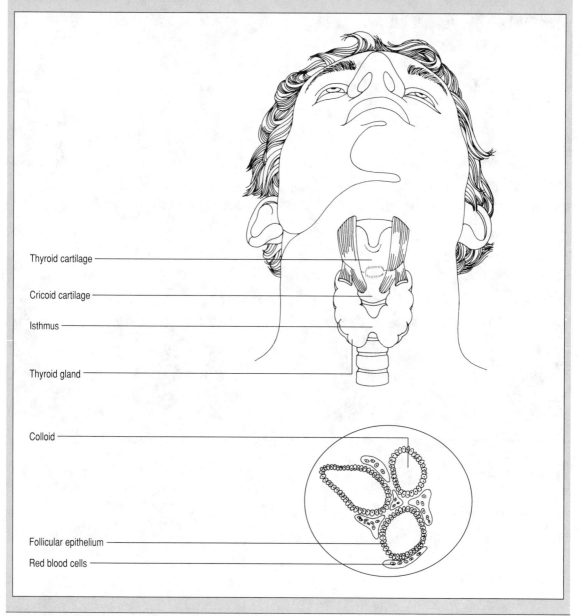

Thyroid cartilage

Cricoid cartilage

Isthmus

Thyroid gland

Colloid

Follicular epithelium

Red blood cells

Why is this test done?

Thyroxine levels may be measured for the following reasons:

- To evaluate thyroid gland activity
- To aid the diagnosis of hyperthyroidism and hypothyroidism (overactive and underactive thyroid activity)
- To monitor response to antithyroid medication in hyperthyroidism or to thyroid replacement therapy in hypothyroidism.

What should you know before the test?

- You don't need to fast or restrict your activities before this test.
- The test requires a blood sample, which takes less than 3 minutes to collect. While the sample is being drawn, you may experience slight discomfort from the needle puncture and tourniquet pressure.
- The doctor or nurse will check your medication history. Any medications that may interfere with test results will usually be withheld before the test. However, if this test is used to monitor thyroid therapy, daily thyroid supplements will be continued.

What happens during the test?

A nurse or medical technician inserts a needle into a vein, usually in your forearm. A blood sample is collected in a tube, which is then sent to a lab for testing.

What happens after the test?

- If swelling develops at the needle puncture site, warm soaks are applied to the area to ease discomfort.
- With the doctor's permission, you may resume taking medications that were discontinued before the test.

What are the normal results?

Normally, total thyroxine levels range from 5 to 13.5 micrograms of hormone per deciliter of blood.

What do abnormal results mean?

Abnormally high levels of thyroxine indicate hyperthyroidism. Subnormal levels suggest hypothyroidism, or may be due to thyroxine suppression. In doubtful cases of hypothyroidism, further hormone tests may be needed. Overt signs of hyperthyroidism likewise require further testing. Normal thyroxine levels don't necessarily indicate normal thyroid activity.

TRIIODOTHYRONINE

This test measures blood levels of triiodothyronine, a hormone secreted by the thyroid. Triiodothyronine is present in the blood in minute quantities, but it has a great impact on a person's metabolism. Results of this test are used to investigate signs of thyroid dysfunction.

Why is this test done?

Triiodothyronine levels may be measured for the following reasons:
- To evaluate thyroid gland activity and to determine the cause of certain symptoms
- To aid diagnosis of triiodothyronine toxicosis (poisoning)
- To aid diagnosis of hypothyroidism and hyperthyroidism (underactive and overactive thyroid activity)
- To monitor a person's response to thyroid replacement therapy for hypothyroidism.

What should you know before the test?

- This test requires a blood sample, which takes less than 3 minutes to collect. While the sample is being drawn, you may experience slight discomfort from the needle puncture and tourniquet pressure.
- The doctor or nurse will check your medication history. Any drugs that may influence thyroid activity, such as steroids, Inderal, and Questran, will usually be withheld before the test.

What happens during the test?

A nurse or medical technician inserts a needle into a vein, usually in your forearm. A blood sample is collected in a tube, which is then sent to a lab for testing.

What happens after the test?

- If swelling develops at the needle puncture site, warm soaks are applied to the area to ease discomfort.
- With the doctor's permission, you may resume taking medications that were discontinued before the test.

What are the normal results?

Triiodothyronine levels normally range from 90 to 230 nanograms per deciliter. These values may vary with the lab performing this test.

What do abnormal results mean?

Triiodothyronine and thyroxine levels usually rise and fall in tandem, except in triiodothyronine toxicosis, when only triiodothyronine levels rise while thyroxine levels remain normal. Triiodothyronine toxicosis occurs with Graves' disease, toxic adenoma, or toxic nodular goiter.

Triiodothyronine levels normally increase during pregnancy.

Low triiodothyronine levels may appear in people with liver or kidney disease, during severe acute illness, or after injury or major surgery. Low triiodothyronine levels sometimes also occur with malnutrition.

THYROXINE-BINDING GLOBULIN

This test measures the level of thyroxine-binding globulin in a blood sample. Thyroxine-binding globulin carries thyroxine and triiodothyronine in the bloodstream. Any condition that affects thyroxine-binding globulin levels also affects the amount of thyroxine and triiodothyronine circulating in the blood. This is significant because these hormones influence many functions in the body, such as metabolism, reproduction, growth, and development.

Why is this test done?

Thyroxine-binding globulin levels may be measured for the following reasons:
- To evaluate thyroid activity
- To supplement tests for triiodothyronine or thyroxine levels
- To identify thyroxine-binding globulin abnormalities.

What should you know before the test?

- This test requires a blood sample, which takes less than 3 minutes to collect. While the sample is being drawn, you may experience slight discomfort from the needle puncture and tourniquet pressure.

- The doctor or nurse will check your medication history. Any drugs that may interfere with the test results are withheld. These may include estrogens, anabolic steroids, Dilantin, or thyroid preparations. If these medications must be continued, the lab is notified. In some cases, the medications may be continued to determine their effect on thyroxine-binding globulin levels.

What happens during the test?

A nurse or medical technician inserts a needle into a vein, usually in your forearm. A blood sample is collected in a tube, which is then sent to a lab for testing.

What happens after the test?

- If swelling develops at the needle puncture site, warm soaks are applied to the area to ease discomfort.
- With the doctor's permission, you may resume taking medications that were discontinued before the test.

What are the normal results?

Normal values for thyroxine-binding globulin range from 10 to 26 micrograms of thyroxine per 100 milliliters of blood. When measured by a method called *radioimmunoassay*, values for thyroxine-binding globulin range from 1.3 to 2 milligrams per deciliter.

What do abnormal results mean?

High thyroxine-binding globulin levels may indicate hypothyroidism, an inherited excess, some forms of liver disease, or a condition known as acute intermittent porphyria. Thyroxine-binding globulin levels normally increase during pregnancy and are high in newborns. Suppressed levels may indicate hyperthyroidism (an overactive thyroid) or an inborn deficiency. This can occur with nephrotic syndrome, malnutrition, acute illness, surgical stress, or active acromegaly, which is abnormal enlargement of the hands, feet, nose, and jaw.

People with thyroxine-binding globulin abnormalities require additional testing to evaluate thyroid activity more precisely.

Any condition that affects thyroxine-binding globulin levels also affects hormones that influence many functions in the body, such as metabolism, reproduction, growth, and development.

TRIIODOTHYRONINE RESIN UPTAKE

This test measures thyroxine levels in the blood. A hormone produced in the thyroid gland, thyroxine influences many functions in the body, such as metabolism, reproduction, growth, and development. This test — which measures thyroxine indirectly — is used less frequently than more rapid tests for the major thyroid hormones.

Why is this test done?

Thyroxine levels may be measured for the following reasons:
- To evaluate thyroid activity
- To diagnose hypothyroidism and hyperthyroidism (deficient or excessive thyroid activity)
- To diagnose abnormal levels of thyroxine-binding globulin, a substance that carries thyroid hormones in the bloodstream.

What should you know before the test?

- This test requires a blood sample, which takes less than 3 minutes to collect. While the sample is being drawn, you may experience slight discomfort from the needle puncture and tourniquet pressure.
- The doctor or nurse will check your medication history, and drugs that may interfere with the test results are withheld. These may include estrogens, androgens, Dilantin, salicylates, or thyroid preparations.

What happens during the test?

A nurse or medical technician inserts a needle into a vein, usually in your forearm. A blood sample is collected in a tube, which is then sent to a lab for testing. The lab requires several days to complete the analysis.

What happens after the test?

- If swelling develops at the needle puncture site, warm soaks are applied to the area to ease discomfort.
- With the doctor's permission, you may resume taking medications that were discontinued before the test.

What are the normal results?

Normally, 25% to 35% of triiodothyronine in a blood sample is absorbed by, or binds to, the resin, a substance that's added to the test sample.

What do abnormal results mean?

A high resin uptake percentage with high thyroxine levels indicates hyperthyroidism. However, a low resin uptake percentage, together with low thyroxine levels, indicates hypothyroidism.

When thyroxine and triiodothyronine resin uptake values are discordant, it suggests that the person has a thyroxine-binding globulin abnormality.

LONG-ACTING THYROID STIMULATOR

This test determines whether a person's blood contains long-acting thyroid stimulator, an abnormal substance that mimics the action of thyroid-stimulating hormone but has more prolonged effects. Long-acting thyroid stimulator causes the thyroid gland to produce and secrete thyroid hormones in excessive amounts.

Why is this test done?

The long-acting thyroid stimulator test may be performed for the following reasons:
- To evaluate thyroid activity
- To confirm diagnosis of Graves' disease.

What should you know before the test?

- This test requires a blood sample, which takes less than 3 minutes to collect. While the sample is being drawn, you may experience slight discomfort from the needle puncture and tourniquet pressure.
- The doctor or nurse will check your medication history. Any drugs that may influence the test results are usually withheld before the test.

What happens during the test?

A nurse or medical technician inserts a needle into a vein, usually in your forearm. A blood sample is collected in a tube, which is then sent to a lab for testing.

What happens after the test?

- If swelling develops at the needle puncture site, warm soaks are applied to the area to ease discomfort.
- With the doctor's permission, you may resume taking medications that were discontinued before the test.

What are the normal results?

Normally, long-acting thyroid stimulator does not appear in the blood.

What do abnormal results mean?

Long-acting thyroid stimulator in a blood sample indicates Graves' disease, with or without signs of hyperthyroidism. About 80% of people with Graves' disease have detectable long-acting thyroid stimulator in their blood.

Long-acting thyroid stimulator is an abnormal substance that mimics the action of the natural hormone but has more prolonged effects.

SCREENING TEST FOR HYPOTHYROIDISM IN INFANTS

This test measures the levels of thyroxine, a thyroid hormone, in the blood of newborn infants. It's used to detect hypothyroidism (deficient thyroid activity).

Congenital hypothyroidism is characterized by low or absent levels of thyroxine at birth and affects roughly 1 in 5,000 newborns. It strikes girls three times more often than boys. If untreated, it can lead to irreversible brain damage by age 3 months. There are few signs of hypothyroidism in newborns, so most cases used to go undetected until a condition called *cretinism* became apparent or the infant died from respiratory distress.

Tests for thyroxine and thyroid-stimulating hormone are not commonly used to screen newborns, but the test is now mandatory in some states.

Why is this test done?

This test may be performed to screen newborns for hypothyroidism.

What should you know before the test?

- This test requires a small blood sample, which is taken from the infant's heel. It's performed before the infant is discharged from the hospital and again 4 to 6 weeks later.
- Another test is sometimes done before the infant is discharged to confirm results.

What happens during the test?

- The infant's heel is cleaned and then dried thoroughly with a gauze pad.
- A nurse or medical technician punctures the infant's heel with a small instrument called a lancet.
- Squeezing the heel gently, the nurse or technician blots a few drops of blood with a special type of paper.
- Gentle pressure is applied with a gauze pad to stop the bleeding at the puncture site.
- When the filter paper is dry, it's sent to the lab for testing.

Congenital hypothyroidism strikes girls three times more often than boys and can lead to irreversible brain damage by age 3 months.

What happens after the test?

- Heel punctures heal readily and require no special care.
- If results of the screening test indicate congenital hypothyroidism, additional testing is necessary to determine the cause of the disorder.
- If a diagnosis is confirmed, replacement therapy can restore normal thyroid gland activity. Such therapy is lifelong, and the dosage will increase until the adult requirement is reached.

What are the normal results?

Immediately after birth, thyroxine levels are considerably higher than normal adult levels. By the end of the first week, however, thyroxine levels decrease markedly:

- 1 to 5 days: 4.9 micrograms or less of thyroxine per deciliter of blood
- 6 to 8 days: 4.0
- 9 to 11 days: 3.5
- 12 to 120 days: 3.0

What do abnormal results mean?

Low thyroxine levels in the newborn's blood indicate a need for additional testing to clarify a diagnosis. A complete thyroid workup — including tests for triiodothyronine, thyroxine-binding globulin, and free thyroxine levels — is necessary to confirm a diagnosis of congenital hypothyroidism before treatment begins.

CALCITONIN

This test measures levels of calcitonin, a hormone that's produced by the thyroid gland. The exact role of calcitonin in the body hasn't been fully defined. However, calcitonin affects other thyroid hormones and lowers calcium levels in the blood. This test is usually performed when a form of thyroid cancer is suspected.

Why is this test done?

Calcitonin levels may be measured for the following reasons:
- To evaluate thyroid activity
- To help diagnose thyroid cancer or tumors.

What should you know before the test?

- You'll be instructed to fast overnight before the test because food may interfere with calcitonin levels.
- This test requires a blood sample, which takes less than 3 minutes to collect. While the sample is being drawn, you may experience slight discomfort from the needle puncture and tourniquet pressure.

What happens during the test?

A nurse or medical technician inserts a needle into a vein, usually in your forearm. A blood sample is collected in a tube, which is then sent to a lab for testing. The lab requires several days to complete the analysis.

What happens after the test?

If swelling develops at the needle puncture site, warm soaks are applied to the area to ease discomfort.

Calcitonin levels in the blood are usually measured when thyroid cancer is suspected.

What are the normal results?

Normal calcitonin levels are 0.155 nanograms or less per milliliter of blood in men; in women, normal levels are 0.105 or less.

Normal results after calcium is provided intravenously are:
- Men: 0.265 nanograms per milliliter of blood
- Women: 0.120.

Normal results after a substance called *pentagastrin* is given intravenously are:
- Men: 0.210 nanograms per milliliter of blood
- Women: 0.105.

What do abnormal results mean?

High calcitonin levels without low calcium levels usually indicate a form of thyroid cancer. Occasionally, high calcitonin levels may be due to certain types of lung or breast cancer.

*P*ARATHYROID HORMONE

Produced by the parathyroid glands, this hormone regulates the amount of calcium and phosphorus in the blood. The overall effect of parathyroid hormone is to raise the levels of calcium while lowering phosphorus levels.

Additional tests for measuring calcium, phosphorus, and creatinine levels along with parathyroid hormone levels are used to analyze abnormal parathyroid activity. Suppression or stimulation tests may help to confirm the findings.

Why is this test done?

Parathyroid hormone levels may be measured to evaluate parathyroid activity and disorders.

What should you know before the test?

- Because food may affect parathyroid hormone levels and interfere with the test results, you'll be instructed to fast overnight before the test.
- This test requires a blood sample, which takes less than 3 minutes to collect. While the sample is being drawn, you may experience slight discomfort from the needle puncture and tourniquet pressure.

What happens during the test?

A nurse or medical technician inserts a needle into a vein, usually in your forearm. A blood sample is collected in a tube, which is then sent to a lab for testing. The lab requires several days to complete the analysis.

What happens after the test?

- If swelling develops at the needle puncture site, warm soaks are applied to the area to ease discomfort.
- With the doctor's permission, you may resume your usual diet.

What are the normal results?

Normal parathyroid hormone levels vary, depending on the lab, and must be interpreted with calcium levels.

What do abnormal results mean?

When considered with calcium levels, abnormally high parathyroid hormone values may indicate hyperparathyroidism. Abnormally low parathyroid hormone levels may result from hypoparathyroidism and from certain malignant diseases.

ADRENAL HORMONES

ALDOSTERONE

This test measures levels of the hormone aldosterone in the blood. (See *The adrenal gland: Hormone production site*, page 460.) In the body, aldosterone helps maintain blood pressure and blood volume and regulate fluid and electrolyte balance. This test helps the doctor detect aldosteronism, a condition caused by too much aldosterone.

Why is this test done?

Aldosterone levels may be measured for the following reasons:
- To determine if a person's symptoms are due to faulty secretion of aldosterone

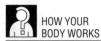

HOW YOUR
BODY WORKS

The adrenal gland: Hormone production site

In the normal human body, two adrenal glands are found — one on top of each kidney. Each adrenal gland consists of the outer cortex, which is composed of three layers, and the medulla, or central portion. The outer layer of the cortex — the zona glomerulosa — produces the hormone aldosterone. The first inner layer — the zona fasciculata — produces the hormone cortisol. The medulla stores the catecholamines, epinephrine, and norepinephrine.

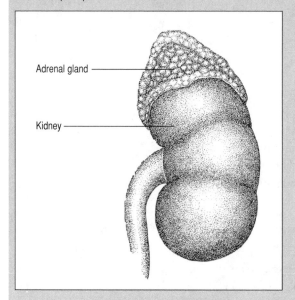

Adrenal gland

Kidney

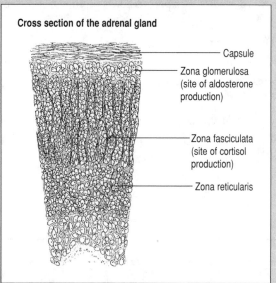

Cross section of the adrenal gland

Capsule

Zona glomerulosa
(site of aldosterone
production)

Zona fasciculata
(site of cortisol
production)

Zona reticularis

- To help diagnose aldosteronism and determine the potential causes of this disorder.

What should you know before the test?
- This test requires two blood samples, each of which takes less than 3 minutes to collect. While the sample is being drawn, you may experience slight discomfort from the needle puncture and tourniquet pressure.
- You'll be instructed to maintain a low-carbohydrate, normal-salt diet for at least 2 weeks or, preferably, for 30 days before the test.
- The doctor or nurse will check your medication history. Any drugs that alter fluid, salt, and potassium balance — especially diuretics, antihypertensives, steroids, cyclic progestational agents, and estro-

gens — will be withheld for at least 2 weeks or, preferably, for 30 days before the test.

- Any drugs that inhibit the secretion of the enzyme renin, such as propranolol, will usually be withheld for 1 week before the test.
- Avoid eating licorice for at least 2 weeks before the test.

What happens during the test?

- The first blood sample is collected while you're still in bed after a night's rest. A nurse or medical technician inserts a needle into a vein, usually in your forearm. A blood sample is collected in a tube, which is then sent to a lab for testing. The lab requires at least 10 days to complete the analysis.
- Another sample is collected 4 hours later, while you're standing and after you've been up and about, to evaluate the effect of a postural change.

What happens after the test?

- If swelling develops at the needle puncture site, warm soaks are applied to the area to ease discomfort.
- With the doctor's permission, you may resume taking medications that were discontinued before the test.
- You may resume your usual diet.

What are the normal results?

Normally, aldosterone levels in a standing, nonpregnant person range from 1 to 16 nanograms of aldosterone per deciliter of blood. However, the range for an adult man or woman who's been standing for at least 2 hours is 4 to 31 nanograms per deciliter. Values for women are variable.

What do abnormal results mean?

Excessive aldosterone secretion may indicate aldosteronism resulting from certain forms of cancer, high blood pressure, congestive heart failure, cirrhosis of the liver, pregnancy, or other conditions.

Depressed serum aldosterone levels may indicate a salt-losing syndrome, toxemia of pregnancy, Addison's disease, or aldosterone deficiency.

You'll be instructed to maintain a low-carbohydrate, normal-salt diet for at least 2 weeks or, preferably, for 30 days before the test.

CORTISOL

This hormone is secreted by the adrenal cortex, or outer layer of the adrenal gland. It helps the body use nutrients, mediate stress, and regulate the immune system. Cortisol secretion normally increases during the early morning hours and peaks around 8 a.m. It declines to very low levels in the evening and during the early phase of sleep. Intense heat or cold, infection, injury, exercise, obesity, and debilitating diseases influence cortisol secretion.

This test, which is used to measure cortisol levels in the blood, is usually ordered for people with signs of dysfunction of the adrenal gland. However, additional tests are generally required to confirm a diagnosis.

> *Cortisol is a hormone that helps the body use nutrients, mediate stress, and regulate the immune system.*

Why is this test done?
Cortisol levels may be measured for the following reasons:
- To determine if a person's symptoms are due to faulty secretion of cortisol
- To help diagnose Cushing's disease or syndrome, Addison's disease, and adrenal insufficiency.

What should you know before the test?
- You'll be instructed to maintain a normal salt diet for 3 days before the test and to fast and limit physical activity for 10 to 12 hours before the test.
- You may be asked to relax and lie down for at least 30 minutes before the test.
- This test requires a blood sample, which takes less than 3 minutes to collect. While the sample is being drawn, you may experience slight discomfort from the needle puncture and tourniquet pressure.
- The doctor or nurse will check your medication history. Any medications that may interfere with plasma cortisol levels — such as estrogens, androgens, and Dilantin — will usually be withheld for 48 hours before the test.

What happens during the test?
- A nurse or medical technician inserts a needle into a vein, usually in your forearm. A blood sample is collected in a tube, which is then

sent to a lab for testing. The lab requires at least 2 days to complete the analysis.

- Another blood sample may be collected later in the day.

What happens after the test?

- If swelling develops at the needle puncture site, warm soaks are applied to the area to ease discomfort.
- With the doctor's permission, you may resume eating your usual diet and taking medications that were discontinued before the test.

What are the normal results?

Normal cortisol levels in the blood range from 7 to 28 micrograms of this hormone per deciliter of blood in the morning and from 2 to 18 micrograms per deciliter in the afternoon. The afternoon level is usually half the morning level.

What do abnormal results mean?

High cortisol levels may indicate Cushing's disease, a rare disease of the pituitary gland, or Cushing's syndrome, which may include a cortisol excess from any cause. With Cushing's syndrome, little or no difference in values is found between morning samples and afternoon samples. Daily variations may also be absent in otherwise healthy people who are under emotional or physical stress.

Decreased cortisol levels may indicate Addison's disease. They may also be an indication of tuberculosis, fungal invasion, or hemorrhage. Low cortisol levels may also occur with impaired corticotropin secretion.

CATECHOLAMINES

This test measures catecholamines in the blood. Catecholamines are hormones, such as epinephrine, norepinephrine, and dopamine, which are secreted by the adrenal gland.

When secreted into the bloodstream, catecholamines prepare the body for the fight-or-flight reaction. They increase the heart rate, constrict blood vessels and redistribute circulating blood, activate energy reserves, and sharpen alertness. Excessive catecholamine secretion by tumors may cause high blood pressure, weight loss, sweating, headache, heart palpitations, and anxiety. (See *Fight or flight: How the body reacts to stress.*)

Catecholamine levels commonly fluctuate in response to stress, diet, smoking, kidney failure, obesity, use of certain drugs, and other conditions. If blood tests reveal high catecholamine levels, these findings must be confirmed by urine sample testing.

This test may be performed in people with high blood pressure or signs of certain adrenal tumors. It may also be performed in people with nerve-related tumors that affect endocrine activity.

Why is this test done?

Catecholamine levels may be measured for the following reasons:

- To determine if high blood pressure or other symptoms are related to improper hormonal secretion
- To rule out pheochromocytoma (a type of tumor that affects the adrenal gland) in people with high blood pressure (See *Is it high blood pressure or a rare tumor?* page 466.)
- To help identify tumors of the central nervous system, called *neuroblastomas, ganglioneuroblastomas,* and *ganglioneuromas*
- To aid diagnosis of autonomic nervous system dysfunction

Catecholamine levels commonly fluctuate in response to stress, diet, smoking, kidney failure, obesity, and use of certain drugs.

What should you know before the test?

- Be sure to strictly follow the instructions you receive before this test. You'll be asked to refrain from using self-prescribed medications, especially cold or allergy remedies, for 2 weeks before the test. You'll be instructed to eliminate certain foods and beverages — such as bananas, avocados, cheese, coffee, tea, cocoa, beer, and Chianti — for 48 hours before the test and to take vitamin C, which is necessary for the formation of catecholamines.
- Don't smoke for 24 hours before the test, and fast for 10 to 12 hours.
- This test requires one or two blood samples. You may feel some discomfort from the needle punctures, but collecting the samples takes less than 20 minutes.
- The doctor or nurse will check your medication history. Any medications that affect catecholamine levels — such as amphetamines, phenothiazines, sympathomimetics, and tricyclic antidepressants — will be withheld before the test.
- Because the stress of a needle puncture may raise catecholamine levels, a device for collecting blood called an *indwelling venous catheter* may be inserted in a vein 24 hours before the test.

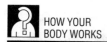 HOW YOUR BODY WORKS

Fight or flight: How the body reacts to stress

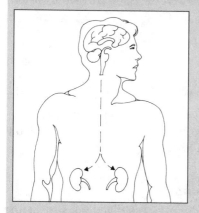

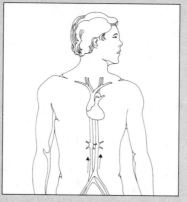

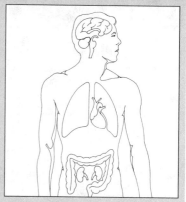

Stress — emotional or physical — causes nerve impulses to begin moving toward the adrenal gland.

Nerve impulses cause the adrenal gland to release catecholamines, primarily epinephrine and norepinephrine, into the bloodstream. This prepares the body for the fight-or-flight reaction to stress.

The fight-or-flight reaction is characterized by the following signs and symptoms:
- increased respiratory rate
- increased blood pressure, pulse rate, and cardiac output
- increased muscle strength
- increased blood supply to major organs: brain, heart, and kidneys
- decreased blood supply to skin and intestines.

- You may be asked to relax and lie down for 45 to 60 minutes before the test.
- You may be given extra blankets to keep you warm because low temperatures stimulate catecholamine secretion.

What happens during the test?

- Between 6 a.m. and 8 a.m., a nurse or medical technician collects a blood sample in a tube, which is then sent to a lab for testing. The lab requires up to 1 week to complete the analysis.
- If a second sample is required, you're asked to stand for 10 minutes before the sample is drawn.

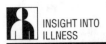

Is it high blood pressure or a rare tumor?

The clonidine suppression test is a simple method for differentiating between essential high blood pressure and pheochromocytoma, an uncommon, but potentially fatal, tumor of the adrenal gland. Both of these conditions cause elevated catecholamine levels.

This test requires the administration of clonidine, a drug used to treat high blood pressure.

How the test is performed

To undergo this test, you're first instructed to lie on a table or bed. A blood sample is drawn to obtain your baseline (pretest) catecholamine levels. Next, you receive a dose of clonidine by mouth.

Another blood sample is collected after 3 hours to measure catecholamine levels again. Finally, the test results are compared.

What results reveal

People with pheochromocytoma show no decrease in catecholamine levels after clonidine administration. In contrast, people with high blood pressure show catecholamine levels that are reduced to normal levels.

What happens after the test?

- If swelling develops at the needle puncture site, warm soaks are applied to the area to ease discomfort.
- With the doctor's permission, you may resume eating your usual foods and taking medications that were discontinued before the test.

What are the normal results?

In one type of analysis, called *fractional analysis,* catecholamine levels range as follows:

- Reclining: epinephrine, 0 to 110 picograms of this hormone per milliliter of blood; norepinephrine, 70 to 750; dopamine, 0 to 30
- Standing: epinephrine, 0 to 140 picograms per milliliter of blood; norepinephrine, 200 to 1,700; dopamine, 0 to 30.

What do abnormal results mean?

High catecholamine levels may indicate several conditions, including pheochromocytoma, neuroblastoma, ganglioneuroblastoma, or ganglioneuroma. Elevations are possible with, but do not confirm, thyroid disorders, low blood sugar, or cardiac disease. Electroshock therapy, shock resulting from hemorrhage, endotoxins, and anaphylaxis also raise catecholamine levels.

In people with normal or low morning catecholamine levels, failure to show an increase in the sample taken after standing suggests autonomic nervous system dysfunction.

ERYTHROPOIETIN

This test measures erythropoietin, a hormone that's secreted by the kidneys and that influences red blood cell production. The test results are used to evaluate anemia (deficient red blood cell production), polycythemia (increased red blood cell production), and kidney tumors. It's also used to evaluate abuse of commercially prepared erythropoietin by athletes who believe the drug enhances performance.

Why is this test done?

Erythropoietin levels may be measured for the following reasons:
- To determine if hormonal secretion is causing changes in red blood cells
- To aid the diagnosis of anemia and polycythemia
- To aid the diagnosis of kidney tumors
- To detect abuse of erythropoietin by athletes.

What should you know before the test?

- You'll be instructed to fast for 8 to 10 hours before the test. You may also be asked to relax and lie down for 30 minutes before the test.
- This test requires a blood sample, which takes less than 3 minutes to collect. While the sample is being drawn, you may experience slight discomfort from the needle puncture and tourniquet pressure.

What happens during the test?

A nurse or medical technician inserts a needle into a vein, usually in your forearm. A blood sample is collected in a tube, which is then sent to a lab for testing. The lab requires up to 4 days to complete the analysis.

What happens after the test?

If swelling develops at the needle puncture site, warm soaks are applied to the area to ease discomfort.

What are the normal results?

The reference range is up to 24 milli-international units of erythropoietin per milliliter of blood.

What do abnormal results mean?

Low levels of erythropoietin may occur in a person with anemia whose hormone production is inadequate or absent. Congenital absence of erythropoietin can occur. Severe kidney disease may decrease the production of erythropoietin.

High levels occur in anemias as the body reestablishes its hormone balance. Inappropriate elevations may be seen in polycythemia and erythropoietin-secreting tumors.

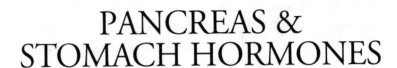

PANCREAS & STOMACH HORMONES

INSULIN

This test measures the levels of the hormone insulin in the blood. Produced in the pancreas, insulin regulates the metabolism and transport of various nutrients in the body.

Insulin secretion reaches peak levels after meals, when metabolism and food storage are greatest. This test is usually performed with tests for glucose levels because glucose, a type of sugar, stimulates insulin secretion. (See *The Pancreas: Site of insulin production.*)

Why is this test done?
Insulin levels may be measured for the following reasons:
- To determine if the pancreas is functioning normally
- To help diagnose hyperinsulinemia (excessive secretion of insulin by the pancreas) or hypoglycemia (low levels of sugar in the blood). These conditions may result from a tumor or abnormal growth of cells in the pancreas, severe liver disease, or a deficiency of substances that regulate sugar levels in the blood.
- To help diagnose diabetes.

What should you know before the test?
- You'll be instructed to fast for 10 to 12 hours before the test.
- You may be asked to relax and lie down for 30 minutes before the test. Agitation or stress may affect insulin levels.
- This test requires a blood sample, which takes less than 3 minutes to collect. While the sample is being drawn, you may experience slight discomfort from the needle puncture and tourniquet pressure.
- The doctor or nurse will check your medication history. Any drugs that may interfere with test results will usually be withheld before the test. Such drugs may include corticotropin, oral contraceptives, thyroid supplements, or epinephrine.
- If the results are uncertain, you may need to undergo a repeat test or a glucose tolerance test.

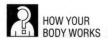

HOW YOUR BODY WORKS

The pancreas: Site of insulin secretion

The pancreas (shown intact, below, and magnified) is a large gland that secretes digestive enzymes and the hormones insulin and glucagon.

Parts of the pancreas
The pancreas is composed of an exocrine portion containing acinar cells that secrete digestive enzymes and an endocrine portion that secretes the hormones insulin and glucagon into the bloodstream in response to changes in blood sugar levels. The islets of Langerhans contain two main types of cells: beta cells, which produce insulin when blood sugar increases, and alpha cells, which produce glucagon when blood sugar decreases. The splenic arteries carry oxygen-rich blood to the pancreas. The mesenteric veins carry insulin and glucagon, in deoxygenated blood, away from the pancreas.

PANCREAS

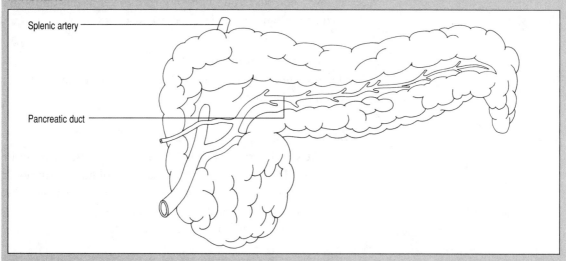

PANCREAS, MAGNIFIED AREA

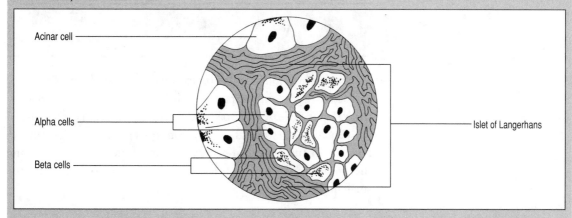

What happens during the test?

A nurse or medical technician inserts a needle into a vein, usually in your forearm. A blood sample is collected in a tube, which is then sent to a lab for testing.

What happens after the test?

- If swelling develops at the needle puncture site, warm soaks are applied to the area to ease discomfort.
- With the doctor's permission, you may resume eating your usual diet and taking medications that were discontinued before the test.

Does the test have risks?

In the person with a pancreatic tumor, fasting for this test may cause severe low blood sugar. Sugar should be readily available during the test to treat low blood sugar levels, if necessary.

What are the normal results?

Insulin levels normally range from 2 to 25 micro-international units of insulin per milliliter of blood.

What do abnormal results mean?

Insulin levels are interpreted with sugar measurements. High insulin and low sugar levels after fasting suggests an insulinoma, a tumor of the pancreas. Prolonged fasting or further testing may be required to confirm a diagnosis. In insulin-resistant diabetes, insulin levels are high; in non-insulin-resistant diabetes, they're low.

GASTRIN

Gastrin is a hormone that's produced and stored in the stomach and, to a lesser degree, in the pancreas. It helps the body digest food by triggering the release of gastric acid. Gastrin also stimulates activity in the pancreas, intestine, and liver. Abnormal secretion of gastrin can result from tumors called *gastrinomas* and from disorders affecting the stomach, pancreas and, less commonly, the esophagus and the small intestine.

This test is used to measure gastrin levels in the blood. It's especially useful in people suspected of having gastrinomas associated with a condition called *Zollinger-Ellison syndrome*. In doubtful situations, additional testing may be needed.

Why is this test done?

Gastrin levels may be measured for the following reasons:

- To determine the cause of a person's gastrointestinal symptoms
- To confirm the diagnosis of a gastrinoma
- To help diagnose some ulcers and anemias.

What should you know before the test?

- You'll be instructed not to drink alcohol for at least 24 hours before the test and to fast for 12 hours before the test, although you may drink water.
- Because stress can increase gastrin levels, you may be asked to relax and lie down for at least 30 minutes before the test.
- This test requires a blood sample, which takes less than 3 minutes to collect. While the sample is being drawn, you may experience slight discomfort from the needle puncture and tourniquet pressure.
- The doctor or nurse will check your medication history, and drugs that may interfere with the test results — especially insulin or anticholinergics, such as atropine and Donnatal — are withheld. If these medications must be continued, the lab is notified.

Gastrin levels may be measured to determine the cause of digestive tract symptoms or to diagnose some ulcers and anemias.

What happens during the test?

A nurse or medical technician inserts a needle into a vein, usually in your forearm. A blood sample is collected in a tube, which is then sent to a lab for testing.

What happens after the test?

- If swelling develops at the needle puncture site, warm soaks are applied to the area to ease discomfort.
- With the doctor's permission, you may resume your usual diet and any medications that were discontinued before the test.

What are the normal results?

Normal gastrin levels are less than 300 picograms of this hormone per milliliter of blood.

What do abnormal results mean?

Gastrin levels greater than 1,000 picograms per milliliter confirm Zollinger-Ellison syndrome.

Increased levels of gastrin may occur in a few people with duodenal ulcers and in people with a condition called *achlorhydria* or with extensive stomach cancer.

SEX HORMONES

ESTROGENS

The ovaries secrete estrogens, the female sex hormones. Estrogens are responsible for the development of some female sex characteristics and for normal menstruation. In women who are in menopause, estrogen secretion drops to a constant, low level.

In this test, a blood sample is examined for levels of estradiol, estrone, and estriol, which are the principal forms of estrogen in the body.

Why is this test done?

Estrogen levels may be measured for the following reasons:
- To determine if secretion of female hormones is normal
- To determine sexual maturation and fertility
- To help diagnose sexual dysfunction, especially early or delayed puberty, menstrual disorders, or infertility
- To determine fetal well-being
- To help diagnose tumors that secrete estrogen.

What should you know before the test?
- You needn't restrict food or fluids before this test.
- This test requires a blood sample, which takes less than 3 minutes to collect. While the sample is being drawn, you may experience slight discomfort from the needle puncture and tourniquet pressure.
- The test may be repeated during the various phases of your menstrual cycle.

- The doctor or nurse will check your medication history. Steroids and other hormones — including estrogens and progestogens — will usually be withheld before the test.

What happens during the test?

A nurse or medical technician inserts a needle into a vein, usually in your forearm. A blood sample is collected in a tube, which is then sent to a lab for testing.

What happens after the test?

- If swelling develops at the needle puncture site, warm soaks are applied to the area to ease discomfort.
- With the doctor's permission, you may resume eating your usual diet and taking medications that were discontinued before the test.

What are the normal results?

Normal estrogen levels for premenopausal women vary widely during the menstrual cycle:
- 1 to 10 days: 24 to 68 picograms of estrogen hormones per milliliter of blood
- 11 to 20 days: 50 to 186
- 21 to 30 days: 73 to 149.

Estrogen levels in men range from 12 to 34 picograms per milliliter of blood. In children under age 6, the normal range is 3 to 10.

What do abnormal results mean?

Low estrogen levels may indicate inadequate activity by a woman's sex organs, or ovarian failure, as in conditions called *Turner's syndrome* or *ovarian agenesis*. Low levels may also occur with menopause or with hypogonadism.

Abnormally high levels may occur with estrogen-producing tumors, in very early puberty, or in severe liver disease such as cirrhosis. High levels may also occur when a person is born with a condition that causes increased conversion of androgens (steroid hormones) to estrogen.

Normal estrogen levels in premenopausal women vary widely. In men, the range is much narrower.

PROGESTERONE

Progesterone is produced by the ovaries when an egg is released, about halfway through the menstrual cycle. This hormone helps the uterine lining prepare for implantation of the egg if conception occurs. Progesterone levels continue to climb, but if pregnancy doesn't occur, they drop sharply and menstruation begins.

During pregnancy, the placenta releases about 10 times the normal monthly amount of progesterone to maintain the pregnancy. Increased secretion begins toward the end of the first trimester (3 months) and continues until delivery of the infant. Progesterone then helps the body increase stored nutrients for the developing fertilized egg.

This test, which measures progesterone levels in a blood sample, provides information for pregnancy and fertility studies. The test may be repeated several times; progesterone can also be monitored through urinalysis.

Testing for plasma progesterone may be repeated at specific times during your menstrual cycle. If you're pregnant, it may be repeated with each prenatal visit.

Why is this test done?
Testing for plasma progesterone may be performed for the following reasons:
- To determine if a woman's female sex hormone secretion is normal
- To help with infertility studies
- To evaluate the activity of the placenta, the tissue that surrounds the fetus during pregnancy
- To help confirm ovulation.

What should you know before the test?
- You needn't restrict food or fluids before this test.
- The test requires a blood sample, which takes less than 3 minutes to collect. While the sample is being drawn, you may experience slight discomfort from the needle puncture and tourniquet pressure.
- The doctor or nurse will check your medication history to determine if you're taking any drugs, including the hormones progesterone or estrogen, that may interfere with test results. Usually, such medications will be discontinued before the test.
- The test may be repeated at specific times during your menstrual cycle. If you're pregnant, it may be repeated with each prenatal visit.

What happens during the test?

A nurse or medical technician inserts a needle into a vein, usually in your forearm. A blood sample is collected in a tube, which is then sent to a lab for testing.

What happens after the test?

- If swelling develops at the needle puncture site, warm soaks are applied to the area to ease discomfort.
- With the doctor's permission, you may resume taking medications that were discontinued before the test.

What are the normal results?

During menstruation, normal results are as follows:

- Follicular phase: less than 150 nanograms of progesterone per deciliter of blood
- Luteal phase: about 300
- Midluteal phase: 2,000.
  During pregnancy, normal values are as follows:
- First trimester: 1,500 to 5,000 nanograms per deciliter of blood
- Second and third trimesters: 8,000 to 20,000.

What do abnormal results mean?

High progesterone levels may indicate ovulation, specific types of tumors, ovarian cysts that produce progesterone, or conditions and tumors that cause progesterone to be produced along with other steroidal hormones.

Low progesterone levels are associated with the absence of normal menstruation due to various causes, certain complications of pregnancy, threatened miscarriage, and fetal death.

TESTOSTERONE

Testosterone is the principal androgen that promotes male characteristics. It's secreted by the testicles. (See *The testicles: Site of testosterone secretion*, page 476.)

Testosterone induces puberty in boys and maintains male secondary sex characteristics, such as facial hair growth. Increased testosterone secretion during puberty stimulates sperm production; it also

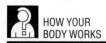

HOW YOUR
BODY WORKS

The testicles: Site of testosterone secretion

In the testicles, several hundred pyramid-shaped lobules contain one or several seminiferous tubules. Within the tissue connecting the tubules are specialized cells, which secrete the potent hormone testosterone. These cells are called *Leydig's cells*.

CROSS SECTION OF A TESTICLE

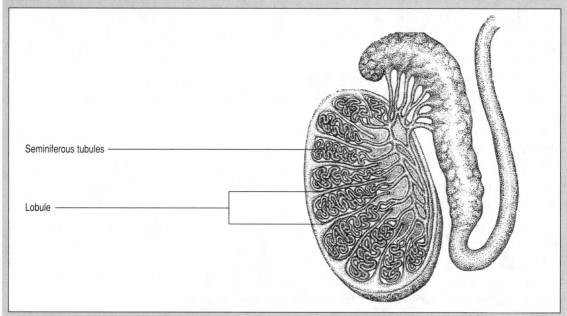

Seminiferous tubules

Lobule

MICROSCOPIC VIEW OF SEMINIFEROUS TUBULES AND LEYDIG'S CELLS

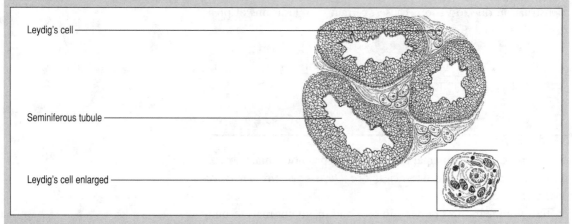

Leydig's cell

Seminiferous tubule

Leydig's cell enlarged

helps enlarge certain muscles, the genitalia, and related sex organs, such as the prostate gland.

Levels of testosterone are low before puberty; they begin to increase at the onset of puberty and continue to increase during adulthood. Production begins to taper off at about age 40, eventually dropping to about one-fifth of the peak level by age 80. In women, the adrenal glands and the ovaries secrete small amounts of testosterone.

This test is used to measure testosterone levels in the blood. When combined with other tests, it helps in the evaluation of sex gland dysfunction in men and women.

Why is this test done?

Testosterone levels may be measured for the following reasons:
- To determine if male sex hormone secretion is adequate
- To help diagnose sexual precocity in boys under age 10
- To help diagnose different forms of hypogonadism (deficient sex gland activity)
- To evaluate male infertility or other sexual dysfunction
- To evaluate abnormal hair growth and masculinization in women.

What should you know before the test?

- You needn't restrict food or fluids before this test.
- The test requires a blood sample, which takes less than 3 minutes to collect. While the sample is being drawn, you may experience slight discomfort from the needle puncture and tourniquet pressure.
- The doctor or nurse may ask you if you've received hormone therapy in the past.

What happens during the test?

A nurse or medical technician inserts a needle into a vein, usually in your forearm. A blood sample is collected in a tube, which is then sent to a lab for testing.

What happens after the test?

If swelling develops at the needle puncture site, warm soaks are applied to the area to ease discomfort.

Normal levels of testosterone in men vary widely. Levels in women are lower and their range is much narrower.

What are the normal results?

Normal levels of testosterone are as follows, although lab values vary slightly:

- Men: 300 to 1,200 nanograms of testosterone per deciliter of blood
- Women: 30 to 95
- Prepubertal children: in boys, less than 100 nanograms per deciliter of blood; in girls, less than 40.

What do abnormal results mean?

High testosterone levels in prepubertal boys may indicate true sexual precocity (early development) or false precocious puberty due to male hormone production by a testicular tumor. They can also indicate other conditions that result in precocious puberty in boys and masculinization in girls.

Increased levels can occur with a benign adrenal tumor or cancer, inadequate thyroid activity, or in the early phases of puberty. In women with ovarian tumors or other disorders, testosterone levels may increase, leading to abnormal hair growth.

Depressed testosterone levels can indicate inadequate sex gland activity, as in conditions called *Klinefelter's syndrome* or *hypogonadotropic eunuchoidism.* Low testosterone levels can also follow removal of the testes, testicular or prostate cancer, delayed male puberty, estrogen therapy, or cirrhosis.

PREGNANCY-TRIGGERED HORMONES

HUMAN CHORIONIC GONADOTROPIN

Human chorionic gonadotropin is a hormone that's produced in the placenta. If conception occurs, a test for human chorionic gonadotropin may detect this hormone in the blood 9 days after ovulation. (See *Human chorionic gonadotropin secretion: An early sign of pregnancy.*)

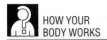

HOW YOUR
BODY WORKS

Human chorionic gonadotropin secretion: An early sign of pregnancy

The hormone human chorionic gonadotropin is secreted if conception takes place. The fertilized egg becomes implanted in the uterine wall. There it begins to develop into the embryo and placenta. Nine days after ovulation, special cells in the tissue that will eventually form the placenta begin secreting human chorionic gonadotropin. These special cells are called *trophoblastic cells*.

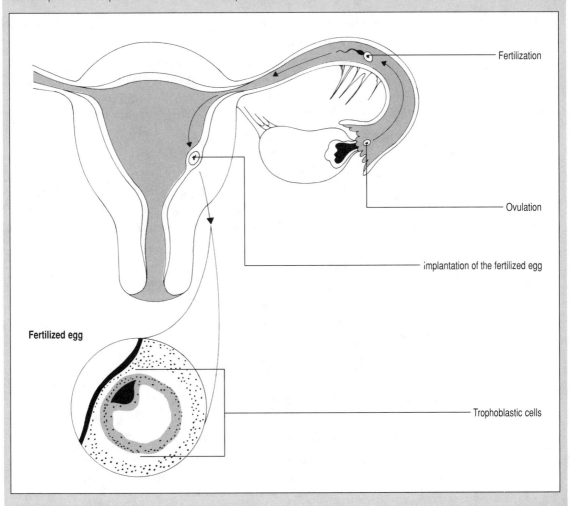

Fertilization

Ovulation

Implantation of the fertilized egg

Fertilized egg

Trophoblastic cells

Production of human chorionic gonadotropin increases steadily during the first trimester (3 months) of pregnancy, peaking around the 10th week. Levels then decrease drastically. About 2 weeks after delivery, the hormone may no longer be detectable.

This test measures the amount of human chorionic gonadotropin in a blood sample. It's more sensitive and costly than the routine pregnancy test using a urine specimen.

Why is this test done?
Human chorionic gonadotropin levels may be measured for the following reasons:
- To detect pregnancy early
- To check hormonal production in high-risk pregnancies
- To help diagnose certain tumors
- To monitor treatment for inducing ovulation and conception.

What should you know before the test?
- You needn't restrict food or fluids before this test.
- This test requires a blood sample, which takes less than 3 minutes to collect. While the sample is being drawn, you may experience slight discomfort from the needle puncture and tourniquet pressure.

What happens during the test?
A nurse or medical technician inserts a needle into a vein, usually in your forearm. A blood sample is collected in a tube, which is then sent to a lab for testing.

What happens after the test?
If swelling develops at the needle puncture site, warm soaks are applied to the area to ease discomfort.

What are the normal results?
Normal values for this hormone are less than 5 international units per liter of blood and can vary in early pregnancy.

What do abnormal results mean?
High human chorionic gonadotropin levels indicate pregnancy; significantly higher concentrations are present in a multiple pregnancy. Increased levels may also suggest several types of tumors that secrete

human chorionic gonadotropin. Low levels may occur in ectopic pregnancy or pregnancy of less than 9 days.

HUMAN PLACENTAL LACTOGEN

This hormone helps prepare a pregnant woman's breasts for lactation (milk secretion) and influences fetal growth. It also indirectly provides energy for maternal metabolism and fetal nutrition. Human placental lactogen is also known as *human chorionic somato-mammotropin.*

Secretion of this hormone begins about the fifth week of gestation and declines rapidly after the baby is delivered. Some experts believe this hormone may not be essential for a successful pregnancy.

This test measures human placental lactogen levels in the blood. It may be required in high-risk pregnancies or in suspected placental tissue dysfunction. Because values vary widely during the last half of pregnancy, several tests performed over several days provide the most reliable test results.

Why is this test done?
Human placental lactogen levels may be measured for the following reasons:
- To assess placental activity and fetal well-being
- To help diagnose certain tumors and to monitor treatment of tumors that secrete human placental lactogen.

What should you know before the test?
- This test requires a blood sample, which takes less than 3 minutes to collect. While the sample is being drawn, you may experience slight discomfort from the needle puncture and tourniquet pressure.
- The test may be repeated during your pregnancy.

What happens during the test?
A nurse or medical technician inserts a needle into a vein, usually in your forearm. A blood sample is collected in a tube, which is then sent to a lab for testing.

What happens after the test?

If swelling develops at the needle puncture site, warm soaks are applied to the area to ease discomfort.

What are the normal results?

For pregnant women, normal human placental lactogen levels are as listed in the chart below.

GESTATION PERIOD	HUMAN PLACENTAL LACTOGEN LEVELS
5 to 27 weeks	Less than 4.6 micrograms of hormone per milliliter of blood
28 to 31 weeks	2.4 to 6.1
32 to 35 weeks	3.7 to 7.7
36 weeks to term	5 to 8.6

At term, a pregnant woman with diabetes may have levels of 9 to 11 micrograms. Normal levels for men and nonpregnant women are 0.5 micrograms.

What do abnormal results mean?

Human placental lactogen levels are correlated with a pregnant woman's gestational stage. For example, after 30 weeks' gestation, levels below 4 micrograms may indicate placental dysfunction. Low human placental lactogen concentrations are also characteristically associated with several pregnancy problems. Declining concentrations may help differentiate incomplete early miscarriage from a threatened miscarriage.

Low human placental lactogen concentrations don't confirm fetal distress. Conversely, concentrations over 4 micrograms after 30 weeks' gestation don't guarantee fetal well-being.

Human placental lactogen measurement over 6 micrograms after 30 weeks' gestation may suggest an unusually large placenta, commonly occurring in people with diabetes, multiple pregnancy, or a condition called *Rh isoimmunization*.

Below-normal concentrations of human placental lactogen may be associated with certain types of tumors and cancers.

13

IMMUNE SYSTEM TESTS:
Studying the Body's Defenses

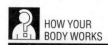

Why some blood types don't mix

All blood group classifications are based on the types of antigens on the surfaces of red blood cells. An antigen is a substance that triggers the body's defenses and produces an antibody to fight another substance. These antigens explain why people need their own type of blood for a transfusion.

The antigen's the thing

In 1930, a doctor identified the most important of the blood classifications — the ABO blood group system. He classified human red blood cells as A, B, AB, or O, depending on the presence or absence of antigens. He found that persons with group A blood have antigens different from people with group B blood. AB blood contains both antigens, and O has neither. Because type O has no antigens, it can be given to anyone in an emergency, with little risk of a bad reaction. The type O person is called a *universal donor.*

The universal recipient

A person with AB blood has both antigens but no anti-A or anti-B antibodies and can receive A, B, or O blood. A type AB person is called a *universal recipient.*

BLOOD COMPATIBILITY

ABO BLOOD TYPE

This test classifies blood according to either type A, type B, type AB, or type O. Different blood types are not compatible, so typing is required before a transfusion to protect the recipient from a lethal reaction.

Why is this test done?

A person's blood type is determined to check the compatibility of a donor's and a recipient's blood before transfusion. If you're scheduled for a transfusion, once your blood type is known, it can be matched with the right donor blood. (See *Why some blood types don't mix* and *Identifying compatible blood types.*)

What should you know before the test?

You won't need to change your diet before the test.

What happens during the test?

▪ A nurse or medical technician inserts a needle into a vein, usually in your forearm. A blood sample is collected in a tube, which is then sent to a lab for testing.
▪ Although you may feel a sting from the needle and pressure from the tourniquet, collecting the sample takes only a few minutes.

What happens after the test?

If swelling develops at the needle puncture site, warm soaks may be applied to ease discomfort.

Identifying compatible blood types

There are four major blood types, and a transfusion is safe and effective if the donor and recipient have compatible types. The top illustration provides a guide to blood type compatibility. The bottom illustration shows the distribution of blood types among different population groups.

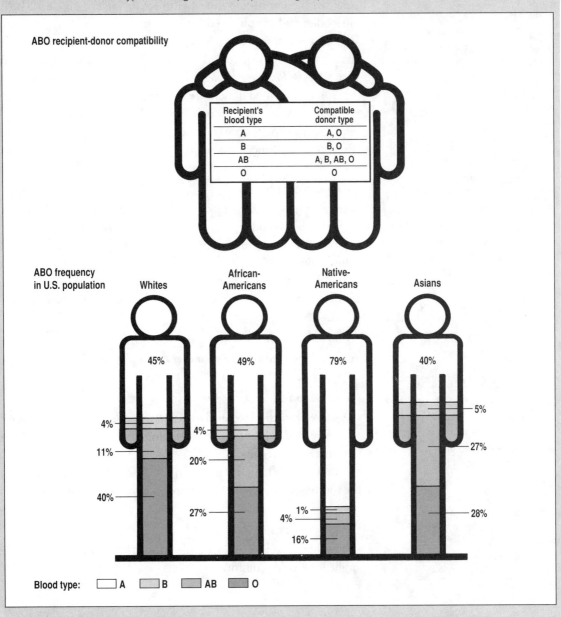

ABO recipient-donor compatibility

Recipient's blood type	Compatible donor type
A	A, O
B	B, O
AB	A, B, AB, O
O	O

ABO frequency in U.S. population

Whites — 45%, 4%, 11%, 40%

African-Americans — 49%, 4%, 20%, 27%

Native-Americans — 79%, 1%, 4%, 16%

Asians — 40%, 5%, 27%, 28%

Blood type: ☐ A ☐ B ☐ AB ☐ O

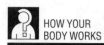

Why the Rh factor matters

More than 85% of people carry the Rh antigen, called the *Rh₀(D) factor*, on their red blood cells. Their blood is classified Rh-positive. The remaining 15% lack this factor and their blood is typed Rh-negative.

Risk factor: Rh-negative blood

The Rh antigen is more likely to stimulate formation of antibodies to fight other blood cells than any other known antigen. Consequently, a person with Rh-positive blood does not carry any anti-Rh antibodies (because they would destroy the red blood cells). A person with Rh-negative blood, however, develops anti-Rh antibodies following exposure to Rh-positive blood (by transfusion or pregnancy). A transfusion reaction does not usually occur in such a person after the first exposure. Instead, anti-Rh antibodies develop slowly, over several weeks, causing the transfusion recipient to become sensitized to the Rh antigen. It takes a second exposure to Rh-positive blood to trigger a reaction. In infants, the reaction is called *hemolytic disease of the newborn*.

Rh TYPE: POSITIVE OR NEGATIVE

The Rh system classifies blood by the presence or absence of the $Rh_o(D)$ antigen on the surface of red blood cells. In this test, a person's red blood cells are mixed with serum containing anti-$Rh_o(D)$ antibodies and are observed for a reaction. If there's a reaction, the $Rh_o(D)$ antigen is present, and the person's blood is typed Rh-positive. If there's no reaction, the person's blood is typed Rh-negative. (See *Why the Rh factor matters*.)

Prospective blood donors are fully tested to exclude the D^u variant of the $Rh_o(D)$ antigen before being classified as Rh-negative. People who have this antigen are considered Rh-positive donors but generally can receive Rh-negative blood.

Why is this test done?

Rh typing may be performed for the following reasons:

- To establish blood type according to the Rh system
- To check compatibility of the donor and recipient and ensure a safe transfusion
- To determine whether the person will require an Rh immune globulin injection to prevent complications in a future pregnancy.

What should you know before the test?

You won't need to change your diet before the test.

What happens during the test?

- A nurse or medical technician inserts a needle into a vein, usually in your forearm. A blood sample is collected in a tube, which is then sent to a lab for testing.
- Although you may feel a sting from the needle and pressure from the tourniquet, collecting the sample takes only a few minutes.

What happens after the test?

- If swelling develops at the needle puncture site, warm soaks may be applied to ease discomfort.

▪ If you're pregnant and your test shows that your blood is Rh-positive, you should carry a card saying that you may need to receive Rh immune globulin.

What are the normal results

Classified as Rh-positive, Rh-negative, or Rh-positive D^u, donor blood may be transfused only if compatible with the recipient's blood.

What do abnormal results mean?

If an Rh-negative woman delivers an Rh-positive baby or aborts a fetus with an unknown Rh-type, she should receive an Rh immune globulin injection within 72 hours to prevent hemolytic disease of the newborn in future births.

FETAL-MATERNAL RED BLOOD CELL TRANSFER

This test — which doctors call the *fetal-maternal erythrocyte distribution test* — measures the number of fetal red blood cells in the mother's blood. Some transfer of red blood cells from the fetus's to the mother's circulation occurs during most spontaneous or elective abortions and most normal deliveries. Usually, the amount of blood transferred is minimal and makes no difference. But transfer of significant amounts of blood from an Rh-positive fetus to an Rh-negative mother can cause the mother to develop anti-Rh-positive antibodies in her blood. During a subsequent pregnancy, the mother's antibodies are potentially fatal to an Rh-positive fetus.

Why is this test done?

The fetal-maternal red blood cell transfer test may be performed for the following reasons:
▪ To detect and measure fetal-maternal blood transfer
▪ To determine the amount of Rh immune globulin needed to keep the mother from developing immunization to the $Rh_o(D)$ antigen
▪ To determine or verify a person's blood group — an important step for a safe transfusion.

What should you know before the test?

- You won't need to change your diet before the test.
- The nurse or technician will ask whether you've recently been given dextran, intravenous contrast dye, or other drugs that may alter test results.

What happens during the test?

- A nurse or medical technician inserts a needle into a vein, usually in your forearm. A blood sample is collected in a tube, which is then sent to a lab for testing.
- Although you may feel a sting from the needle and pressure from the tourniquet, collecting the sample takes only a few minutes.

What happens after the test?

If swelling develops at the needle puncture site, warm soaks may be applied to ease discomfort.

What are the normal results?

Normally, the mother's blood contains no fetal red blood cells.

What do abnormal results mean?

If a pregnant woman has too many fetal red blood cells in her blood, she must have several doses of Rh immune globulin to keep her from developing antibodies.

Rh immune globulin should be given to an unsensitized Rh-negative mother as soon as possible (no later than 72 hours) after the birth of an Rh-positive infant or after a spontaneous or elective abortion. The Rh immune globulin prevents complications in future pregnancies. Most doctors now give Rh immune globulin as a preventive measure at 28 weeks' gestation to women who are Rh-negative but have no detectable Rh antibodies.

Who should be screened?

The following people should be screened for Rh isoimmunization or irregular antibodies: all Rh-negative mothers during their first prenatal visit and at 28 weeks' gestation and all Rh-positive mothers with histories of transfusion, a jaundiced infant, stillbirth, cesarean delivery, abortion, or miscarriage.

CROSSMATCHING

Crossmatching establishes compatibility or incompatibility of the donor's and the recipient's blood. It's the best antibody detection test available for avoiding lethal transfusion reactions. The test is available in major and minor forms.

After both the donor's and recipient's ABO blood types and Rh factor types are known, *major crossmatching* determines the compatibility of the donor's red blood cells and the recipient's serum. *Minor crossmatching* determines the compatibility of the donor's serum and the recipient's red blood cells. Because the antibody-screening test is routinely performed on all blood donors, minor crossmatching is often omitted.

Why is this test done?

Crossmatching may be performed to serve as the final check for compatibility of the donor's blood and the recipient's blood and to avoid a transfusion reaction.

What should you know before the test?

You won't need to change your diet before the test.

What happens during the test?

- The nurse or technician asks whether you've recently been given Dextran, intravenous contrast dye, or drugs that may alter test results.
- A nurse or medical technician inserts a needle into a vein, usually in your forearm. A blood sample is collected in a tube, which is then sent to a lab for testing.
- Although you may feel a sting from the needle and pressure from the tourniquet, collecting the sample takes only a few minutes.

What happens after the test?

- If swelling develops at the needle puncture site, warm soaks may be applied to ease discomfort.
- You should carry an ABO group identification card. Such identification is helpful but doesn't replace crossmatching before a transfusion.

What are the normal results?

The absence of clumping indicates compatibility of the donor's and the recipient's blood, which means that the transfusion may proceed.

What do abnormal results mean?

A positive crossmatch (clumping) means the donor and recipient are incompatible and there is an antigen-antibody reaction. The donor's blood must be withheld and the crossmatch continued to determine the cause of the incompatibility and to identify the antibody.

DIRECT ANTIGLOBULIN TEST

The direct antiglobulin test (or direct Coombs' test) detects immunoglobulins (antibodies) on the surfaces of red blood cells. These immunoglobulins coat red blood cells when they become sensitized to an antigen, such as the Rh factor.

Why is this test done?

Direct antiglobulin testing may be performed for the following reasons:
- To diagnose a blood compatibility problem called *hemolytic disease of the newborn*
- To investigate blood transfusion reactions
- To help the doctor diagnose specific anemias that may be inherited, caused by drugs, or caused by an immune system reaction.

What should you know before the test?

You won't need to change your diet before the test.

What happens during the test?

- For a newborn, the nurse draws a sample from the umbilical cord after it's clamped and cut.
- For an adult, a nurse or medical technician inserts a needle into a vein, usually in your forearm. A blood sample is collected in a tube, which is then sent to a lab for testing.
- Although you may feel a sting from the needle and pressure from the tourniquet, collecting the sample takes only a few minutes.

What happens after the test?

▪ An infant with hemolytic disease of the newborn will need more testing to monitor anemia.

▪ If swelling develops at the needle puncture site, warm soaks may be applied to ease discomfort.

What are the normal results?

A negative test, in which neither antibodies nor complement (another component of the immune system) appears on the red blood cells, is normal.

What do abnormal results mean?

A positive test on a newborn's umbilical cord blood indicates that the mother's antibodies have crossed the placenta and have coated fetal red blood cells, causing hemolytic disease of the newborn. The infant may need a transfusion of compatible blood, without the antigens that have been built against the mother's antibodies, to keep from being anemic.

In an adult, a positive test result may indicate hemolytic anemia and help the doctor decide whether the anemia is caused by drugs or linked to an underlying disease, such as lymphoma. A positive test can also indicate infection. Or, a weakly positive test (showing relatively less cell agglutination) may mean the person's antibodies are reacting to transfused blood.

ANTIBODY SCREENING TEST

Also called the *indirect Coombs' test,* this test detects unexpected circulating antibodies in the person's blood. This screening test detects 95% to 99% of the circulating antibodies; another, more specific test can isolate the exact antibodies in the person's blood.

Why is this test done?

Antibody screening tests may be performed for the following reasons:

▪ To detect unexpected circulating antibodies to red cell antigens in the recipient's or donor's blood before transfusion

- To determine the presence of Rh-positive antibodies in a mother's blood
- To learn whether a pregnant mother needs Rh immune globulin
- To help the doctor diagnose acquired hemolytic anemia or some other form of anemia
- To help the doctor evaluate the possibility of a transfusion reaction.

What should you know before the test?

You won't need to change your diet before the test.

What happens during the test?

- A nurse or medical technician inserts a needle into a vein, usually in your forearm. A blood sample is collected in a tube, which is then sent to a lab for testing.
- Although you may feel a sting from the needle and pressure from the tourniquet, collecting the sample takes only a few minutes.

What happens after the test?

If swelling develops at the needle puncture site, warm soaks may be applied to ease discomfort.

What are the normal results?

Normally, there's no clumping, indicating that your blood contains no circulating antibodies other than anti-A and anti-B.

What do abnormal results mean?

A positive result indicates the presence of unexpected circulating antibodies to red cell antigens. Such a reaction demonstrates donor and recipient incompatibility.

If you're pregnant and Rh-negative, a positive result may show antibodies to the Rh factor from a previous transfusion with incompatible blood or from a previous pregnancy with an Rh-positive fetus. If the positive result is strong, the fetus may develop hemolytic disease of the newborn. In that case, you'll need to have repeated tests throughout your pregnancy to evaluate your antibody levels.

WHITE CELL ANTIBODIES TEST

This test detects leukoagglutinins — antibodies that react with white blood cells — which may cause a transfusion reaction. These antibodies usually develop after a person has been exposed to foreign white cells through transfusions, pregnancies, or a graft of tissue from an unrelated donor. The doctor will use a microscope to examine the person's blood for these antibodies.

Why is this test done?

White cell antibodies tests may be performed for the following reasons:

- To detect leukoagglutinins in blood recipients who develop transfusion reactions and to distinguish this reaction from other transfusion reactions
- To detect leukoagglutinins in blood donors after transfusion of the donor's blood causes a reaction in the recipient.

What should you know before the test?

You won't need to change your diet before the test.

What happens during the test?

- A nurse or medical technician inserts a needle into a vein, usually in your forearm. A blood sample is collected in a tube, which is then sent to a lab for testing.
- Although you may feel a sting from the needle and pressure from the tourniquet, collecting the sample takes only a few minutes.

What happens after the test?

If swelling develops at the needle puncture site, warm soaks may be applied to ease discomfort.

What are the normal results?

Normally, test results are negative: The blood doesn't clump because it contains no antibodies.

What do abnormal results mean?

If the recipient has a positive white cell antibodies test, continued transfusions will require premedication with acetaminophen 1 to 2 hours before the transfusion, transfusion of specially prepared leukocyte-poor blood, or the use of leukocyte removal blood filters to prevent further reactions.

If the donor's blood shows a positive result, indicating the presence of leukoagglutinins, it means the recipient's transfusion reaction is caused by acute, noncardiogenic pulmonary edema.

IMMUNE SYSTEM COMPONENTS

T- AND B-CELL COUNTS

This test measures T cells, B cells, and so-called "null" cells to find evidence of several diseases that influence their numbers in the blood. T cells and B cells are two important types of lymphocytes — white blood cells that can recognize antigens or foreign cells through special receptors on their surfaces. Null cells alone have little diagnostic significance.

The lab marks the cell types, then counts them and compares their numbers with normal baselines.

Why is this test done?

These lymphocyte tests may be performed for the following reasons:
- To help the doctor diagnose immunodeficiency diseases
- To distinguish benign from malignant lymphocyte-producing diseases
- To monitor a person's response to therapy.

What should you know before the test?

You won't need to change your diet before the test.

What happens during the test?

▪ A nurse or medical technician inserts a needle into a vein, usually in your forearm. A blood sample is collected in a tube, which is then sent to a lab for testing.

▪ Although you may feel a sting from the needle and pressure from the tourniquet, collecting the sample takes only a few minutes.

What happens after the test?

If swelling develops at the needle puncture site, warm soaks may be applied to ease discomfort.

What are the normal results?

Currently, T-cell and B-cell counts are being standardized, and values may differ from one lab to another, depending on the test technique. Generally, normal results, measured as a percentage of the total white blood cell count, are as follows:

▪ T cells: 68% to 75%

▪ B cells: 10% to 20%

▪ Null cells: 5% to 20%.

Normal T-cell and B-cell counts don't necessarily mean the person's immune system is strong. In autoimmune diseases, such as lupus and rheumatoid arthritis, T cells and B cells may be present in normal numbers but may not function well.

What do abnormal results mean?

An abnormal T-cell or B-cell count suggests, but doesn't confirm, specific diseases. If your cell count is abnormal, the doctor starts looking for additional signs of diseases, including:

▪ an elevated B-cell count, which occurs in a form of leukemia, multiple tumors, and some kinds of anemia

▪ a decreased B-cell count, found in acute lymphocytic leukemia and in certain inherited or acquired immunoglobulin deficiency diseases

▪ an increased T-cell count, which occurs occasionally in infectious mononucleosis but more often in multiple tumors and acute lymphocytic leukemia

▪ a decreased T-cell count, which occurs in some inherited T-cell deficiency diseases, chronic lymphocytic leukemia, and AIDS.

HOW YOUR BODY WORKS

Natural weapons against bacteria

A group of white blood cells called *neutrophils* are the body's main bacteria fighters. They engulf and destroy bacteria and foreign particles by a process called *phagocytosis*.

In people who have recurrent bacterial infections, neutrophil function tests show whether these cells can kill offending bacteria or can move toward the infection site.

Measuring neutrophil effectiveness

The *nitroblue tetrazolium test* measures the killing ability of neutrophils. It looks for the enzymes and toxins that neutrophils make during phagocytosis.

Another test evaluates luminescence (light-emitting ability) of neutrophils, which shows how well the neutrophils are working. Finally, the neutrophils' ability to find bacteria can also be measured by placing them in separate parts of a chamber and observing their rate of migration from one area to another.

LYMPHOCYTE TRANSFORMATION TESTS

Transformation tests evaluate lymphocyte (white blood cell) function, which is crucial to the immune system. These tests don't require injecting foreign cells into the skin, which eliminates the risk of immune reactions.

The lab tests match the person's white blood cells with foreign cells and evaluate what doctors call the *mitotic response,* the *antigen assay,* and the *mixed lymphocyte culture assay.* The last test is useful in matching transplant recipients and donors.

Why are these tests done?

Lymphocyte transformation tests may be performed for the following reasons:

- To assess and monitor genetic and acquired immune deficiencies
- To check compatibility of both tissue transplant recipients and donors
- To see if a person has been exposed to diseases, such as malaria, hepatitis, and mycoplasmal pneumonia.

What should you know before the tests?

You won't need to change your diet before the tests.

What happens during the tests?

- A nurse or medical technician inserts a needle into a vein, usually in your forearm. A blood sample is collected in a tube, which is then sent to a lab for testing.
- Although you may feel a sting from the needle and pressure from the tourniquet, collecting the sample takes only a few minutes.

What happens after the tests?

If swelling develops at the needle puncture site, warm soaks may be applied to ease discomfort.

What are the normal results?

Results depend on the antigens and mitogens the doctor used.

What do abnormal results mean?

In the mitogen and antigen assays, a low response or no response shows that the person has a depressed or defective immune system. An additional series of tests can monitor the effectiveness of therapy in a person with an immunodeficiency disease.

In the mixed lymphocyte culture test, if the person's white blood cells show a high reaction to a specific pathogen, it may show that he or she has been exposed to malaria, hepatitis, mycoplasmal pneumonia, periodontal disease, and certain viral infections where the person no longer has antibodies in the blood. (See *Natural weapons against bacteria.*)

IMMUNOGLOBULINS G, A, AND M

This test measures a person's disease-fighting antibodies by checking three important types of immunoglobulins. Immunoglobulins are proteins that function as specific antibodies to neutralize foreign cells. Deviations from normal immunoglobulin percentages are characteristic in many immune disorders, including cancer, liver disorders, rheumatoid arthritis, and lupus.

The test identifies immunoglobulin G, immunoglobulin A, and immunoglobulin M in a blood sample.

Why is this test done?

Immunoglobulins G, A, and M may be tested for the following reasons:
- To diagnose such conditions as multiple tumors and blood disorders
- To detect diseases, such as cirrhosis and hepatitis, that are linked to abnormally high immunoglobulin levels
- To check the effectiveness of chemotherapy or radiation therapy.

What should you know before the test?

You'll have to go without food and fluids, except for water, for 12 to 14 hours before the test.

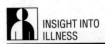

Why your insulin may not work

An insulin antibodies test can detect insulin antibodies in the blood of people who receive insulin for treatment of diabetes mellitus. Most insulin preparations are derived from the pancreas of beef or pork and contain insulin-related peptides (impurities that are the major causes of immune reactions to the medicine). Immunoglobulin G antibodies that form in response to these peptides neutralize the insulin so that it cannot regulate sugar metabolism.

What happens during the test?

- A nurse or medical technician inserts a needle into a vein, usually in your forearm. A blood sample is collected in a tube, which is then sent to a lab for testing.
- Although you may feel a sting from the needle and pressure from the tourniquet, collecting the sample takes only a few minutes.

What happens after the test?

- If swelling develops at the needle puncture site, warm soaks may be applied to ease discomfort.
- You may resume your normal diet.

What are the normal results?

When the lab uses a method called *nephelometry,* immunoglobulin levels for adults range as follows:

- Immunoglobulin G: 700 to 1,800 milligrams per deciliter
- Immunoglobulin A: 70 to 440 milligrams per deciliter
- Immunoglobulin M: 60 to 290 milligrams per deciliter.

What do abnormal results mean?

In people with inherited and acquired blood diseases or tumors, the findings confirm the doctor's diagnosis. In liver and autoimmune diseases, leukemias, and lymphomas, they just support other tests, such as biopsies and white blood cell measures and physical examination. Some people can develop antibodies to their medications. (See *Why your insulin may not work.*)

If your test results are to high or too low, the doctor will discuss the following;

- If you have abnormally low immunoglobulin levels (especially of immunoglobulin G or immunoglobulin M) you must protect yourself against bacterial infection. It helps to learn to watch for signs of infection, such as fever, chills, rash, or skin ulcers.
- If you have abnormally high immunoglobulin levels and symptoms of a blood disorder, the doctor will urge you to report bone pain and tenderness, signs of kidney failure, and frequent bone fractures.

IMMUNE COMPLEX TEST

This test checks your immune system by looking for what doctors call *immune complexes*. When immune complexes are produced faster than they can be cleared by the lymph system, the person who has been ill gets sick again. For example, a person may develop an illness after recovering from an infection or after undergoing a transfusion. In some people, the presence of immune complexes leads to drug sensitivity, rheumatoid arthritis, or lupus.

Why is this test done?
An immune complex test may be performed for the following reasons:
- To evaluate the immune system by finding circulating immune complexes in the blood
- To monitor a person's response to therapy
- To estimate the severity of disease.

What should you know before the test?
You won't need to change your diet before the test.

What happens during the test?
- A nurse or medical technician inserts a needle into a vein, usually in your forearm. A blood sample is collected in a tube, which is then sent to a lab for testing.
- Although you may feel a sting from the needle and pressure from the tourniquet, collecting the sample takes only a few minutes.

What happens after the test?
If swelling develops at the needle puncture site, warm soaks may be applied to ease discomfort.

What are the normal results?
Under normal circumstances, immune complexes are not detectable.

What do abnormal results mean?
The presence of detectable immune complexes in blood usually prompts the doctor to use other tests to diagnose a condition such as drug sensitivity, rheumatoid arthritis, or lupus.

COMPLEMENT TESTS

These tests measure a group of proteins that fight infection. *Complement* is a collective term for a system of at least 20 blood proteins that interact to destroy foreign cells and to help remove foreign materials. A complement deficiency can increase a person's susceptibility to infection and diseases.

Why are these tests done?
Complement tests may be performed for the following reasons:
- To help the doctor detect diseases that are affected by the immune system
- To check for an inherited deficiency in these proteins
- To monitor effectiveness of therapy.

What should you know before the tests?
You won't need to change your diet before the tests.

What happens during the tests?
- A nurse or medical technician inserts a needle into a vein, usually in your forearm. A blood sample is collected in a tube, which is then sent to a lab for testing.
- Although you may feel a sting from the needle and pressure from the tourniquet, collecting the sample takes only a few minutes.

What happens after the tests?
If swelling develops at the needle puncture site, warm soaks may be applied to ease discomfort.

What are the normal results?
Normal values for complement range are:
- Total complement: 330 to 730 CH_{50} units
- C1 esterase inhibitor: 7.8 to 23.4 milligrams per deciliter
- C3: 57 to 125 milligrams per deciliter
- C4: 10 to 54 milligrams per deciliter.

What do abnormal results mean?

Complement abnormalities may be genetic or acquired, but acquired abnormalities are the most common. A person with depressed total complement levels (more important than elevated levels) may have an imbalance between his production of antigen-antibody complexes and his body's ability to get rid of them. The doctor uses this information to track down the disorder in a long list of possible problems.

IMMUNE SYSTEM REACTIONS

ALLERGY TEST

This test — which doctors call the *radioallergosorbent test (RAST)* — is used to determine what causes an allergic reaction. It measures immunoglobulin E antibodies in blood and identifies specific allergens that cause rashes, asthma, hay fever, drug reactions, or other skin complaints. The radioallergosorbent test is easier to perform and more specific than skin testing; it's also less painful and less dangerous. Skin tests, however, are still the most common allergy tests.

Why is this test done?

The allergy test may be performed to identify allergens that affect the person.

What should you know before the test?

You won't need to change your diet before the test.

What happens during the test?

■ A nurse or medical technician inserts a needle into a vein, usually in your forearm. A blood sample is collected in a tube, which is then sent to a lab for testing.

■ Although you may feel a sting from the needle and pressure from the tourniquet, collecting the sample takes only a few minutes.

The radioallergosorbent test can tell what's causing your rashes, asthma, hay fever, drug reactions, or other skin problems. It's easier, less painful, and more reliable than the old skin tests.

What happens after the test?

If swelling develops at the needle puncture site, warm soaks may be applied to ease discomfort.

What are the normal results?

Radioallergosorbent test results are interpreted in relationship to a control or reference serum that differs among laboratories.

What do abnormal results mean?

Higher-than-normal immunoglobulin E levels in the blood suggest hypersensitivity to the specific allergen or allergens used.

WHITE BLOOD CELL ANTIGEN TEST

This test — which doctors call the *human leukocyte antigen test* — identifies a group of antigens present on the surfaces of all live cells but most easily detected on white blood cells. There are four types of human leukocyte antigens: HLA-A, HLA-B, HLA-C, and HLA-D. These antigens are essential to immunity and determine the degree of compatibility between transplant recipients and donors.

Why is this test done?

The white blood cell antigen test may be performed for the following reasons:
- To match tissue recipients and donors
- To aid genetic counseling
- To aid paternity testing.

What should you know before the test?

You won't need to change your diet before the test.

What happens during the test?

- A nurse or medical technician inserts a needle into a vein, usually in your forearm. A blood sample is collected in a tube, which is then sent to a lab for testing.
- Although you may feel a sting from the needle and pressure from the tourniquet, collecting the sample takes only a few minutes.

What happens after the test?

If swelling develops at the needle puncture site, warm soaks may be applied to ease discomfort.

What are the normal results?

In HLA-A, HLA-B, and HLA-C testing, white blood cells that react with the test antiserum break down and absorb a marker dye, which can be detected microscopically. In HLA-D testing, white blood cell incompatibility is marked by cellular and other changes.

What do abnormal results mean?

Incompatible HLA-A, HLA-B, HLA-C, or HLA-D groups may cause unsuccessful tissue transplantation. Many diseases have a strong association with certain types of human leucocyte antigens, and information from testing may help with diagnosis.

In paternity testing, if the HLA dye markers in a possible father's blood do not match the child's, it proves that he's no relation. If the man's human leukocyte antigen test shows a match with the child's, then the probability that he's the father is quite high.

This test helps predict whether an organ transplant will be successful. It's also used in paternity testing.

ANTIBODIES TO CELL NUCLEI

This test — called the *antinuclear antibodies test* — is done to evaluate the immune system. In conditions such as lupus, scleroderma, and certain infections, the body's immune system may treat portions of its own cell nuclei as if they were foreign substances and produce antinuclear antibodies against them.

Because they don't penetrate living cells, antinuclear antibodies are harmless. Sometimes, though, they form antigen-antibody complexes that cause tissue damage (as in systemic lupus erythematosus). Because several organs could be involved, the test results are used to support other evidence. Further testing is usually required for a diagnosis.

Why is this test done?

The test for antibodies to cell nuclei may be done for the following reasons:

- To screen for systemic lupus erythematosus (failure to detect antinuclear antibodies essentially rules out active systemic lupus erythematosus)
- To monitor the effectiveness of therapy for systemic lupus erythematosus.

What should you know before the test?

You won't need to change your diet before the test.

What happens during the test?

- A nurse or medical technician inserts a needle into a vein, usually in your forearm. A blood sample is collected in a tube, which is then sent to a lab for testing.
- Although you may feel a sting from the needle and pressure from the tourniquet, collecting the sample takes only a few minutes.

What happens after the test?

- If swelling develops at the needle puncture site, warm soaks may be applied to ease discomfort.
- You should keep a clean, dry bandage over the site for at least 24 hours.

What are the normal results?

Normally, the test is negative if the concentration of antinuclear antibodies is below a certain level.

What do abnormal results mean?

Low concentrations of antinuclear antibodies may point to disorders such as viral diseases, chronic liver disease, collagen vascular disease, and autoimmune diseases. The higher the concentration, the more likely it is that the person has lupus. Besides the concentration of antinuclear antibodies, patterns of antibodies that indicate other diseases can also be identified.

ANTIBODIES TO CELL MITOCHONDRIA

This test — called the *antimitochondrial antibodies test* — evaluates liver function. It's usually performed with the test for anti-smooth-muscle antibodies. Determining results requires searching for the antimitochondrial antibodies in blood samples with a microscope. These antibodies show up in several liver diseases, although their role is unknown and there's no evidence they cause liver damage. Most commonly, they're linked to cirrhosis of the liver and, sometimes, chronic active hepatitis and drug-induced jaundice. Anti-mitochondrial antibodies are also linked to autoimmune diseases, such as lupus, rheumatoid arthritis, pernicious anemia, and a disease of the adrenal glands called Addison's disease.

Why is this test done?

A test for antibodies to cell mitochondria may be performed for the following reasons:

- To aid diagnosis of biliary cirrhosis
- To distinguish between jaundice caused by something outside the liver and biliary cirrhosis.

What should you know before the test?

You won't need to change your diet before the test.

What happens during the test?

- A nurse or medical technician inserts a needle into a vein, usually in your forearm. A blood sample is collected in a tube, which is then sent to a lab for testing.
- Although you may feel a sting from the needle and pressure from the tourniquet, collecting the sample takes only a few minutes.

What happens after the test?

- If swelling develops at the needle puncture site, warm soaks may be applied to ease discomfort.
- Because people with liver disease may bleed excessively, the nurse will apply pressure to the venipuncture site until bleeding stops.

What are the normal results?

The blood test should show no antimitochondrial antibodies.

What do abnormal results mean?

Although antimitochondrial antibodies appear in 79% to 94% of people with primary biliary cirrhosis, this test alone doesn't confirm the diagnosis. The autoantibodies also appear in some people with chronic active hepatitis, drug-induced jaundice, and cirrhosis of unknown origins.

ANTIBODIES TO SMOOTH MUSCLE

This test — called the *anti–smooth-muscle antibodies test* — helps evaluate liver function. It measures the relative concentration of anti–smooth-muscle antibodies in blood and is usually performed with the test for antimitochondrial antibodies.

Anti–smooth-muscle antibodies appear in several liver diseases, especially chronic active hepatitis and, less often, cirrhosis of the liver. Although anti–smooth-muscle antibodies are most commonly linked to liver diseases, their role is unknown, and there's no evidence that they cause liver damage.

This test helps the doctor evaluate liver disease, especially chronic active hepatitis and cirrhosis of the liver.

Why is this test done?

A test for anti–smooth-muscle antibodies may be done to aid diagnosis of chronic active hepatitis and cirrhosis of the liver.

What should you know before the test?

You won't need to change your diet before the test.

What happens during the test?

- A nurse or medical technician inserts a needle into a vein, usually in your forearm. A blood sample is collected in a tube, which is then sent to a lab for testing.
- Although you may feel a sting from the needle and pressure from the tourniquet, collecting the sample takes only a few minutes.

What happens after the test?

If swelling develops at the needle puncture site, warm soaks may be applied to ease discomfort.

What are the normal results?

Normal concentration of anti–smooth-muscle antibodies in serum is less than 1 part to 20 of serum.

What do abnormal results mean?

The test for anti–smooth-muscle antibodies is not very specific. The antibodies appear in about 66% of people with chronic active hepatitis and 30% to 40% of people with cirrhosis of the liver.

Anti–smooth-muscle antibodies may also be present in people with infectious mononucleosis, acute viral hepatitis, malignant tumor of the liver, and asthma.

ANTITHYROID ANTIBODIES

The antithyroid antibodies test is done to evaluate thyroid function. In immune system disorders, such as Hashimoto's thyroiditis and Graves' disease (an overactive thyroid), the thyroid gland releases thyroglobulin into the blood. Because thyroglobulin is not normally released into circulation, antithyroglobulin antibodies are produced to attack this foreign substance. The resulting immune response may damage the thyroid gland.

Why is this test done?

A test for antithyroid antibodies may be performed to detect circulating antithyroglobulin antibodies in a person whose symptoms indicate Hashimoto's thyroiditis, Graves' disease, or other thyroid diseases.

What should you know before the test?

You won't need to change your diet before the test.

What happens during the test?

- A nurse or medical technician inserts a needle into a vein, usually in your forearm. A blood sample is collected in a tube, which is then sent to a lab for testing.
- Although you may feel a sting from the needle and pressure from the tourniquet, collecting the sample takes only a few minutes.

What happens after the test?

If swelling develops at the needle puncture site, warm soaks may be applied to ease discomfort.

What are the normal results?

The normal concentration of antithyroglobulin antibodies is less than 1 part per 100. Low levels of these antibodies are normal in 10% of the general population and in 20% or more of people age 70 or older.

What do abnormal results mean?

The presence of antithyroglobulin antibodies in blood can indicate autoimmune thyroid disease, Graves' disease, or myxedema (a drying and thickening of the skin). High concentrations strongly suggest Hashimoto's thyroiditis.

THYROID-STIMULATING FACTOR

This test — called the *thyroid-stimulating immunoglobulin test* by doctors — checks the function of the thyroid, a butterfly-shaped gland located in the neck. Thyroid-stimulating factor appears in the blood of most people with Graves' disease (an overactive thyroid). This disease stimulates the thyroid gland to produce and excrete excessive amounts of thyroid hormones.

Why is this test done?

The test for thyroid-stimulating factor may be done for the following reasons:

- To help diagnose suspected thyroid disease
- To aid diagnosis of suspected thyroid overproduction.

What should you know before the test?

You won't need to change your diet before the test.

What happens during the test?

- A nurse or medical technician inserts a needle into a vein, usually in your forearm. A blood sample is collected in a tube, which is then sent to a lab for testing.
- Although you may feel a sting from the needle and pressure from the tourniquet, collecting the sample takes only a few minutes.

What happens after the test?

If swelling develops at the needle puncture site, warm soaks may be applied to ease discomfort.

What are the normal results?

Thyroid-stimulating factor doesn't normally appear in blood. However, it may be present in 5% of people who don't have the disease.

What do abnormal results mean?

Increased thyroid-stimulating factor levels are linked to several thyroid diseases, including exophthalmos, Graves' disease, and recurrence of an underactive thyroid.

This test looks for antibodies that are attacking the thyroid gland, responding to a compound that the diseased gland would not normally release into the blood.

LUPUS TEST

A procedure called the *lupus erythematosus cell preparation* may be used to diagnose systemic lupus erythematosus, commonly known as lupus. (See *Facts about systemic lupus erythematosus*, page 512.)

Why is this test done?

The lupus test may be done for the following reasons:

- To aid diagnosis of lupus
- To monitor treatment of lupus. (About 60% of successfully treated people show no lupus erythematosus cells after 4 to 6 weeks of therapy.)

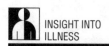

INSIGHT INTO
ILLNESS

Facts about systemic lupus erythematosus

Who does it strike?
Systemic lupus erythematosus usually strikes black women ages 15 to 30. It occurs in 10 times as many women as men (15 times as many women of childbearing age) and most often in blacks.

What is it?
Lupus is a chronic inflammatory connective tissue disease of unknown cause that affects the skin, joints, and muscles. It may cause death from failure of vital organs, especially the kidneys, but it's not always fatal. Here are some of the symptoms:

- facial rash
- hair loss
- sensitivity to light
- anemia
- positive antinuclear antibody or lupus erythematosus cell test
- false-positive blood test for syphilis
- stiff joints
- mental problems or seizures.

What should you know before the test?
You won't need to change your diet before the test.

What happens during the test?
- A nurse or medical technician inserts a needle into a vein, usually in your forearm. A blood sample is collected in a tube, which is then sent to a lab for testing.
- Although you may feel a sting from the needle and pressure from the tourniquet, collecting the sample takes only a few minutes.

What happens after the test?
- If swelling develops at the needle puncture site, warm soaks may be applied to ease discomfort.
- Because many people with lupus have damaged immune systems, you must keep a clean, dry bandage over the puncture site for at least 24 hours.

What are the normal results?
Normally, no lupus erythematosus cells are present.

What do abnormal results mean?

The presence of at least two lupus erythematosus cells may indicate lupus. Such cells may also be detected in chronic active hepatitis, rheumatoid arthritis, scleroderma, and drug reactions.

CARDIOLIPIN ANTIBODIES

This test evaluates concentrations of immunoglobulin G or M antibodies in the person's blood relative to a phospholipid called *cardiolipin*. The antibodies appear in the blood of some people with lupus and others who do not have all the signs of lupus but who experience recurrent episodes of spontaneous blood clots or miscarriages.

Why is this test done?

The test for cardiolipin antibodies may be done to aid diagnosis of cardiolipin antibody syndrome in people with or without lupus who have repeated blood clots or miscarriages.

What should you know before the test?

You won't need to change your diet before the test.

What happens during the test?

- A nurse or medical technician inserts a needle into a vein, usually in your forearm. A blood sample is collected in a tube, which is then sent to a lab for testing.
- Although you may feel a sting from the needle and pressure from the tourniquet, collecting the sample takes only a few minutes.

What happens after the test?

If swelling develops at the needle puncture site, warm soaks may be applied to ease discomfort.

What are the normal results?

If serum dilution levels are low, cardiolipin antibodies aren't a problem.

What do abnormal results mean?

A high serum dilution level, along with a history of blood clots or miscarriages suggests cardiolipin antibody syndrome. The doctor may prescribe anticoagulants or platelet-inhibitor therapy to stop blood clots.

Rheumatoid Arthritis Test

The most useful immune system test for confirming rheumatoid arthritis is called the *rheumatoid factor test*. In this disease, "renegade" immunoglobulin G antibodies, produced by lymphocytes in the synovial joints, react with other immunoglobulins to produce immune complexes, complement activation, and tissue destruction. How immunoglobulin G molecules become antigenic is still unknown, but they may be altered by aggregating with viruses or other antigens. Techniques for detecting rheumatoid factor include the sheep cell agglutination test and the latex fixation test.

This test detects immune complexes formed by "renegade" immunoglobulin G antibodies that interact with other immunoglobulins, complement, and other substances. These complexes are a sign of rheumatoid arthritis.

Why is this test done?

The rheumatoid factor test may be done to help confirm a diagnosis of the disease.

What should you know before the test?

You won't need to change your diet before the test.

What happens during the test?

- A nurse or medical technician inserts a needle into a vein, usually in your forearm. A blood sample is collected in a tube, which is then sent to a lab for testing.
- Although you may feel a sting from the needle and pressure from the tourniquet, collecting the sample takes only a few minutes.

What happens after the test?

- If swelling develops at the needle puncture site, warm soaks may be applied to ease discomfort.

- Because a person with rheumatoid arthritis may have a damaged immune system from the disease or from corticosteroid therapy, it's important to keep the puncture site covered with a clean, dry bandage for 24 hours.

What are the normal results?

The normal rheumatoid factor concentration is less than 1 part per 20 of serum.

What do abnormal results mean?

High rheumatoid factor concentrations are found in 80% of people with rheumatoid arthritis. But because people with some rheumatoid factor in their blood have other diseases and people with rheumatoid factor don't always have rheumatoid arthritis, the test isn't conclusive.

COLD ANTIBODIES TO BLOOD CELLS

Called the *cold agglutinins test* by doctors, this test detects cold agglutinins (antibodies, usually of the immunoglobulin M type) that cause red blood cells to clump at low temperatures. They may occur in small amounts in healthy people. Short-term elevations of these antibodies develop during certain infectious diseases, such as pneumonia. This test reliably detects such pneumonia within 1 to 2 weeks after infection.

Why is this test done?

A cold antibodies test may be done for the following reasons:
- To help confirm a diagnosis of one type of pneumonia
- To provide additional diagnostic evidence for cold agglutinin disease that is linked to many viral infections or lymph gland cancer.

What should you know before the test?

You won't need to change your diet before the test.

What happens during the test?

- A nurse or medical technician inserts a needle into a vein, usually in your forearm. A blood sample is collected in a tube, which is then sent to a lab for testing.
- Although you may feel a sting from the needle and pressure from the tourniquet, collecting the sample takes only a few minutes.

What happens after the test?

- If swelling develops at the needle puncture site, warm soaks may be applied to ease discomfort.
- If cold agglutinin disease is suspected, the nurse will urge you to keep warm. If you're exposed to low temperatures, blood-clumping may occur within hand and foot blood vessels, possibly leading to frostbite, anemia or, rarely, gangrene.

What are the normal results?

Normal concentrations are less than 1 part in 32 of serum but may be higher in elderly people.

What do abnormal results mean?

High concentrations of cold antibodies may show up independently (as with cold agglutinin disease) or with infections, lymph gland cancer, and many other diseases. Chronically high concentrations are most commonly linked to pneumonia and lymph gland cancer.

COLD SENSITIVITY ANTIBODIES

This test — which doctors call the *cryoglobulin test* — detects antibodies that may cause people to be sensitive to low temperatures. Cryoglobulins are abnormal proteins in the blood that precipitate at low temperatures and redissolve after being warmed. Their presence in the blood (called *cryoglobulinemia*) is usually, but not always, linked to immune system disease. If people with cryoglobulinemia are subjected to cold, they may experience pain and coldness of the fingers and toes (Raynaud's disease symptoms).

Why is this test done?

The cold sensitivity antibodies test may be done to detect cryoglobulinemia in people with Raynaud-like circulation symptoms.

What should you know before the test?

You'll fast for 4 to 6 hours before the test.

What happens during the test?

- A nurse or medical technician inserts a needle into a vein, usually in your forearm. A blood sample is collected in a tube, which is then sent to a lab for testing.
- Although you may feel a sting from the needle and pressure from the tourniquet, collecting the sample takes only a few minutes.

What happens after the test?

- If swelling develops at the needle puncture site, warm soaks may be applied to ease discomfort.
- You may resume your usual diet.
- If the test is positive for cryoglobulins, you should avoid cold temperatures or contact with cold objects.

People with cold-sensitive disease have to keep warm to avoid a blood-clumping reaction that can clog their blood vessels, leading to frostbite.

What are the normal results?

Normally, the blood test shows no cryoglobulins.

What do abnormal results mean?

The presence of cryoglobulins in the blood confirms cryoglobulinemia. However, this finding doesn't always mean the presence of a disease.

MYASTHENIA GRAVIS TEST

This immune system test — which doctors call the *acetylcholine receptors antibodies test* — confirms a diagnosis of myasthenia gravis. The acetylcholine receptor antibodies test is the most useful immune system test for confirming the disease, a disorder of neuromuscular transmission. In myasthenia gravis, antibodies block and destroy acetylcholine receptor sites, causing muscle weakness.

Why is this test done?

The myasthenia gravis test may be done to confirm a diagnosis of the disease and to monitor the effectiveness of therapy.

What should you know before the test?

You won't need to change your diet before the test.

What happens during the test?

- A nurse or medical technician inserts a needle into a vein, usually in your forearm. A blood sample is collected in a tube, which is then sent to a lab for testing.
- Although you may feel a sting from the needle and pressure from the tourniquet, collecting the sample takes only a few minutes.

What happens after the test?

- If swelling develops at the needle puncture site, warm soaks may be applied to ease discomfort.
- Keep a clean, dry bandage over the site for at least 24 hours.

What are the normal results?

Normal blood has no acetylcholine receptor antibodies or only a tiny concentration.

What do abnormal results mean?

Acetylcholine receptor antibodies in the blood of an adult with symptoms confirms the diagnosis of myasthenia gravis.

VIRUSES

RUBELLA TEST

This blood test diagnoses or evaluates a person's susceptibility to rubella, which is also known as *German measles*. Although rubella is generally a mild viral infection in children and young adults, it can produce severe infection in a fetus, resulting in spontaneous abortion, stillbirth, or inherited rubella syndrome. Because rubella infection normally stimulates production of immunoglobulin G and immunoglobulin M antibodies, measuring rubella antibodies can identify a current infection or an immunity resulting from past infection.

Why is this test done?

The test for rubella antibodies may be performed for the following reasons:

- To diagnose rubella, especially inherited infection in infants
- To determine susceptibility to rubella in children and in women of childbearing age.

What should you know before the test?

You won't need to change your diet before the test.

What happens during the test?

- A nurse or medical technician inserts a needle into a vein, usually in your forearm. A blood sample is collected in a tube, which is then sent to a lab for testing.
- Although you may feel a sting from the needle and pressure from the tourniquet, collecting the sample takes only a few minutes.

What happens after the test?

- If swelling develops at the needle puncture site, warm soaks may be applied to ease discomfort.
- If a current infection is suspected, a second blood sample will be needed in 2 to 3 weeks.

What are the normal results?

A high concentration of antibodies shows the person has adequate protection against rubella. The antibodies normally appear 2 to 4 days after the measles rash, peak in 2 to 3 weeks, then slowly decline but remain detectable for life.

What do abnormal results mean?

A low concentration means the person is susceptible to rubella and should be treated according to these guidelines:

- If a woman of childbearing age is found susceptible to the disease, vaccination can prevent rubella. But she must wait at least 3 months after the vaccination before becoming pregnant, or she risks permanent damage to or death of the fetus.

If the test confirms rubella in a pregnant woman, she may need counseling to deal with permanent damage to or the loss of the fetus.

▪ If a pregnant woman is found susceptible to rubella, she should have a follow-up rubella antibody test to detect possible subsequent infection.

▪ If the test confirms a current rubella infection in a pregnant woman, she may need counseling to deal with permanent damage to or the loss of her fetus.

What do the results mean in an infant?

Because maternal antibodies cross the placenta and persist in the infant's blood for up to 6 months, inherited rubella can be detected only after this period. A high concentration of antibodies in an infant age 6 months or older, who hasn't been exposed to rubella since birth, confirms a diagnosis of inherited rubella.

HEPATITIS B SCREENING TEST

This test helps identify a type of viral hepatitis by screening blood for hepatitis B surface antigen. Hepatitis B surface antigen appears in the blood of people with hepatitis B virus. It can be detected by the lab during the extended incubation period, during the first 3 weeks of acute infection, or if the person is a carrier.

Because transmission of hepatitis is one of the gravest complications linked to blood transfusion, all donors must be screened for hepatitis B before their blood is stored. This screening, required by the Food and Drug Administration's Bureau of Biologics, has helped reduce the incidence of hepatitis. However, this test doesn't screen for hepatitis A virus (infectious hepatitis).

Why is this test done?

The test for hepatitis B may be done for the following reasons:

▪ To screen blood donors for hepatitis B

▪ To screen people at high risk for contracting hepatitis B, such as hemodialysis nurses

▪ To help determine which type of viral hepatitis a person has.

What should you know before the test?

You won't need to change your diet before the test.

What happens during the test?

- A nurse or medical technician inserts a needle into a vein, usually in your forearm. A blood sample is collected in a tube, which is then sent to a lab for testing.
- Although you may feel a sting from the needle and pressure from the tourniquet, collecting the sample takes only a few minutes.

What happens after the test?

- If swelling develops at the needle puncture site, warm soaks may be applied to ease discomfort.
- If you're a blood donor, you'll be notified that you're positive for the antigen.
- A report of confirmed viral hepatitis will be made to public health authorities. This is a reportable disease in most states.

What are the normal results?

Normal blood shows no hepatitis B surface antigen.

What do abnormal results mean?

The presence of hepatitis B surface antigen in a person with hepatitis confirms hepatitis B. Hepatitis B surface antigen also may show up in about 5% of people with certain diseases other than hepatitis, such as hemophilia, Hodgkin's disease, and leukemia. Blood samples that test positive should be retested because inaccurate results do occur.

INFECTIOUS MONONUCLEOSIS TESTS

Called the *heterophil agglutination tests* by doctors, these tests can detect infectious mononucleosis. They're used to identify antibodies in human blood that react against foreign red blood cells. There are two types of these antibodies: Epstein-Barr virus antibodies and Forssman antibodies. Because the two types of antibodies react the same way, it takes one test to find them (the Paul-Bunnell test) and another (Davidsohn's test) to distinguish between them. (See *Spot test for mononucleosis,* page 522.)

Spot test for mononucleosis

The doctor may use one of several screening tests to diagnose mononucleosis (popularly known as *mono*). The simplest of these tests is Monospot, a rapid slide test. Monospot relies on agglutination (clumping) of horse red blood cells by mononucleosis antibodies presumed to be in the patient's serum. To confirm this reaction, serum is also mixed with a spot of guinea pig kidney cell antigen on one end of a glass slide and a spot of beef red blood cell antigen on the other end. Only the beef cell antigen is specific for mononucleosis. When horse red blood cells are added to the serum sample on each spot, clumping that occurs only on the beef cell end of the slide confirms the diagnosis.

Quick but not perfect

Monospot rivals the classic heterophil agglutination test for sensitivity. However, false-positive results may occur if the person has lymphoma, hepatitis A or B, leukemia, or pancreatic cancer.

Why are these tests done?

These tests may be performed to help distinguish infectious mononucleosis from other disorders.

What should you know before the tests?

You won't need to change your diet before the test.

What happens during the tests?

- A nurse or medical technician inserts a needle into a vein, usually in your forearm. A blood sample is collected in a tube, which is then sent to a lab for testing.
- Although you may feel a sting from the needle and pressure from the tourniquet, collecting the sample takes only a few minutes.

What happens after the tests?

- If swelling develops at the needle puncture site, warm soaks may be applied to ease discomfort.
- If the titer is positive and infectious mononucleosis is confirmed, instruct the person in the treatment plan.
- If the titer is positive but infectious mononucleosis isn't confirmed, or if the titer is negative but symptoms persist, explain that additional testing will be necessary in a few days or weeks to confirm diagnosis and plan effective treatment.

What are the normal results?

Normally, the concentration of heterophil antibodies is less than 1 part in 56, but it may be higher in elderly people.

What do abnormal results mean?

Although heterophil antibodies are present in the blood of approximately 80% of people with infectious mononucleosis 1 month after onset, a high concentration of them does not confirm this disorder. For example, a high concentration can also be caused by lupus or syphilis. A gradual increase in antibody concentration during week 3 or 4 of the illness, followed by a gradual decrease during weeks 4 to 8, proves most conclusive for infectious mononucleosis.

EPSTEIN-BARR VIRUS TEST

This test is used to diagnose infectious mononucleosis if other tests are inconclusive. Epstein-Barr virus causes infectious mononucleosis, Burkitt's lymphoma, and nose and throat cancers. This test measures Epstein-Barr virus antibodies, which combat the virus during an active infection. These antibodies can be measured precisely by a method called *indirect immunofluorescence.*

Why is this test done?
The Epstein-Barr test may be performed for the following reasons:
- To provide a laboratory diagnosis of mononucleosis missed by the Monospot test
- To determine the antibody status to Epstein-Barr virus of a person with a suppressed immune system and lymph gland involvement.

What should you know before the test?
You won't need to change your diet before the test.

What happens during the test?
- A nurse or medical technician inserts a needle into a vein, usually in your forearm. A blood sample is collected in a tube, which is then sent to a lab for testing.
- Although you may feel a sting from the needle and pressure from the tourniquet, collecting the sample takes only a few minutes.

What happens after the test?
If swelling develops at the needle puncture site, warm soaks may be applied to ease discomfort.

What are the normal results?
People who have never been infected with Epstein-Barr virus will have no detectable antibodies to the virus.

What do abnormal results mean?
Epstein-Barr virus infection can be ruled out if the person's blood has no Epstein-Barr virus antigens in the indirect immunofluorescence test. An indirect immunofluorescence test that is either immuno-

globulin M–positive or Epstein-Barr nuclear antigen–negative indicates acute Epstein-Barr virus infection.

RESPIRATORY VIRUS TEST

An immune system test called the *respiratory syncytial virus test* detects a respiratory infection that's often found in children. Respiratory syncytial virus is the major viral cause of severe lower respiratory tract disease in infants, but may cause infections in people of any age. Respiratory syncytial virus infections are most common and produce the most severe disease during the first 6 months of life.

In this test, immunoglobulin G and immunoglobulin M class antibodies to the virus are measured, using a method doctors call *indirect immunofluorescence*.

Why is this test done?
The respiratory virus test may be performed to diagnose infections caused by respiratory syncytial virus.

What should you know before the test?
You or your child won't need to change your diet before the test.

What happens during the test?
- A nurse or medical technician inserts a needle into a vein, usually in your forearm. A blood sample is collected in a tube, which is then sent to a lab for testing.
- Although you may feel a sting from the needle and pressure from the tourniquet, collecting the sample takes only a few minutes.

What happens after the test?
If swelling develops at the needle puncture site, warm soaks may be applied to ease discomfort.

What are the normal results?
Blood from people who have never been infected with respiratory syncytial virus will have no detectable antibodies to the virus.

What do abnormal results mean?

The presence of immunoglobulin M or a 400% or greater increase in immunoglobulin G antibodies indicates active respiratory syncytial virus infection. In infants, blood-test diagnosis of respiratory syncytial virus infections is difficult because of the presence of the mother's immunoglobulin G antibodies. That makes the presence of immunoglobulin M antibodies most significant.

HERPES SIMPLEX VIRUS TEST

Herpes simplex virus causes various severe conditions, including genital lesions, inflammation of the eye, generalized skin lesions, and pneumonia. Severe herpes is linked to intrauterine or neonatal infections and encephalitis, especially in people with suppressed immune systems.

There are two closely related types of herpes virus. Type 1 usually causes infections above the waistline. Type 2 infections predominantly involve the external sex organs. People usually first contract this virus in early childhood as sores around the mouth or, more commonly, as a hidden infection.

Why is this test done?

This test is performed to confirm infections caused by the herpes simplex virus.

What should you know before the test?

You won't need to change your diet before the test.

What happens during the test?

- A nurse or medical technician inserts a needle into a vein, usually in your forearm. A blood sample is collected in a tube, which is then sent to a lab for testing.
- Although you may feel a sting from the needle and pressure from the tourniquet, collecting the sample takes only a few minutes.

What happens after the test?

If swelling develops at the needle puncture site, warm soaks may be applied to ease discomfort.

What are the normal results?

Blood from people who have never been infected with herpes simplex virus will have no detectable antibodies.

What do abnormal results mean?

The presence of antibodies suggests infection with herpes simplex. The presence of immunoglobulin M or a 400% or greater increase in immunoglobulin G antibodies indicates active herpes simplex virus infection. Reactivated infections caused by herpes simplex virus can be recognized in blood tests only by a sharp increase in immunoglobulin G antibodies.

> *Of the two types of herpes, Type 1 usually strikes above the waistline. Type 2 infections usually affect the genitalia.*

TRANSPLANT REACTION SCREENING TEST

An immune system test called the *cytomegalovirus antibody screening test* is used to protect a person from transfusion or transplant reactions.

After an infection, cytomegalovirus remains latent in white blood cells. In a person with a damaged immune system, cytomegalovirus can come back to cause active infection. In some cases, blood or tissue from a donor with cytomegalovirus antibodies may cause active infection in recipients or in infants, especially those born prematurely.

Why is this test done?

The transplant reaction screening test may be performed for the following reasons:

- To detect previous cytomegalovirus infection in organ or blood donors and recipients
- To screen for cytomegalovirus infection in infants who require blood transfusion or tissue transplants
- To detect previous cytomegalovirus infection in people with damaged immune systems.

What should you know before the test?

You won't need to change your diet before the test.

What happens during the test?

- A nurse or medical technician inserts a needle into a vein, usually in your forearm. A blood sample is collected in a tube, which is then sent to a lab for testing.
- Although you may feel a sting from the needle and pressure from the tourniquet, collecting the sample takes only a few minutes.

What happens after the test?

If swelling develops at the needle puncture site, warm soaks may be applied to ease discomfort.

What are the normal results?

People who have never been infected with cytomegalovirus have no detectable antibodies to the virus.

What do abnormal results mean?

A blood sample positive for the cytomegalovirus antibody shows that the person has been infected with cytomegalovirus and that his or her blood could infect someone with a damaged immune system.

*H*IV INFECTION TESTS

These tests detect human immunodeficiency virus (HIV) infection. HIV is the virus that causes acquired immunodeficiency syndrome (AIDS). This virus may be transmitted when contaminated blood or blood products are exchanged from one person to another, during sexual intercourse with an infected partner, when intravenous drugs are shared, and during pregnancy or breast-feeding (passed from an infected mother to her child).

HIV is usually first identified by a test called the *enzyme-linked immunosorbent assay* (ELISA) and then confirmed by the Western blot or immunofluorescence test. Both of these tests detect antibodies to HIV, rather than the virus itself.

SELF-HELP

Ensuring an accurate AIDS test result

Tests that measure antibodies to HIV, the virus that causes AIDS, have been licensed by the Food and Drug Administration and are now commercially available. These tests are used to screen donated blood for AIDS to prevent contamination of the nation's blood supply. They also confirm that a person has been exposed to HIV.

Confirmation needed

The initial screening test for HIV is commonly called the *enzyme-linked immunosorbent assay* (ELISA). This test isn't 100% accurate, however, and sometimes gives false results. Because test sensitivity varies among labs, a negative result doesn't necessarily mean that no HIV antibodies are present.

On the other hand, a false-positive result may also reflect a lab error. As a result, the U.S. Public Health Service recommends that the doctor confirm any positive result *before* the person is notified. To confirm, the Western Blot test is used. This test is more reliable than the ELISA test, but it's technically more difficult.

Why are these tests done?

The tests may be performed for the following reasons:

- To screen for HIV infection (see *Ensuring an accurate AIDS test result* and *How HIV destroys immunity*)
- To screen donated blood for HIV infection.

What should you know before the tests?

You won't need to fast or restrict fluids before the test to ensure reliable results. More important, the test results are confidential and will be revealed to no one without your permission.

What happens during the tests?

- A nurse or medical technician inserts a needle into a vein, usually in your forearm. A blood sample is collected in a tube, which is then sent to a lab for testing.
- Although you may feel a sting from the needle and pressure from the tourniquet, collecting the sample takes only a few minutes.

What happens after the tests?

- If swelling develops at the needle puncture site, warm soaks may be applied to ease discomfort.
- Assume that you can transmit HIV to others until conclusively proven otherwise. To prevent possible contagion, use safe-sex precautions.
- If the results are positive, get medical follow-up care, even if you have no symptoms. You should be on the lookout for early signs of AIDS, such as fever, weight loss, swollen lymph glands, rash, and persistent cough or diarrhea. Women should also report gynecologic symptoms.
- If you're found to be HIV-positive, don't share razors, toothbrushes, or utensils (which may be contaminated with blood) and clean such items with household bleach diluted 1 part to 10 in water. Practice safe sex to prevent giving HIV to another person. Don't donate blood, tissues, or an organ. Inform your doctor and dentist about your condition so that they can take the proper precautions.

What are the normal results?

The ELISA test should be negative, which means that it shows no HIV antibodies. However, this result, while certainly favorable,

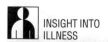

INSIGHT INTO
ILLNESS

How HIV destroys immunity

The difference between a normal and a damaged immune system is that a healthy person has the right cells to fight off infections. To understand how HIV affects immunity, consider first how a healthy immune system functions.

Normal immune function

When viruses enter the bloodstream, they're identified as foreign bodies (antigens) by cells called *macrophages*. The macrophages process the antigens and present them to T cells and B cells.

The antigen-activated T cells multiply and form several kinds of T cells. For example:
- Helper T cells stimulate B cells.
- Suppressor T cells balance them, controlling the extent of T-cell help for B cells.
- Lymphokine-producing T cells are involved in delayed hypersensitivity and other immune reactions.
- Cytotoxic, or killer, T cells directly destroy antigens.
- Memory T cells are stored to recognize and attack a reinvading antigen.

The B cells multiply, forming memory cells and plasma cells that produce antigen-specific antibodies, which then attack and kill the invading virus.

Impaired immune function

HIV selectively infects the helper T cells, impairing their ability to recognize antigens. Thus the virus is free to multiply, causing abnormal immune system function and progressive destruction.

As the person's immunity weakens, he or she becomes vulnerable to potentially fatal protozoal, viral, and fungal infections and to certain forms of cancer. Meanwhile, many more HIV particles are released and invade other T cells, further weakening the immune system.

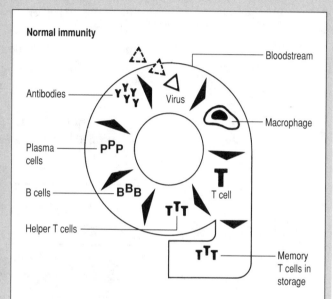

Normal immunity

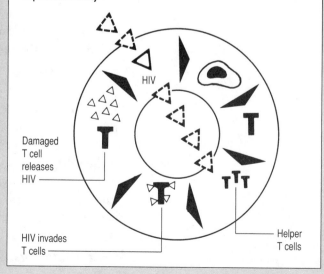

Impaired immunity

doesn't guarantee that a person is free from HIV infection. That's because the test doesn't identify people who've been exposed to HIV but whose bodies haven't yet created antibodies to the virus. This lag time typically varies from a few weeks to months. During this period, an HIV-infected person will test negative for HIV antibodies.

What do abnormal results mean?

A positive ELISA test indicates exposure to HIV. A positive test can't determine whether a person harbors the actively growing virus or when the person will show symptoms of AIDS. Many apparently healthy people have been exposed to HIV and have circulating antibodies. What's more, people in the later stages of AIDS may show no detectable antibodies in their blood because they can no longer mount an antibody response.

If an ELISA test is positive, the test should be repeated and then confirmed by the Western blot or an immunofluorescence test.

BACTERIA & FUNGI

STREP TEST

Called the *antistreptolysin-O test* by doctors, this test detects the immune system's response to bacteria called *streptococci* (popularly known as *strep*). It measures the relative concentrations of antibodies developed against *streptolysin O,* an antigen produced by the streptococcus bacteria.

Why is this test done?

The strep test may be performed for the following reasons:
- To confirm recent or ongoing infection with strep bacteria
- To help diagnose suspected rheumatic fever and kidney disease that may follow a strep infection
- To distinguish between rheumatic fever and rheumatoid arthritis when the person has joint pains.

What should you know before the test?

You won't need to change your diet before the test.

What happens during the test?

- A nurse or medical technician inserts a needle into a vein, usually in your forearm. A blood sample is collected in a tube, which is then sent to a lab for testing.
- Although you may feel a sting from the needle and pressure from the tourniquet, collecting the sample takes only a few minutes.

What happens after the test?

- If swelling develops at the needle puncture site, warm soaks may be applied to ease discomfort.
- The test may be repeated at regular intervals to identify active and inactive diseases by measuring changes in antibody levels.

What are the normal results?

Even healthy people have some detectable antistreptolysin-O concentration because of antibodies from previous minor strep infections.

What do abnormal results mean?

High antistreptolysin-O concentrations usually show up only after prolonged or recurrent infections. Doctors use the antibody levels from a series of tests to track down diseases. Roughly 15% to 20% of people with a disease that follows strep don't have elevated antistreptolysin-O concentrations, so this test is just one of the methods used to diagnose such diseases.

FEVER EVALUATION TESTS

Called *febrile agglutination tests* by doctors, these tests provide important diagnostic information regarding bacterial infections (such as tularemia, brucellosis, and disorders caused by salmonella) and rickettsial infections (such as Rocky Mountain spotted fever and typhus) that sometimes cause fevers of undetermined origin. In such conditions, causative organisms are difficult to isolate from blood or excretions.

Why are these tests done?

Fever evaluation tests may be performed for the following reasons:
- To support clinical findings in diagnosis of disorders caused by *Salmonella*, *Rickettsia*, *Francisella tularensis*, or *Brucella* organisms
- To identify the cause of fevers of undetermined origin.

These tests help pinpoint disorders that are hard to diagnose and that cause fevers of unknown origin.

What should you know before the tests?

You won't need to change your diet before the tests.

What happens during the tests?

- A nurse or medical technician inserts a needle into a vein, usually in your forearm. A blood sample is collected in a tube, which is then sent to a lab for testing.
- Although you may feel a sting from the needle and pressure from the tourniquet, collecting the sample takes only a few minutes.

What happens after the tests?

- If swelling develops at the needle puncture site, warm soaks may be applied to ease discomfort.
- This test requires a series of blood samples to detect a pattern of concentrations that is characteristic of the suspected disorder. Remember that a positive concentration only suggests a disorder.
- In fevers of undetermined origin and suspected infection, the hospital may have to isolate the person.

What are the normal results?

Normal antibody dilution values are as follows:
- Salmonella antibody: less than 1:80
- Brucellosis antibody: less than 1:80
- Tularemia antibody: less than 1:40
- Rickettsial antibody: less than 1:40.

What do abnormal results mean?

The doctor has to check the rise and fall of antibody dilutions to detect an active infection. If this is not possible, certain dilution levels may suggest the disorder. For all febrile agglutinins, a 400% increase in concentration is strong evidence of infection.

FUNGAL INFECTION TESTS

Blood tests (fungal serology) help the doctor diagnose specific fungal infections. Most fungi enter the body as spores inhaled into the lungs or through wounds in the skin or mucous membranes. If the body's defenses can't destroy the organisms quickly, the fungi multiply to form lesions. The person's blood and lymph vessels may then spread the fungus throughout the body. Most healthy people easily overcome a new fungal infection, but elderly people and people with deficient immune systems are more susceptible to acute or chronic infections.

Why are these tests done?
The tests may be used for the following reasons:
- To help diagnose fungal infection
- To monitor the effectiveness of therapy for fungal infection.

What should you know before the tests?
You'll restrict food and fluids for 12 to 24 hours before the test.

What happens during the tests?
- A nurse or medical technician inserts a needle into a vein, usually in your forearm. A blood sample is collected in a tube, which is then sent to a lab for testing.
- Although you may feel a sting from the needle and pressure from the tourniquet, collecting the sample takes only a few minutes.

What happens after the tests?
If swelling develops at the needle puncture site, warm soaks may be applied to ease discomfort.

What are the normal results?
Depending on the test method (complement fixation or cell agglutination procedures), a negative finding, or a normal concentration, usually indicates the absence of any fungal infection.

What do abnormal results mean?

Abnormal findings may indicate one of the following fungal infections:

- blastomycosis, a fungal condition that usually affects the lungs and produces bronchopneumonia
- coccidioidomycosis, a fungal condition that usually causes a respiratory infection but may spread throughout the body
- histoplasmosis, a fungal infection that occurs in three forms: *primary acute histoplasmosis, progressive disseminated histoplasmosis,* and *chronic pulmonary histoplasmosis,* with varying signs and symptoms
- aspergillosis, a fungal infection that occurs in four major forms: *aspergilloma* (which affects the lungs), *allergic aspergillosis* (a hypersensitive asthmatic reaction), *aspergillosis endophthalmitis* (an infection of the eye), and *disseminated aspergillosis* (an acute infection that produces blood poisoning and blood clots)
- sporotrichosis, a chronic condition that may affect the skin or lungs or may spread to the joints
- cryptococcosis, which usually starts as a lung infection without symptoms but may spread to other body regions.

CANDIDIASIS TEST

Candida albicans is a type of yeast that's commonly present in the body. It can cause an infection when the person's immune defenses have been significantly weakened.

Infection with this organism is called *candidiasis.* Candidiasis is usually limited to the skin and mucous membranes but may cause life-threatening systemic infection. Risk factors include recent antibacterial, antimetabolic, or corticosteroid therapy; immune system defects; diabetes; a debilitating disease; pregnancy; or obesity. Oral candidiasis is common and benign in children. In adults, it may be an early indication of AIDS.

When other methods fail, the doctor may use an immune system test to look for the *Candida* antibody to spot systemic candidiasis. Be aware that blood testing for these antibodies is not reliable. Medical experts continue to disagree about its usefulness.

Why is this test done?

The candidiasis test may be performed to help diagnose the infection when a culture or tissue study can't confirm it.

What should you know before the test?

You won't need to change your diet before the test.

What happens during the test?

■ A nurse or medical technician inserts a needle into a vein, usually in your forearm. A blood sample is collected in a tube, which is then sent to a lab for testing.
■ Although you may feel a sting from the needle and pressure from the tourniquet, collecting the sample takes only a few minutes.

What happens after the test?

If swelling develops at the needle puncture site, warm soaks may be applied to ease discomfort.

What are the normal results?

A normal test result is negative for the *Candida* antigen.

What do abnormal results mean?

A positive test for *Candida albicans* antigen is common in people with widespread candidiasis. However, this test yields a significant percentage of false-positive results.

When cultures and blood studies aren't definitive, doctors may look for the Candida antibody. But the test isn't considered reliable, and investigators still disagree about its usefulness.

BACTERIAL MENINGITIS TEST

Called the *bacterial meningitis antigen test,* this test can detect specific antigens of *Streptococcus pneumoniae, Neisseria meningitidis,* and *Haemophilus influenzae* type B, all of which are the major bacteria that cause meningitis. Lab technicians can use samples of blood, spinal fluid, urine, lung fluid, or joint fluid to perform the test.

Why is this test done?

The bacterial meningitis test may be performed for the following reasons:

- To identify the specific bacteria causing meningitis
- To aid diagnosis of bacterial meningitis.

What should you know before the test?

- You'll be told whether this test requires a urine specimen or a specimen of spinal fluid collected by a procedure called a *lumbar puncture.*
- If spinal fluid is to be collected, you'll be given a local anesthesic before the test, but you may feel short-term discomfort from the needle puncture.

What happens during the test?

- If a specimen of spinal fluid is required, a doctor performs the lumbar puncture procedure. This method requires insertion of a needle between the vertebrae of the lower spine. It takes about 20 minutes.
- If a urine specimen is required, you're instructed to urinate into a sterile container, which is then sent to a lab for testing.

What happens after the test?

A headache is the most common effect of lumbar puncture but your cooperation during the test minimizes the possibility of this reaction.

What are the normal results?

The test should be negative for bacterial antigens.

What do abnormal results mean?

Positive results identify the specific bacteria causing the infection: *Streptococcus pneumoniae, Neisseria meningitidis, Haemophilus influenzae* type B, or group B streptococci.

LYME DISEASE TEST

This test helps determine whether a person's symptoms are caused by Lyme disease. Lyme disease affects the skin, nervous system, heart, and joints as it goes through its various stages. It's caused by *Borrelia burgdorferi,* a bacterium commonly carried by wood ticks.

This blood test measures the antibody response to the bacteria and can identify 50% of people with early-stage Lyme disease. It can also identify all people with later complications of carditis, neuritis, and arthritis and all people who are in remission from these effects.

Why is this test done?
The test may be performed to confirm the doctor's diagnosis of Lyme disease.

What should you know before the test?
You'll have to fast for 12 hours before the blood sample is drawn, but you can drink fluids as usual.

What happens during the test?
- A nurse or medical technician inserts a needle into a vein, usually in your forearm. A blood sample is collected in a tube, which is then sent to a lab for testing.
- Although you may feel a sting from the needle and pressure from the tourniquet, collecting the sample takes only a few minutes.

What happens after the test?
If swelling develops at the needle puncture site, warm soaks may be applied to ease discomfort.

What are the normal results?
Normally, the test finds no Lyme disease antibodies. If there's a trace of antibodies, you may need repeat testing in 4 to 6 weeks.

What do abnormal results mean?
A positive test can help confirm the doctor's diagnosis, but it's not definitive. Other similar diseases and high rheumatoid factor concentrations can cause false-positive results. More than 15% of people with Lyme disease fail to develop antibodies.

This test measures the antibody response to the organism that causes Lyme disease; it can identify early stages of the disease in 50% of cases.
It's not definitive, however, because 15% of people with Lyme disease don't develop antibodies.

MISCELLANEOUS TESTS

VDRL TEST FOR SYPHILIS

The Venereal Disease Research Laboratory (VDRL) test is widely used to diagnose syphilis. Usually, a blood sample is used in the VDRL test, but this test may also be performed on a specimen of spinal fluid to test for tertiary syphilis, the stage marked by skin eruptions.

Why is this test done?
The VDRL test may be performed for the following reasons:
- To screen for syphilis
- To confirm syphilis in the presence of syphilitic lesions
- To monitor the infected person's response to treatment.

What should you know before the test?
You won't need to change your diet, but you shouldn't have any alcohol for 24 hours before the test.

What happens during the test?
- A nurse or medical technician inserts a needle into a vein, usually in your forearm. A blood sample is collected in a tube, which is then sent to a lab for testing.
- Although you may feel a sting from the needle and pressure from the tourniquet, collecting the sample takes only a few minutes.

What happens after the test?
- If swelling develops at the needle puncture site, warm soaks may be applied to ease discomfort.
- If the test is nonreactive or borderline but syphilis hasn't been ruled out, you should return for follow-up testing. Borderline test results don't necessarily mean you're free of the disease.

- If the test is reactive, you'll need antibiotic therapy. Also, there will be mandatory inquiries from public health authorities.
- If the test is reactive but you show no signs of syphilis, you'll need more specific tests to rule out the disease. Many uninfected people show false-positive reactions.

What are the normal results?

Normal blood shows no flocculation (thickening) when mixed with the required antigen complex and is reported as a nonreactive test.

What do abnormal results mean?

Definite flocculation is reported as a reactive test. Slight flocculation is reported as a weakly reactive test. A reactive VDRL test occurs in about 50% of people with primary syphilis and in nearly all people with secondary syphilis.

If you have syphilitic lesions, a reactive VDRL test confirms the diagnosis. If there are no lesions it means you must be repeatedly tested. However, biological false-positive reactions can be caused by conditions unrelated to syphilis; for example, infectious mononucleosis, malaria, leprosy, hepatitis, lupus, and rheumatoid arthritis.

Delayed-reaction

A nonreactive test doesn't rule out syphilis because it causes no detectable changes in the blood for 14 to 21 days after infection. However, the doctor can use a microscopic examination of matter from suspicious lesions to identify the bacteria.

A reactive VDRL test performed on spinal fluid indicates neurosyphilis, which can follow the other stages of the disease in people who don't get treatment.

*F*TA TEST FOR SYPHILIS

The fluorescent treponemal antibody (FTA) absorption test for syphilis is more exact than other syphilis tests. It detects antibodies to the bacteria in the blood that causes syphilis.

Why is this test done?

The FTA absorption test may be performed for the following reasons:

- To confirm primary or secondary stage syphilis
- To screen for suspected false-positive results of the VDRL test.

What should you know before the test?

You won't need to change your diet before the test.

What happens during the test?

- A nurse or medical technician inserts a needle into a vein, usually in your forearm. A blood sample is collected in a tube, which is then sent to a lab for testing.
- Although you may feel a sting from the needle and pressure from the tourniquet, collecting the sample takes only a few minutes.

What happens after the test?

- If swelling develops at the needle puncture site, warm soaks may be applied to ease discomfort.
- If the test is reactive, you'll need antibiotic treatment, and your sexual partners should also receive treatment.
- Because the disease must be reported, be prepared for inquiries from the public health authorities.
- If the test is nonreactive or findings are borderline, but syphilis has not been ruled out, you'll need to return for follow-up testing. Inconclusive results don't necessarily mean you're free of the disease.

What are the normal results?

Normally, reaction to the test is negative (no fluorescence).

What do abnormal results mean?

Antibodies in your blood — a reactive test result — do not indicate the stage or the severity of the infection. Elevated antibody levels appear in 80% to 90% of people with primary syphilis and in 100% of people with secondary syphilis. Higher antibody levels persist for several years, with or without treatment.

The absence of antibodies doesn't necessarily rule out syphilis because the infection doesn't cause detectable immunologic changes in the blood for 14 to 21 days. The doctor may find organisms earlier by examining suspicious lesions with a microscope. If you have borderline findings, the doctor may recommend repeated testing.

Possible sources of confusion
Although the FTA test is specific, some people with other conditions (such as lupus, genital herpes, or increased or abnormal globulins) and pregnant women may show slightly reactive levels. In addition, the test doesn't always distinguish between the organism that causes syphilis and related organisms.

CANCER SCREENING TEST

Also called the *carcinoembryonic antigen test*, this procedure detects and measures a special protein that's not normally present in adults. Carcinoembryonic antigen is secreted onto the lining of the fetus's digestive tract during the first 6 months of fetal life. Normally, this antigen is not produced after birth, but tumor growth can cause it to reappear in the blood later in life.

Because carcinoembryonic antigen levels are also raised by bile duct obstruction, alcoholic hepatitis, chronic heavy smoking, and other conditions, this test can't be used as a general indicator of cancer, but it can help the doctor stage and monitor treatment of certain cancers.

Why is this test done?
The cancer screening test may be performed for the following reasons:
- To monitor the effectiveness of cancer therapy
- To assist in preoperative staging of colon and rectum cancers, check the adequacy of surgical resection, and to test for the return of the cancers.

What should you know before the test?
You won't need to change your diet before the test.

What happens during the test?

- A nurse or medical technician inserts a needle into a vein, usually in your forearm. A blood sample is collected in a tube, which is then sent to a lab for testing.
- Although you may feel a sting from the needle and pressure from the tourniquet, collecting the sample takes only a few minutes.

What happens after the test?

If swelling develops at the needle puncture site, warm soaks may be applied to ease discomfort.

What are the normal results?

Normal blood carcinoembryonic antigen values are less than 5 nanograms per milliliter in healthy nonsmokers. However, about 5% of the population has above-normal concentrations.

What do abnormal results mean?

Persistent elevation of carcinoembryonic antigen levels suggests that the person has residual or recurrent tumor. If levels exceed normal before surgical resection, chemotherapy, or radiation therapy, their return to normal within 6 weeks suggests successful treatment.

High carcinoembryonic antigen levels show up various malignant conditions, particularly certain tumors of the gastrointestinal organs and the lungs, and in certain nonmalignant conditions, such as benign hepatic disease, hepatic cirrhosis, alcoholic pancreatitis, and inflammatory bowel disease. They also may appear in people with breast cancer or ovarian cancer.

This test is used for preoperative staging of colon and rectum cancers. It also sheds light on lung cancers as well as some nonmalignant liver, pancreas, and bowel diseases.

BIRTH DEFECT AND CANCER THERAPY MONITORING

Doctors call this the *alpha-fetoprotein test*. It monitors a person's response to cancer therapy by measuring a specific blood protein. It also detects birth defects in a developing fetus, often leading to more testing, such as amniocentesis and ultrasound. Alpha-fetoprotein is produced by fetal tissue and by tumors. During fetal development, alpha-fetoprotein levels in blood and the amniotic fluid in the womb increase. Alpha-fetoprotein crosses the placenta and appears in the mother's blood.

Why is this test done?

The alpha-fetoprotein test may be performed for the following reasons:

- To monitor the effectiveness of therapy in certain cancers, such as hepatomas and germ cell tumors, and in certain nonmalignant conditions
- To determine the need for amniocentesis or high-resolution ultrasound in a pregnant woman.

What should you know before the test?

You won't need to change your diet before the test.

What happens during the test?

- A nurse or medical technician inserts a needle into a vein, usually in your forearm. A blood sample is collected in a tube, which is then sent to a lab for testing.
- Although you may feel a sting from the needle and pressure from the tourniquet, collecting the sample takes only a few minutes.

What happens after the test?

If swelling develops at the needle puncture site, warm soaks may be applied to ease discomfort.

What are the normal results?

Alpha-fetoprotein values are low to nonexistent in men and nonpregnant women.

What do abnormal results mean?

High alpha-fetoprotein in a pregnant woman's blood may suggest a neural tube defect or other spinal abnormalities in a fetus after 14 weeks' gestation. Alpha-fetoprotein levels increase sharply in approximately 90% of fetuses with no developing brain and in 50% of those with spina bifida. Definitive diagnosis requires ultrasound and amniocentesis. High alpha-fetoprotein levels may indicate that the fetus has died.

High levels in nonpregnant people may indicate a long list of digestive system cancers. Short-term, modest elevations can mean alcoholic cirrhosis and acute or chronic hepatitis.

TORCH TEST

This test helps detect exposure to pathogens involved in inherited infections in infants. TORCH is an acronym for *toxoplasmosis, rubella, cytomegalovirus, syphilis,* and *herpes simplex.* These problems are not readily apparent in newborns and may cause severe central nervous system damage. The TORCH test detects specific antibodies to these pathogens in the infant's blood.

Why is this test done?

The TORCH test may be performed to aid diagnosis of acute infections that are present in an infant at birth.

What happens during the test?

- The test requires a sample of your infant's blood.
- A nurse or a medical technician will take the sample, either with a needle or from the umbilical cord of a newborn.
- Although your infant may feel short-term discomfort, collecting the sample takes less than 3 minutes.

What are the normal results?

A normal test result is negative for TORCH agents.

What do abnormal results mean?

Depending on what antibodies are found, the doctor will use more tests to be sure of the correct diagnosis. For example, both toxoplasmosis and rubella are diagnosed by an increase in antibody concentration over time.

TUBERCULOSIS TESTS

Tuberculin skin tests help detect tuberculosis. They screen for previous infection by the tubercle bacillus. They're routinely performed in children, young adults, and other people whose X-rays suggest tuberculosis. In both the old tuberculin and purified protein derivative tests, injection of the tuberculin antigen under the skin causes a delayed hypersensitivity reaction in people with active or dormant tuberculosis. (See *Who's at risk for tuberculosis?* page 546.)

Why are these tests done?

Tuberculin skin tests may be done for the following reasons:

- To distinguish tuberculosis from other diseases, including blastomycosis, coccidioidomycosis, and histoplasmosis
- To identify persons who need to checked further for tuberculosis.

What should you know before the test?

- The tests require an injection under your skin, which may cause short-term discomfort.
- The nurse will check your history for active tuberculosis, the results of previous skin tests, or hypersensitivities. If you've had tuberculosis, the nurse won't perform the test.
- If you've had an allergic reaction to acacia, you won't be given the old tuberculin test because this product contains acacia.

What happens during the tests?

- You sit and support your extended arm on a flat surface while the nurse cleans your upper forearm with alcohol and allows the area to dry completely.
- For a Mantoux test, the needle is inserted under your skin and you feel a sting.
- For a multipuncture test, a four-pronged device punctures your skin and releases materials.

What happens after the tests?

- For either test, the nurse makes an appointment for you to return to have the skin test read — generally 48 to 72 hours later.
- A positive reaction to a skin test appears as a red, hard, raised area at the injection site. Although the area may itch, don't scratch it.

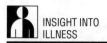

INSIGHT INTO
ILLNESS

Who's at risk for tuberculosis?

Researchers may argue about the causes behind the increased incidence of tuberculosis, but they do agree that tuberculosis is on the rise. And they can identify people with the highest risk.

Generally at risk

- People disadvantaged by crowded, poorly ventilated, unsanitary living conditions (such as those in some prisons, tenement housing, or shelters for the homeless)
- Men (tuberculosis is twice as common in men than in women)
- Nonwhites (tuberculosis is four times as common in nonwhites than in whites; the typical newly diagnosed tuberculosis patient is a single, homeless, nonwhite man)
- People in close contact with a recently diagnosed tuberculosis patient
- Individuals who've previously had tuberculosis
- People with weak immune systems

Specifically at risk

- Black and Hispanic men between ages 25 and 44
- People with multiple sexual partners
- Recent immigrants from Africa, Asia, Mexico, and South America
- People who've had a gastrectomy
- People afflicted by silicosis, diabetes, malnutrition, cancer, and diseases affecting the immune system
- Drug and alcohol abusers
- People in institutions for the chronically or mentally ill
- Nursing home residents (who are 10 times more likely to contract tuberculosis than anyone in the general populace)

- Remember that a positive reaction doesn't always indicate active tuberculosis.

Do the tests have risks?

- Tuberculin skin tests are dangerous for people with current reactions to smallpox vaccinations, any rash, skin disorder, or active tuberculosis. You should tell the doctor or nurse if you have any of those conditions.
- The nurse or technician will have epinephrine available to treat a possible acute hypersensitivity reaction.

What are the normal results?

In tuberculin skin tests, normal findings show minimal or no reactions.

What do abnormal results mean?

A positive tuberculin reaction indicates previous infection by tubercle bacilli. It doesn't distinguish between an active and dormant infection, nor does it provide a definitive diagnosis. If you have a positive reaction, a sputum smear and culture and a chest X-ray are necessary for further information.

DELAYED HYPERSENSITIVITY SKIN TESTS

These tests evaluate a person's immune system after application or injection of small doses of antigens. Skin testing is used to evaluate the immune response of people with severe recurrent infection, infection caused by unusual organisms, or suspected disorders associated with delayed hypersensitivity. Because diminished, delayed hypersensitivity may be linked to a poor chance of recovery from certain malignancies, this test may help the doctor estimate the prognosis for some cancer patients.

Why are these tests done?

Delayed hypersensitivity skin tests may be performed for the following reasons:
- To evaluate the person's immune responses
- To measure the effectiveness of immunotherapy when the person's immune response is being boosted
- To diagnose fungal diseases, bacterial diseases, and viral diseases
- To monitor the course of certain diseases.

What should you know before the tests?

You won't need to change your diet before the tests.

What happens during the tests?

- You sit and support your arm on a flat surface.
- A nurse or medical technician injects or applies the antigens.
- Although you may feel a sting from the needle, the discomfort is short-term.
- It takes about 10 minutes for each antigen to be administered.

What happens after the tests?

- Reactions should appear in 48 to 72 hours.
- Some antigens are given again after 2 weeks or, if the test is negative, a stronger dose of antigen may be given.

Do the tests have risks?

- If hypersensitivity to the antigens is suspected, they're first applied in low concentrations.
- The nurse watches for signs of a severe allergic reaction: hives, respiratory distress, and low blood pressure. If such signs develop, you're given epinephrine.

What are the normal results?

In a test called the *DNCB test,* a positive reaction (swelling, hardness, redness) appears 48 to 96 hours after the second (challenge) dose in 95% of the population. In the *recall antigen test,* a positive response (a significant reaction at the test site) appears 48 hours after injection.

What do abnormal results mean?

In the DNCB test, failure to react to the challenge dose indicates diminished, delayed hypersensitivity. In the recall antigen test several things demonstrate diminished, delayed hypersensitivity: a positive response to less than two of the six test antigens, a persistent unresponsiveness to an under-the-skin injection of higher-strength antigens, or a generalized diminished reaction.

Diminished, delayed hypersensitivity can be caused by many conditions: Hodgkin's disease; sarcoidosis; liver disease; inherited immune disease, such as DiGeorge's syndrome and Wiskott-Aldrich syndrome; uremia; acute leukemia; viral diseases, such as influenza, infectious mononucleosis, measles, mumps, and rubella; fungal diseases, such as coccidioidomycosis and cryptococcosis; bacterial diseases, such as tuberculosis; and terminal cancer. Diminished, delayed hypersensitivity can also result from immunosuppressive or steroid drugs or viral vaccination.

URINE TESTS:
Examining the Body's Excess Fluids

ANALYSIS OF URINE

ROUTINE URINALYSIS

These tests help diagnose kidney or urinary tract disease and evaluate your overall body function. (See *The kidneys and urine formation,* page 552.) The tests use several techniques, including:
- visual examination for physical characteristics (color, odor, and opacity) of urine
- refractometry to determine specific gravity and pH
- chemical tests to detect and measure protein, glucose, and ketone bodies
- microscopic inspection of sediment for blood cells, casts, and crystals.

Why is this test done?
Routine urinalysis may be performed for the following reasons:
- To screen your urine for kidney or urinary tract disease
- To help the doctor detect metabolic or systemic disease unrelated to kidney disorders.

What should you know before the test?
- You won't need to change your diet before the test.
- The nurse will ask about any current or recent medication use; many drugs may affect test results.

What happens during the test?
- You use a clean container to collect a urine specimen of at least 15 milliliters.
- Collect a specimen from your first voiding in the morning, if possible.

What are the normal results?
Harmless variations in normal values may result from diet, non-threatening conditions, specimen collection time, and other factors. The doctor looks for the following normal characteristics:
- Color: straw
- Odor: slightly aromatic

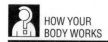

HOW YOUR
BODY WORKS

The kidneys and urine formation

The kidneys, through the activity of the nephrons, continuously remove metabolic wastes, drugs, and other foreign substances. They filter excess fluids, inorganic salts, and acid and base substances from the blood for eventual excretion in the urine.

The nephron: Master filter

Each kidney has approximately 1 million nephrons. Each of these nephrons consists of an ultrafilter, called a *glomerulus*, and a tubule — a lined conduit that works to reabsorb recyclable matter and secrete foreign and waste substances.

Each tubule is made up of four sections: the proximal convoluted tubule, loop of Henle, distal convoluted tubule, and collecting tubule. As the filtrate from the glomerulus travels through the renal tubules, resorption and secretion modify it to meet the body's needs. The end result is urine.

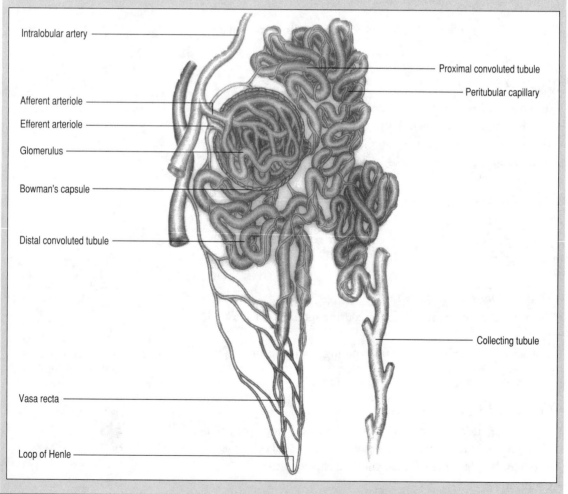

Intralobular artery

Afferent arteriole

Efferent arteriole

Glomerulus

Bowman's capsule

Distal convoluted tubule

Vasa recta

Loop of Henle

Proximal convoluted tubule

Peritubular capillary

Collecting tubule

- Appearance: clear
- Specific gravity (the ratio of the density of urine to the density of water): 1.005 to 1.035
- pH: 4.5 to 8.0
- Sugars: none
- Epithelial cells: few
- Casts: none, except occasional translucent casts
- Crystals: present
- Yeast cells: none.

What do abnormal results mean?

The following abnormal findings generally suggest diseased conditions:

- Color: Color change can result from diet, drugs, and many diseases.
- Odor: In diabetes mellitus, starvation, and dehydration, a fruity odor accompanies formation of ketone bodies. In urinary tract infections, a fetid odor commonly is associated with *Escherichia coli*. Maple syrup, urine disease, and phenylketonuria also cause distinctive odors.
- Turbidity: Turbid urine may contain red or white cells, bacteria, fat, or chyle and may reflect kidney infection.
- Specific gravity: Low specific gravity (less than 1.005) is characteristic of diabetes insipidus, nephrogenic diabetes insipidus, acute tubular necrosis, and pyelonephritis. Fixed specific gravity, in which values remain 1.010 regardless of fluid intake, occurs in chronic glomerulonephritis with severe kidney damage. High specific gravity (more than 1.035) occurs in nephrotic syndrome, dehydration, acute glomerulonephritis, congestive heart failure, liver failure, and shock.
- pH: Alkaline urine pH may result from Fanconi's syndrome, urinary tract infection, and metabolic or respiratory alkalosis. Acid urine pH is associated with kidney tuberculosis, fever, phenylketonuria, alkaptonuria, and acidosis.
- Protein: Protein in the urine suggests kidney failure or disease (including nephrosis, glomerulosclerosis, glomerulonephritis, nephrolithiasis, and polycystic kidney disease) or, possibly, multiple tumors.
- Sugars: Glycosuria usually indicates diabetes mellitus, but may be caused by a long list of diseases, including pheochromocytoma, Cushing's syndrome, impaired tubular reabsorption, advanced kidney disease, and increased intracranial pressure. Fructosuria, galacto-

The color of urine can be affected by a person's diet, use of drugs, or a long list of diseases.

suria, and pentosuria generally suggest rare hereditary metabolic disorders (except for lactosuria during pregnancy and lactation).

- Ketone bodies: Ketonuria occurs in diabetes mellitus or in starvation and following diarrhea or vomiting.
- Bilirubin: Bilirubin in urine may occur in liver disease caused by obstructive jaundice, hepatotoxic drugs, or toxins or by fibrosis of the biliary canaliculi (which may occur in cirrhosis).
- Urobilinogen: Bilirubin is changed into urobilinogen in the duodenum by intestinal bacteria. The liver reprocesses the remainder into bile. Increased urobilinogen in the urine may indicate liver damage, hemolytic disease, or severe infection. Decreased levels may occur with biliary obstruction, inflammatory disease, antimicrobial therapy, severe diarrhea, or kidney insufficiency.
- Cells: Bloody urine indicates bleeding within the genitourinary tract, possibly caused by a long list of problems: infection, obstruction, inflammation, trauma, tumors, glomerulonephritis, kidney hypertension, lupus nephritis, kidney tuberculosis, kidney vein thrombosis, kidney stones, hydronephrosis, pyelonephritis, scurvy, malaria, parasitic infection of the bladder, subacute bacterial endocarditis, polyarteritis nodosa, and hemorrhagic disorders.

Strenuous exercise or exposure to toxic chemicals may also cause blood in the urine. An excess of white cells in urine usually implies urinary tract inflammation. White cells and white cell casts in urine suggest kidney infection. Numerous epithelial cells suggest kidney tubular degeneration.

- Casts (plugs of gelled proteinaceous material): Casts form in the kidney's tubules and collecting ducts by agglutination of protein cells or cellular debris and are flushed loose by urine flow. Excessive numbers of casts indicate kidney disease.
- Crystals: Some crystals normally appear in urine, but numerous calcium oxalate crystals suggest hypercalcemia. Cystine crystals (cystinuria) reflect an inborn error of metabolism.
- Other components: Bacteria, yeast cells, and parasites in urinary sediment reflect genitourinary tract infection or contamination of external genitalia. Yeast cells, which may be mistaken for red cells, are identifiable by their oval shape, lack of color, variable size, and frequently, signs of budding. The most common parasite in sediment is *Trichomonas vaginalis,* which causes vaginitis, urethritis, and prostatovesiculitis.

KIDNEY STONE TEST

This test checks you for kidney stones. Lab analysis will reveal their composition. Kidney stones are insoluble substances most commonly formed of these mineral salts: calcium oxalate, calcium phosphate, magnesium ammonium phosphate, urate, or cystine. They may appear anywhere in the urinary tract and range in size from microscopic to several centimeters.

How kidney stones develop

You can get kidney stones from reduced urine output, increased excretion of mineral salts, holding urine, pH changes, and decreased protective substances. Stones usually form in the kidney, pass into the ureter, and are excreted in the urine. Because not all stones pass spontaneously, they may require surgical extraction. Kidney stones don't always cause symptoms, but when they do, blood in the urine is most common. If stones obstruct the ureter, they may cause severe flank pain, difficulty urinating, and urinary retention, frequency, and urgency.

The most common symptom of kidney stones is blood in the urine.

Why is this test done?

The test for kidney stones may be performed to detect and identify stones in the urine.

What should you know before the test?

- Your urine will be collected and strained.
- You don't have to restrict your diet.
- Your symptoms will go away immediately after you get rid of any stones.
- You can have medication to control pain.

What happens during the test?

- You void into the strainer.
- The strainer is carefully inspected because the stones may be tiny; they look like gravel or sand.

What are the normal results?

Normally, stones are not present in urine.

Detecting diabetes insipidus with the dehydration test

The dehydration test checks your urine to measure your kidneys' concentrating capacity after a period of dehydration and after an injection of the pituitary hormone vasopressin. Comparison of the two samples is a reliable diagnosis of diabetes insipidus, a metabolic disorder marked by vasopressin (antidiuretic hormone) deficiency.

How the test is done
If you have this test, you'll have no fluids the evening before and the morning of the test. Your urine will be collected at hourly intervals in the morning for analysis, to see if you are dehydrated enough for the second part of the test. When you're dry enough, you'll be injected with vasopressin and the nurse will take one more urine specimen within an hour. That specimen will be used to check for diabetes and other diseases.

What do abnormal results mean?

More than half of all kidney stones in urine are of mixed composition, containing two or more mineral salts; calcium oxalate is the most common component. When the composition of kidney stones is determined, it helps identify various metabolic disorders.

KIDNEY FUNCTION TESTS

Two tests called the *urine concentration test* and the *dilution test* help the doctor to evaluate your kidney function. The kidneys normally concentrate or dilute urine according to your fluid intake. When intake is excessive, the kidneys excrete more water in the urine. When intake is limited, they excrete less. These tests measure your kidneys' capacity to concentrate urine in response to fluid deprivation or to dilute it in response to fluid overload.

Why are these tests done?

The concentration and dilution tests may be performed to evaluate the kidneys' tubular function and detect kidney damage. (See *Detecting diabetes insipidus with the dehydration test.*)

What should you know before the tests?

- The tests require multiple urine specimens. The nurse will explain how many specimens will be collected and at what intervals.
- You should discard any urine voided during the night.
- If you're using diuretics, they should be stopped.

Concentration test
- You should have a high-protein meal and only 200 milliliters of fluid the night before the test.
- You'll limit your food and fluids for at least 14 hours before the test. (Some concentration tests require that water be withheld for 24 hours but permit relatively normal food intake.)
- Limit salt at your evening meal to prevent excessive thirst.

Dilution test
Generally, this test directly follows the concentration test and requires no additional preparation. If you're just having this test done, you'll only need to skip breakfast.

What happens during the tests?

Concentration test

You're asked to urinate into a special container at specific times: 6 a.m., 8 a.m., and 10 a.m.

Dilution test

- You should first void and discard the urine.
- You're given 1,500 milliliters of water to drink within 30 minutes.
- You're then asked to urinate into a special container. Urine specimens are collected every half hour or every hour for 4 hours thereafter.

Both tests

- You should have a balanced meal or a snack after collecting the final specimen.
- The nurse checks to make sure you void within 8 to 10 hours after the test.

What are the normal results?

In the *concentration test,* specific gravity ranges from 1.025 to 1.032, and osmolality rises above 800 milliosmols per kilogram of water in people with normal kidney function.

In the *dilution test,* specific gravity falls below 1.003 and osmolality below 100 milliosmols per kilogram for at least one specimen; 80% or more of the ingested water is eliminated in 4 hours. In elderly persons, depressed values can be associated with normal kidney function.

What do abnormal results mean?

Decreased kidney capacity to concentrate urine in response to fluid deprivation or to dilute urine in response to fluid overload may indicate tubular epithelial damage, decreased kidney blood flow, loss of functional nephrons, or pituitary or heart dysfunction.

PHOSPHATE REABSORPTION BY THE KIDNEYS

This test — which doctors call the *tubular reabsorption of phosphate test* — evaluates the parathyroid gland and measures its hormone levels. Parathyroid hormone helps maintain optimum blood levels of calcium and controls the kidneys' excretion of calcium and phosphate.

In this test, levels of phosphate and creatinine in the urine and blood are measured and these values are used to calculate the reabsorption of phosphate by tubules in the kidney.

Why is this test done?

The tubular reabsorption test may be performed for the following reasons:

- To evaluate parathyroid function
- To help the doctor diagnose primary hyperparathyroidism
- To distinguish between hypercalcemia (calcium excess) due to hyperparathyroidism and hypercalcemia due to other causes.

What should you know before the test?

- The test requires a blood sample and urine collection over a 24-hour period.
- You'll be instructed to maintain a normal phosphate diet for 3 days before the test because low phosphate intake (less than 500 milligrams per day) may elevate tubular reabsorption values and a high-phosphate diet (3,000 milligrams per day) may lower them. Common nutritional sources of phosphorus include legumes, nuts, milk, egg yolks, meat, poultry, fish, cereals, and cheese. These foods should be eaten in moderate amounts.
- You must fast after midnight the night before the test.

The doctor needs one blood sample and a container of urine collected over a 24-hour period.

What happens during the test?

- For the blood test, a nurse or medical technician inserts a needle into a vein, usually in your forearm. A blood sample is collected in a tube, which is then sent to a lab for testing.
- You're asked to urinate into a special container over a 24-hour period.
- Void and discard the urine, and then begin 24-hour collection with the next voiding.

- After you place the first specimen in the container, add the preservative given to you by the nurse or medical technician.
- Add each voiding to the container immediately. If any urine is lost, restart the test.
- Plan the start of your test so that collection ends at a time that the lab is open.
- Just before the end of the test period, make an effort to void and add that urine to the container.
- Be sure not to contaminate the specimen with toilet paper or stools.
- Occasionally, a 4-hour collection is ordered instead.

What happens after the test?

- You can eat and should drink fluids to maintain adequate urine flow after the blood test.
- If swelling develops at the needle puncture site, apply warm soaks.
- You may resume your usual diet.

What are the normal results?

Kidney tubules normally reabsorb 80% or more of phosphate.

What do abnormal results mean?

Reabsorption of less than 74% of phosphate strongly suggests primary hyperparathyroidism. Hypercalcemia is the most common manifestation of primary hyperparathyroidism. However, a person with hypercalcemia may still require additional testing to confirm primary hyperparathyroidism as the cause.

Depressed reabsorption occurs in a small number of people with kidney stones who don't have parathyroid tumor. Also, about one-fifth of people with parathyroid tumor exhibit normal reabsorption. Increased reabsorption of phosphate may be caused by uremia, kidney tubular disease, osteomalacia, sarcoidosis, and tumors.

AMYLASE

This test evaluates the function of your pancreas and salivary glands. Amylase is a starch-splitting enzyme produced primarily in the pancreas and salivary glands. It's usually secreted into the digestive tract and absorbed into the blood. Small amounts of amylase are also absorbed into the blood directly from these sources. Following glomerular filtration, amylase is excreted in the urine.

If your kidneys are working correctly, blood and urine levels of amylase usually increase together. However, within 2 or 3 days of onset of acute pancreatitis, blood amylase levels fall to normal, but elevated urine amylase persists for 7 to 10 days. One method for determining urine amylase levels is the dye-coupled starch method.

To find out how well your pancreas and salivary glands are working, doctors may examine the amount of the amylase enzyme in a urine specimen.

Why is this test done?
The amylase test may be performed for the following reasons:
- To diagnose acute pancreatitis when blood amylase levels are normal or borderline
- To help the doctor diagnose chronic pancreatitis and salivary gland disorders.

What should you know before the test?
- You won't need to change your diet before the test.
- The test requires urine collection for 2, 6, 8, or 24 hours.
- If a woman is menstruating, the test may have to be rescheduled.
- The lab requires 2 days to complete the analysis.
- If you're taking medications, some may be stopped before the test because continued use may interfere with accurate test results.

What happens during the test?
- Your urine is collected over a 2-, 6-, 8-, or 24-hour period.
- Void and discard the urine, and then begin collection with the next voiding.
- After you place the first specimen in the container, add any preservative given to you by the nurse or medical technician.
- Add each voiding to the container immediately. If any urine is lost, restart the test.
- Plan the start of your test so that collection ends at a time that the lab is open.
- Just before the end of the test period, make an effort to void and add that urine to the container.
- Be sure not to contaminate the specimen with toilet tissue or stools.

What are the normal results?
The Mayo Clinic reports urinary excretion of 10 to 80 amylase units per hour as normal.

What do abnormal results mean?

Elevated amylase levels occur in acute pancreatitis; obstruction of the pancreatic duct, intestines, or salivary duct; cancer of the head of the pancreas; mumps; acute injury of the spleen; kidney disease, with impaired absorption; perforated peptic or duodenal ulcers; and gallbladder disease. Depressed levels occur in pancreatitis, physical wasting and malnutrition, alcoholism, cancer of the liver, cirrhosis, hepatitis, and liver abscess.

ARYLSULFATASE A

This test measures an enzyme that's present throughout your body. Arylsulfatase A (ARSA) is a lysosomal enzyme found in every cell except the mature red blood cell. It's principally active in the liver, the pancreas, and the kidneys, where substances such as drugs are detoxified into sulfates. Urine ARSA levels increase in bladder cancer, colorectal cancer, and leukemia.

Why is this test done?

The arylsulfatase A test may be performed to aid diagnosis of bladder, colon, or rectal cancer; of myeloid (granulocytic) leukemia; and of an inherited lipid storage disease.

What should you know before the test?

- You won't need to change your diet before the test.
- If a woman is menstruating, her test may have to be rescheduled.
- The test requires urine collection over a 24-hour period.
- The test results are generally available in 2 or 3 days.

What happens during the test?

- You're asked to urinate into a special container over a 24-hour period.
- Void and discard the urine, and then begin 24-hour collection with the next voiding.
- After you place the first specimen in the container, add the preservative given to you by the nurse or medical technician.
- Add each voiding to the container immediately. If any urine is lost, restart the test.

- Plan the start of your test so that collection ends at a time that the lab is open.
- Just before the end of the test period, make an effort to void and add that urine to the container.
- Be sure not to contaminate the specimen with toilet paper or stools.

What are the normal results?

Normal arylsulfatase A values are as follows:
- Men: 1.4 to 19.3 international units per liter
- Women: 1.4 to 11 international units per liter
- Children: over 1 international unit per liter.

What do abnormal results mean?

Elevated ARSA levels may be caused by cancer of the bladder, the colon, or the rectum, or from myeloid leukemia.

LYSOZYME

This test evaluates your kidney function and your immune system. Lysozyme is a low-molecular-weight enzyme present in mucus, saliva, tears, skin secretions, and various internal body cells and fluids. This enzyme lyses (splits) the cell walls of some bacteria and, with other blood factors, acts to destroy them.

Lysozyme seems to be created in certain blood cells, and it first appears in blood after destruction of those cells. When blood lysozyme levels exceed three times normal, the enzyme appears in the urine. However, since kidney tissue also contains lysozyme, kidney injury alone can cause measurable excretion of this enzyme.

Why is this test done?

The lysozyme test may be performed for the following reasons:
- To aid diagnosis of acute monocytic or granulocytic leukemia and to monitor the progression of these diseases
- To evaluate kidney tubular function and to diagnose kidney damage
- To detect rejection or loss of blood supply to a transplanted kidney.

What should you know before the test?

- You won't need to change your diet before the test.
- If a woman is menstruating, she may have to reschedule the test for a later date.
- Test results should be available in 1 day.

What happens during the test?

- You're asked to urinate into a special container over a 24-hour period.
- Void and discard the urine, and then begin 24-hour collection with the next voiding.
- After you place the first specimen in the container, add the preservative given to you by the nurse or medical technician.
- Add each voiding to the container immediately. If any urine is lost, restart the test.
- Plan the start of your test so that collection ends at a time that the lab is open.
- Just before the end of the test period, make an effort to void and add that urine to the container.
- Be sure not to contaminate the specimen with toilet paper or stools.

Lysozyme is an enzyme that helps your body fight bacteria. But when it shows up in urine, that sets off alarms.

What are the normal results?

Normally, urine lysozyme values are less than 3 milligrams per 24 hours.

What do abnormal results mean?

Elevated urine lysozyme levels may indicate impaired kidney tubular reabsorption, acute pyelonephritis, nephrotic syndrome, tuberculosis of the kidney, severe extrarenal infection, or rejection or stopped blood supply to a transplanted kidney.

Urine levels increase markedly after acute onset or relapse of monocytic or myelomonocytic leukemia and increase moderately after acute onset or relapse of granulocytic (myeloid) leukemia.

HORMONES

ALDOSTERONE

This test evaluates hormonal balance by checking the urine levels of the hormone aldosterone. Aldosterone promotes retention of sodium and excretion of potassium by the kidneys, thereby helping to regulate blood pressure and fluid and electrolyte balance. In turn, aldosterone secretion is controlled by the renin-angiotensin system. This feedback mechanism is vital to maintaining fluid and electrolyte balance.

Why is this test done?
The aldosterone test may be performed to aid diagnosis of primary and secondary aldosteronism, which may be a factor in high blood pressure.

What should you know before the test?
- You should maintain normal levels of salt in your diet (3 grams per day) before the test and avoid high-salt foods, such as bacon, barbecue sauce, corned beef, bouillon cubes or powder, and olives.
- Avoid strenuous physical exercise and stressful situations during the collection period.
- If you're taking medications, some may be stopped or restricted before the test.

Aldosterone is one hormone that helps your body maintain its fluid and electrolyte balance.

What happens during the test?
- You're asked to urinate into a special container over a 24-hour period.
- Void and discard the urine, and then begin 24-hour collection with the next voiding.
- After you place the first specimen in the container, add the preservative given to you by the nurse or medical technician.
- Add each voiding to the container immediately. If any urine is lost, restart the test.
- Plan the start of your test so that collection ends at a time that the lab is open.
- Just before the end of the test period, make an effort to void and add that urine to the container.

- Be sure not to contaminate the specimen with toilet paper or stools.

What happens after the test?

- You can resume any medications withheld during the test.
- You can resume normal physical activity.

What are the normal results?

Normally, urine aldosterone levels range from 2 to 16 micrograms per 24 hours.

What do abnormal results mean?

Elevated urine aldosterone levels suggest primary or secondary aldosteronism. Disorders that may cause secondary aldosteronism are severe high blood pressure, congestive heart failure, cirrhosis of the liver, nephrotic syndrome, and idiopathic cyclic edema.

Low urine aldosterone levels may be caused by Addison's disease, salt-losing syndrome, and toxemia of pregnancy.

TEST FOR CUSHING'S SYNDROME

A hormone test called the *free cortisol test* helps evaluate your adrenal gland function. It's one of the best diagnostic tools for detecting Cushing's syndrome, a disorder marked by excessive secretion of hormones by the cortex of the adrenal gland.

Why is this test done?

The test for free cortisol may be performed to aid diagnosis of Cushing's syndrome.

What should you know before the test?

You won't need to change your diet before the test, but you should avoid stressful situations and excessive physical exercise during the collection period.

What happens during the test?

- You're asked to urinate into a special container over a 24-hour period.
- Void and discard the urine, and then begin 24-hour collection with the next voiding.
- After you place the first specimen in the container, add the preservative given to you by the nurse or medical technician.
- Add each voiding to the container immediately. If any urine is lost, restart the test.
- Plan the start of your test so that collection ends at a time when the lab is open.
- Just before the end of the test period, make an effort to void and add that urine to the container.
- Be sure not to contaminate the specimen with toilet paper or stools.

What happens after the test?

You can resume your normal activities and resume taking any medications you discontinued for the test.

What are the normal results?

Normally, free cortisol values range from 24 to 108 micrograms per 24 hours.

What do abnormal results mean?

Elevated free cortisol levels may indicate Cushing's syndrome, caused by adrenal hyperplasia, adrenal or pituitary tumor, or ectopic corticotropin production. Liver disease and obesity, which can raise plasma cortisol levels, generally don't affect urine levels of free cortisol. Low levels have little significance.

*E*PINEPHRINE, NOREPINEPHRINE, AND DOPAMINE

This test evaluates adrenal gland function by measuring urine levels of the major hormones epinephrine, norepinephrine, and dopamine. These hormones are known as *catecholamines*. Epinephrine is secreted by the adrenal gland; dopamine, by the central nervous system; and norepinephrine, by both.

Catecholamines help regulate metabolism and prepare the body for the fight-or-flight response to stress. Certain tumors can also secrete catecholamines.

Why is this test done?

The test for catecholamines may be performed for the following reasons:

- To aid the diagnosis of pheochromocytoma in a person with unexplained high blood pressure
- To aid the diagnosis of neuroblastoma, ganglioneuroma, and malfunction of the autonomic nervous system.

What should you know before the test?

- You won't need to change your diet before the test, but you should avoid stressful situations and excessive physical activity during the collection period.
- Either a specimen collected over 24 hours or a random specimen may be required.

What happens during the test?

- You're asked to urinate into a special container over a 24-hour period. (If a random specimen is ordered, collect it immediately after a high blood pressure episode.)
- Void and discard the urine, and then begin 24-hour collection with the next voiding.
- After you place the first specimen in the container, add the preservative given to you by the nurse or medical technician.
- Add each voiding to the container immediately. If any urine is lost, restart the test.
- Plan the start of your test so that collection ends at a time the lab is open.
- Just before the end of the test period, make an effort to void and add that urine to the container.
- Be sure not to contaminate the specimen with toilet paper or stools.

What happens after the test?

You can resume any activity or medications restricted during the test.

Catecholamines help regulate metabolism and prepare the body for the fight-or-flight response to stress.

What are the normal results?

Normally, urine catecholamine values range from undetectable to 135 micrograms per 24 hours or from undetectable to 18 micrograms per deciliter of urine in a random specimen.

What do abnormal results mean?

In people with undiagnosed high blood pressure, elevated urine catecholamine levels following an episode of high blood pressure usually indicate a tumor. If tests indicate a tumor, the person may also be tested for multiple endocrine neoplasia.

Elevated catecholamine levels, without marked high blood pressure, may be due to brain tumors. Myasthenia gravis and progressive muscular dystrophy commonly cause urine catecholamine levels to rise above normal, but this test is rarely performed to diagnose these disorders.

ESTROGENS

The total urine estrogens test helps evaluate functioning of the ovaries or the testicles. For a pregnant woman, measuring urine estrogens helps to monitor fetal development and placental function. For a man, this test helps evaluate testicular function.

The test measures total urine levels of estradiol, estrone, and estriol — the major estrogens present in significant amounts in urine. (See *Changes in estrogen levels during the menstrual cycle.*)

Why is this test done?

The total urine estrogens test may be performed for the following reasons:

- To evaluate ovarian activity and help determine why a woman isn't menstruating and has an overproduction of estrogen
- To aid diagnosis of ovarian, adrenocortical, or testicular tumors
- To check the status of a fetus and the surrounding placenta.

What should you know before the test?

- The test requires collection of urine over a 24-hour period.
- You won't need to change your diet before the test.

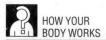

HOW YOUR BODY WORKS

Changes in estrogen levels during the menstrual cycle

The quantity of total estrogens in the urine tells the doctor about the functioning of the ovaries. Estrogen excretion levels during a normal menstrual cycle show a major peak at midpoint in the cycle (ovulatory phase), and another smaller increase (luteal or premenstrual phase) just before menstruation starts.

Peaks in pregnancy
Urine estrogens rise slowly in the first trimester (3 months) of pregnancy, and then increase rapidly to reach high levels as term approaches. With menopause, the cyclical pattern fluctuates and eventually flattens out to a constant low level.

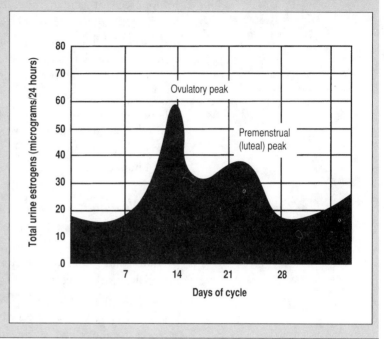

What happens during the test?

- You're asked to urinate into a special container over a 24-hour period.
- Void and discard the urine, and then begin 24-hour collection with the next voiding. After you place the first specimen in the container, add the preservative given to you by the nurse or medical technician.
- Add each voiding to the container immediately. If any urine is lost, restart the test.
- Plan the start of your test so that collection ends at a time when the lab is open.
- Just before the end of the test period, make an effort to void and add that urine to the container.
- Be sure not to contaminate the specimen with toilet paper or stools.
- If you're pregnant, the nurse will note the approximate week of development on the lab slip. If you're a nonpregnant woman, the nurse will note the stage of your menstrual cycle.

What happens after the test?

You can resume any medications withheld before the test.

What are the normal results?

In nonpregnant women, total urine estrogen levels rise and fall during the menstrual cycle, peaking shortly before midcycle, decreasing immediately following ovulation, increasing just before menstruation, and decreasing greatly as menstruation begins.

Normal values for nonpregnant women are as follows: preovulatory phase, 5 to 25 micrograms per 24 hours; ovulatory phase, 24 to 100 micrograms per 24 hours; shedding phase, 12 to 80 micrograms per 24 hours. In postmenopausal women, values are less than 10 micrograms per 24 hours. In men, values are from 4 to 25 micrograms per 24 hours.

What do abnormal results mean?

Decreased total urine estrogen levels may reflect poor ovarian development, primary ovarian insufficiency (due to a flaw), or secondary ovarian insufficiency (due to pituitary or adrenal hypofunction or metabolic disturbances).

Elevated total estrogen levels in nonpregnant women may indicate tumors of ovarian or adrenocortical origin, adrenocortical hyperplasia, or a metabolic or liver disorder. In men, elevated total estrogen levels are associated with testicular tumors. Elevated total urine estrogen levels are normal during pregnancy.

*P*REGNANCY TEST

The human chorionic gonadotropin test determines whether a woman is pregnant or the status of her pregnancy. Also, the test functions as a screen for some types of cancer. Analysis of urine levels of human chorionic gonadotropin allows detection of pregnancy as early as 10 days after a missed menstrual period. Production of human chorionic gonadotropin begins after conception. During the first trimester (3 months), human chorionic gonadotropin levels increase steadily and rapidly, peaking around the tenth week of gestation and subsequently tapering off to less than 10% of peak levels.

Why is this test done?

The test for human chorionic gonadotropin may be performed for the following reasons:
- To detect and confirm pregnancy
- To aid diagnosis of a certain kind of mole or human chorionic gonadotropin-secreting tumors.

What should you know before the test?

- You won't need to change your diet before the test.
- The test uses your first urine voided in the morning or urine collection over a 24-hour period, depending on whether the doctor orders a test that is qualitative or quantitative.
- The nurse will ask about any medications that might affect human chorionic gonadotropin levels.

What happens during the test?

- For verification of pregnancy (qualitative analysis), you collect a first-voided morning specimen. If this isn't possible, collect a random specimen.
- For quantitative analysis of human chorionic gonadotropin, you're asked to urinate into a special container over a 24-hour period.
- Void and discard the urine, and then begin 24-hour collection with the next voiding.
- After you place the first specimen in the container, add the preservative given to you by the nurse or medical technician.
- Add each voiding to the container immediately. If any urine is lost, restart the test.
- Plan the start of your test so that collection ends at a time when the lab is open.
- Just before the end of the test period, make an effort to void and add that urine to the container.
- Be sure not to contaminate the specimen with toilet paper or stools.

What happens after the test?

You can resume any medications withheld during the test.

What are the normal results?

In qualitative analysis, if agglutination (a clumping of cells) fails to occur, test results are positive, indicating pregnancy. In quantitative

SELF-HELP

Over-the-counter pregnancy tests

You can get early confirmation of pregnancy through over-the-counter home pregnancy tests. These tests confirm pregnancy by detecting the presence of human chorionic gonadotropin in the urine.

Options and features
Several different kits are available. Some have a second test to use if levels of the hormone aren't immediately detectable. Each kit contains instructions for performing the test. It lists health conditions or drugs that may affect results. Remember that false-positive or false-negative results can occur. Many kits include toll-free numbers for questions about the kits or the results. Follow-up care with a doctor is recommended for all positive results.

analysis, urine human chorionic gonadotropin levels in the first trimester of a normal pregnancy may be as high as 500,000 international units per 24 hours. In the second trimester, they range from 10,000 to 25,000 international units per 24 hours, and in the third trimester, from 5,000 to 15,000 international units per 24 hours. After delivery, human chorionic gonadotropin levels decline rapidly and within a few days are undetectable.

Measurable human chorionic gonadotropin levels don't normally appear in the urine of men or nonpregnant women.

Besides lab testing, some home pregnancy test kits are also available. (See *Over-the-counter pregnancy tests,* page 571.)

What do abnormal results mean?

During pregnancy, elevated urine human chorionic gonadotropin levels may indicate multiple pregnancy or a fetus with a birth defect.

Depressed urine human chorionic gonadotropin levels may indicate threatened abortion or ectopic pregnancy.

Measurable levels of human chorionic gonadotropin in men and nonpregnant women may indicate some cancers, ovarian or testicular tumors, other tumors, or stomach, liver, pancreatic, or breast cancer.

To confirm that you're pregnant, collect the first urine of the morning for the test.

PLACENTAL ESTRIOL

This test helps determine if a pregnant woman's placenta is functioning properly, which is essential to the health of the fetus. It measures urine levels of placental estriol, the predominant estrogen excreted in urine during pregnancy. A steady increase in estriol reflects a properly functioning placenta and, in most cases, a healthy, growing fetus.

Normally, estriol is secreted in much smaller amounts by the ovaries in nonpregnant women, by the testes in men, and by the adrenal cortex in both sexes.

Why is this test done?

The test for placental estriol is performed to check the status of the fetus and the placenta, especially in a high-risk pregnancy, such as one complicated by the mother's high blood pressure, diabetes, pre-eclampsia, toxemia, or a history of stillbirth.

What should you know before the test?

- You won't need to change your diet before the test.
- This test requires urine collection over a 24-hour period.
- The nurse will ask about any medications that might affect the test and may tell you to discontinue them.

What happens during the test?

- You're asked to urinate into a special container over a 24-hour period.
- Void and discard the urine, and then begin 24-hour collection with the next voiding.
- After you place the first specimen in the container, add the preservative given to you by the nurse or medical technician.
- Add each voiding to the container immediately. If any urine is lost, restart the test.
- Plan the start of your test so that collection ends at a time when the lab is open.
- Just before the end of the test period, make an effort to void and add that urine to the container.
- Be sure not to contaminate the specimen with toilet paper or stools.

What happens after the test?

You can resume any medications withheld during the test.

What are the normal results?

Normal values vary considerably, but a series of measurements of urine estriol levels taken during the pregnancy, when plotted on a graph, should describe a steadily rising curve. (See *Changes in estriol levels during pregnancy,* page 574.)

What do abnormal results mean?

A 40% drop from baseline values that shows up on 2 consecutive days strongly suggests the placenta isn't functioning well and the fetus will be in distress. A 20% drop over 2 weeks or failure of consecutive estriol levels to increase in a normal curve also shows a problem. These developments may require a cesarean section, depending on the mother's condition and other apparent signs of fetal distress.

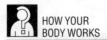

HOW YOUR BODY WORKS

Changes in estriol levels during pregnancy

Levels of estriol in urine rise during the course of pregnancy, as shown in the graph below. Over a period of days, any significant changes in results during a series of lab tests may suggest abnormal conditions that require prompt medical care.

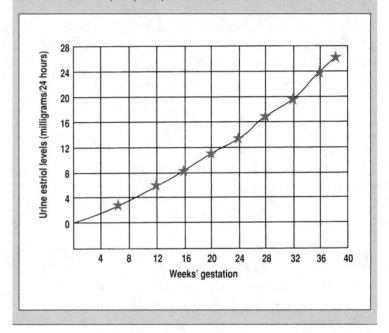

A check for birth defects

A chronically low urine estriol curve may be caused by fetal adrenal insufficiency, major birth defects, blood Rh-factor problems, or a placental sulfatase deficiency. Or, a high estriol level may simply indicate twins.

A high-risk pregnancy in which the mother's kidney function decreases may cause a low-normal estriol curve. Such a pregnancy may occur in a woman with high blood pressure or diabetes, for example. The pregnancy may continue, as long as no complications develop and estriol levels continue to increase.

*P*REGNANETRIOL

This test helps to evaluate the body's secretion of hormones. It checks urine levels of pregnanetriol, which is normally excreted in the urine in minute amounts. Elevated urine pregnanetriol levels suggest adrenogenital syndrome, a condition marked by excessive adrenal gland secretion of androgen. This condition may cause problems in the development of sexual characteristics.

Why is this test done?
The test for pregnanetriol may be performed for the following reasons:
- To aid the diagnosis of adrenogenital syndrome
- To monitor some types of hormone replacement therapy.

What should you know before the test?
You won't need to change your diet before the test.

What happens during the test?
- You're asked to urinate into a special container over a 24-hour period.
- Void and discard the urine, and then begin 24-hour collection with the next voiding.
- After you place the first specimen in the container, add the preservative given to you by the nurse or medical technician.
- Add each voiding to the container immediately. If any urine is lost, restart the test.
- Plan the start of your test so that collection ends at a time when the lab is open.
- Just before the end of the test period, make an effort to void and add that urine to the container.
- Be sure not to contaminate the specimen with toilet paper or stools.

Too much pregnanetriol at birth may cause changes in a child's physical and sexual development.

What are the normal results?
The normal rate of pregnanetriol excretion is as follows:
- Adults: less than 3.5 milligrams per 24 hours
- Children ages 7 to 16: 0.3 to 1.1 milligrams per 24 hours
- Children younger than age 6 (including infants): up to 0.2 milligrams per 24 hours.

What do abnormal results mean?

Elevated urine pregnanetriol levels suggest adrenogenital syndrome, a condition marked by excessive adrenal gland secretion of androgen. Females with this condition fail to develop normal breasts or genitalia and show marked masculinization of external genitalia at birth. Males usually appear normal at birth but later develop signs of premature physical and sexual development.

VANILLYLMANDELIC ACID

This test evaluates the urine levels of vanillylmandelic acid, a metabolite that's normally most prevalent in the urine. Vanillylmandelic acid levels in the urine reflect production of major catecholamines (adrenal gland secretions) and help to detect catecholamine-secreting tumors — for example, a tumor called a *pheochromocytoma*. They also help evaluate the function of the adrenal medulla, the primary site of catecholamine production.

Why is this test done?

The test for vanillylmandelic acid may be performed for the following reasons:

■ To help detect pheochromocytoma (a tumor), neuroblastoma (a malignant soft-tissue tumor that develops in infants and young children), or ganglioneuroma (a tumor of the sympathetic nervous system that develops in older children and adolescents and rarely spreads)

■ To evaluate the function of the adrenal medulla.

What should you know before the test?

■ You'll have to restrict foods and beverages containing phenolic acid, such as coffee, tea, bananas, citrus fruits, chocolate, and vanilla, for 3 days before the test.

■ Avoid stressful situations and excessive physical activity during the urine collection period.

■ The nurse will ask about medications that may affect the test.

What happens during the test?

- You're asked to urinate into a special container over a 24-hour period.
- Void and discard the urine, and then begin 24-hour collection with the next voiding.
- After you place the first specimen in the container, add the preservative given to you by the nurse or medical technician.
- Add each voiding to the container immediately. If any urine is lost, restart the test.
- Plan the start of your test so that collection ends at a time when the lab is open.
- Just before the end of the test period, make an effort to void and add that urine to the container.
- Be sure not to contaminate the specimen with toilet paper or stools.

What happens after the test?

- You can resume any medications withheld before the test.
- You may resume your normal diet and activities.

What are the normal results?

Normally, urine vanillylmandelic acid values range from 0.7 to 6.8 milligrams per 24 hours.

What do abnormal results mean?

Elevated urine vanillylmandelic acid levels may result from a catecholamine-secreting tumor. The doctor may find that more testing is necessary for a precise diagnosis.

Certain foods and situations affect the test results, including stressful situations and excessive physical activity.

HOMOVANILLIC ACID

This test measures urine levels of homovanillic acid, which is a metabolite of dopamine, one of the three major catecholamines (hormones secreted by the adrenal gland). Synthesized primarily in the brain, dopamine is a precursor to epinephrine and norepinephrine, the other principal catecholamines. The liver breaks down most dopamine into homovanillic acid for eventual excretion; a minimal amount of dopamine appears in the urine.

Why is this test done?

The test for homovanillic acid may be performed for the following reasons:

- To aid the diagnosis of neuroblastoma, a malignant soft-tissue tumor that develops in infants and young children, and ganglioneuroma, a tumor of the sympathetic nervous system that develops in older children and adolescents and rarely spreads
- To rule out the diagnosis of pheochromocytoma, a tumor.

What should you know before the test?

- You won't need to change your diet before the test, but avoid stressful situations and excessive physical exercise during the collection period.
- The nurse will ask about any medications that might affect the test and then notify the doctor, who may want you to stop these medications before the test.

What happens during the test?

- You're asked to urinate into a special container over a 24-hour period.
- Void and discard the urine, and then begin 24-hour collection with the next voiding.
- After you place the first specimen in the container, add the preservative given to you by the nurse or medical technician.
- Add each voiding to the container immediately. If any urine is lost, restart the test.
- Plan the start of your test so that collection ends at a time when the lab is open.
- Just before the end of the test period, make an effort to void and add that urine to the container.
- Be sure not to contaminate the specimen with toilet paper or stools.

What happens after the test?

- You can resume taking any medications withheld before the test.
- You may resume activity restricted during the test.

What are the normal results?

Normally, the urine homovanillic acid value for adults is less than 8 milligrams per 24 hours. The range of normal urine homovanillic acid values in children varies with age.

What do abnormal results mean?

Elevated urine homovanillic acid levels suggest neuroblastoma, a malignant tumor of soft-tissues that occurs in infants and young children, or ganglioneuroma, a tumor of the sympathetic nervous system that occurs in older children and adolescents and rarely affects other body systems. Homovanillic acid levels don't usually increase in people with pheochromocytoma because this tumor secretes mainly epinephrine, which metabolizes primarily into vanillylmandelic acid. Thus, an abnormally high urine homovanillic acid level generally rules out pheochromocytoma.

HYDROXYINDOLEACETIC ACID

The analysis of urine levels of 5-hydroxyindoleacetic acid is used mainly to screen for carcinoid tumors (called *argentaffinomas*). Such tumors, found generally in the intestine or appendix, secrete an excessive amount of serotonin, which is reflected by high 5-hydroxyindoleacetic acid levels. (See *Where serotonin comes from,* page 580.)

Why is this test done?

The test for 5-hydroxyindoleacetic acid may be performed to aid diagnosis of argentaffinomas.

What should you know before the test?

- You'll be told not to eat foods containing serotonin, such as bananas, plums, pineapples, avocados, eggplants, tomatoes, or walnuts, for 4 days before the test.
- The nurse will ask about your recent use of drugs that may affect test results. The doctor may want you to discontinue their use.

What happens during the test?

- You're asked to urinate into a special container over a 24-hour period.
- Void and discard the urine, and then begin 24-hour collection with the next voiding.
- After you place the first specimen in the container, add the preservative given to you by the nurse or medical technician.
- Add each voiding to the container immediately. If any urine is lost, restart the test.

Four days before the test, you'll have to give up certain foods, including bananas, avocados, tomatoes, and walnuts.

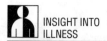

INSIGHT INTO
ILLNESS

Where serotonin comes from

The illustration below shows a microscopic view of the lining of the small intestine. Argentaffin cells in the crypts of Lieberkühn are located in the indentations between the villi in the mucous membrane of the small intestine. These cells produce serotonin. The serotonin metabolizes into 5-hydroxyindoleacetic acid. High levels of this acid in the urine can signal the presence of serotonin-secreting argentaffinomas, a type of carcinoid tumor.

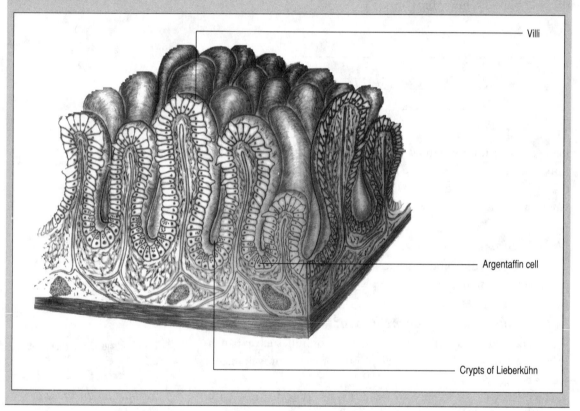

Villi

Argentaffin cell

Crypts of Lieberkühn

- Plan the start of your test so that collection ends at a time when the lab is open.
- Just before the end of the test period, make an effort to void and add that urine to the container.
- Be sure not to contaminate the specimen with toilet paper or stools.

What happens after the test?

You can resume your normal diet and any medications withheld before the test.

What are the normal results?

Normally, urine 5-hydroxyindoleacetic acid values are less than 6 milligrams per 24 hours.

What do abnormal results mean?

Marked elevation of urine 5-hydroxyindoleacetic acid levels, possibly as high as 200 to 600 milligrams per 24 hours, indicates a carcinoid tumor. However, because these tumors vary in their capacity to store and secrete serotonin, some people with carcinoid syndrome (spreading carcinoid tumors) may not show elevated levels.

Repeated testing is often necessary.

PREGNANEDIOL

When evaluating placental or ovarian function, the doctor may order a urine test that measures levels of pregnanediol, the chief metabolite of progesterone. The amount of pregnanediol in the urine provides information about production of its parent hormone, progesterone.

Progesterone is produced in nonpregnant women by the uterine lining during the latter half of each menstrual cycle, preparing the uterus for implantation of a fertilized egg. If implantation doesn't occur, progesterone secretion drops sharply. If implantation does occur, the uterine lining secretes more progesterone to further prepare the uterus for pregnancy and to begin development of the placenta. Toward the end of the first trimester (3 months), the placenta becomes the primary source of progesterone secretion, producing the progressively larger amounts needed to maintain pregnancy.

Why is this test done?

The test for pregnanediol may be performed for the following reasons:
- To evaluate placental function in pregnant women
- To evaluate ovarian function in nonpregnant women.

What should you know before the test?

- You won't need to change your diet before the test.
- If you're pregnant, this test may be repeated several times to get a sequence of measurements.
- The nurse will ask about medications that might affect the test.

What happens during the test?

- You're asked to urinate into a special container over a 24-hour period.
- Void and discard the urine, and then begin 24-hour collection with the next voiding.
- After you place the first specimen in the container, add the preservative given to you by the nurse or medical technician.
- Add each voiding to the container immediately. If any urine is lost, restart the test.
- Plan the start of your test so that collection ends at a time when the lab is open.
- Just before the end of the test period, make an effort to void and add that urine to the container.
- Be sure not to contaminate the specimen with toilet paper or stools.

What are the normal results?

In nonpregnant women, urine pregnanediol values normally range from 0.5 to 1.5 milligrams per 24 hours during the proliferative phase of the menstrual cycle. Within 24 hours after ovulation, pregnanediol levels begin to increase and continue to rise for 3 to 10 days as the uterus lining develops. During this phase, normal urine pregnanediol values range from 2 to 7 milligrams per 24 hours. In the absence of fertilization, levels drop sharply as the uterus lining degenerates and menstruation begins.

During pregnancy, urine pregnanediol levels increase markedly, peaking around the 36th week of gestation and returning to prepregnancy levels by between 5 and 10 days after childbirth. Normal postmenopausal values range from 0.2 to 1 milligram per 24 hours. In males, urine pregnanediol levels rarely rise above 1.5 milligrams per 24 hours.

Low urine pregnanediol levels in nonpregnant women may indicate stopped ovulation, stopped menstruation, or other menstrual problems.

What do abnormal results mean?

During pregnancy, a decrease in urine pregnanediol levels may indicate placental insufficiency and requires immediate investigation. A sharp drop in pregnanediol values may suggest fetal distress — for example, threatened abortion or fetal death. However, pregnanediol measurements are not reliable indicators of fetal viability because levels can remain normal even after fetal death, as long as the mother's circulation to the placenta remains adequate.

In nonpregnant women, abnormally low urine pregnanediol levels may occur with stopped ovulation, stopped menstruation, or other menstrual abnormalities. Elevations may indicate some types of tumors or ovarian cancer that's spreading to other parts of the body. Adrenal gland problems or bile duct obstruction may raise urine pregnanediol values in men or women. Some forms of primary liver disease produce abnormally low levels in both sexes.

PROTEINS & SUGARS

PROTEINS

This test detects proteins in your urine. Normally, the kidneys allow only proteins of low molecular weight to enter the filtrate. The kidneys' tubules then reabsorb most of these proteins. A damaged kidney allows excretion of proteins in the urine. (See *The first step in urine formation,* page 584.) A qualitative screening often precedes this test. A positive result requires quantitative analysis of a 24-hour urine specimen.

Why is this test done?
The test for proteins may be performed to aid diagnosis of illnesses marked by protein in the urine, primarily kidney disease.

What should you know before the test?
- You won't need to change your diet before the test.
- The test usually requires urine collection over a 24-hour period.
- The nurse will ask about medications that might affect the test. The doctor may want to restrict them before the test.

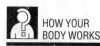

HOW YOUR BODY WORKS

The first step in urine formation

The nephron, the functional unit of the kidney, is the site of glomerular filtration and tubular reabsorption and secretion. Filtration begins when a small artery carries blood to the glomeruli, extremely porous capillaries enclosed by Bowman's capsule.

Pressure works the filter

Strong hydrostatic pressure in the glomeruli forces small molecules of water, sugar, nutrients, metabolites, and amino acids through the arterial walls into Bowman's capsules. Heavier red blood cells and proteins (such as albumin) that cannot pass through the arterial walls remain unfiltered.

Wastes in the loop

The glomerular filtrate collected by Bowman's capsule joins organic wastes and excess salts secreted from surrounding kidney tissues. The wastes flow through the convoluted proximal and distal tubules that make up Henle's loop, into the straight collecting tubule.

What happens during the test?

- You're asked to urinate into a special container over a 24-hour period.
- Void and discard the urine, and then begin 24-hour collection with the next voiding.
- After you place the first specimen in the container, add the preservative given to you by the nurse or medical technician.
- Add each voiding to the container immediately. If any urine is lost, restart the test.
- Plan the start of your test so that collection ends at a time when the lab is open.
- Just before the end of the test period, make an effort to void and add that urine to the container.
- Be sure not to contaminate the specimen with toilet paper or stools.

What happens after the test?

You can resume any medications withheld before the test.

What are the normal results?

Normal values show up to 150 milligrams of protein excreted in 24 hours.

What do abnormal results mean?

Protein in the urine is a chief characteristic of kidney disease. When protein shows up in a single specimen, 24-hour urine collection is required to identify specific kidney problems.

What are the subtle differences?

Slight changes in the amount of protein in the urine suggest the following disorders:

- Persistent protein: kidney disease caused by increased glomerular permeability
- Minimal protein in the urine (less than 0.5 gram per 24 hours): kidney diseases in which glomerular involvement is not a major factor such as chronic pyelonephritis
- Moderate protein (0.5 to 4 grams per 24 hours): kidney diseases such as acute or chronic glomerulonephritis, amyloidosis, toxic nephropathies — or in diseases in which kidney failure often develops as a late complication (diabetes or heart failure, for example)
- Heavy proteinuria (more than 4 grams per 24 hours): nephrotic syndrome

■ Protein in the urine plus elevated white blood cell count: urinary tract infection

■ Protein and blood in the urine: local or diffuse urinary tract disorders. Other disorders (infections and lesions of the central nervous system, for example) can also cause detectable amounts of protein in the urine.

Many drugs damage the kidneys, causing protein in the urine. This makes the routine evaluation of urine proteins essential during drug treatments.

Not all forms of protein in the urine have health significance; some can be caused by changes in body position. Others are linked to exercise, as well as emotional or physiologic stress, and are usually short-term.

BENCE JONES PROTEIN

This test can detect an abnormal protein in the urine. Bence Jones proteins are abnormal immunoglobulins that appear in the urine of 50% to 80% of people with multiple tumors and in most people with a disorder called *Waldenström's macroglobulinemia.*

Screening tests, such as blood coagulation by heat and one called *Bradshaw's test,* can detect Bence Jones proteins, but urine testing is usually the doctor's choice. Both urine and blood studies are frequently used for people who may have multiple tumors.

Why is this test done?
The Bence Jones protein test may be performed to confirm the presence of multiple tumors in people with symptoms such as bone pain (especially in the back and thorax) and persistent anemia and fatigue.

What should you know before the test?
The test requires an early-morning urine specimen; the nurse will teach you how to collect a clean-catch specimen. (See *How to catch a midstream specimen,* page 586.)

SELF-HELP

How to catch a midstream specimen

To minimize contamination by organisms outside your urinary tract, you must get what is called a *clean-catch, midstream specimen*. To collect this specimen, follow the instructions below.

Procedure for women

- If you're menstruating, inform the doctor. He or she may want to postpone the test to avoid contamination. Or, insert a tampon to protect the specimen.
- Kneel or squat over a bedpan or straddle the toilet bowl to separate the folds of skin that cover the urinary opening.
- Separate the labia with your thumb and forefinger and clean the area around the urinary opening with three antiseptic-moistened swabs: one for each side of the opening and the third for the opening itself. Wipe with a front-to-back motion. Use another swab to dry.
- Begin voiding, and without interrupting the flow, catch about 1 ounce (30 milliliters) of urine in a sterile specimen container.

- Replace the lid of the specimen container. If you're not going to the lab immediately, refrigerate the specimen.

Procedure for men

- Be sure your bladder is full. This minimizes the risk of contamination by prostatic fluid.
- Retract your foreskin and clean the tip of your penis with an antiseptic-moistened swab, wiping in a circular motion away from the urinary opening. Use another swab to dry.
- Begin voiding into a toilet and, without interrupting the flow, catch about 1 ounce (30 milliliters) of urine in a sterile specimen container.

What happens during the test?

- You're asked to provide an early-morning urine specimen of at least 50 milliliters.
- Be careful not to contaminate the urine specimen with toilet tissue or stools.

What are the normal results?

Normal urine should contain no Bence Jones proteins.

What do abnormal results mean?

The presence of Bence Jones proteins in urine suggests multiple tumors or Waldenström's macroglobulinemia. Very low levels, in the absence of other symptoms, may be benign.

AMINO ACID DISORDERS SCREEN

This test uses chromatography to help detect amino acid disorders. Abnormal metabolism may cause an excess of one or more amino acids to appear in blood and, as the kidneys' processing capacity is exceeded, in urine. Two types of amino acid disorders are primary (overflow) and secondary (kidney).

To screen newborns, children, and adults for inherited amino acid disorders, the doctor may use blood or urine specimens. The blood test is better for the overflow type. Urine is used to monitor certain disorders and to screen for the kidney type.

Testing for specific amino acid levels is also necessary for infants or young children with acidosis, severe vomiting and diarrhea, and abnormal urine odor. Such testing is especially important in newborns because an early diagnosis and prompt treatment of amino acid problems may prevent mental retardation.

Why is this test done?

The test for amino acids may be performed for the following reasons:
- To screen for kidney amino acid problems
- To follow up on blood-test findings when results of these tests suggest overflow amino acid problems.

What should you know before the test?

- You or your child won't need to change your diet before the test.
- The test requires a urine specimen.
- The nurse will ask about medications that might interfere with the test. (If the test is for your breast-fed infant, the nurse will ask about any drugs you're taking.)

What happens during the test?

- You're asked to urinate into a special container.
- Be sure not to contaminate the specimen with toilet paper or stools.
- If the test is for your infant, the nurse teaches you how to apply and use a pediatric urine collector.

What are the normal results?

Patterns on thin-layer chromatography are reported as normal.

What do abnormal results mean?

If thin-layer chromatography shows gross changes or abnormal patterns, blood and 24-hour urine tests are performed to identify specific amino acid abnormalities and to differentiate overflow and kidney amino acid problems.

CREATININE

This test helps evaluate your kidney function by measuring urine levels of a substance called *creatinine*. The body produces this substance in proportion to total body muscle mass. Creatinine is removed from the blood primarily by the kidneys and is excreted in the urine. Because the body doesn't recycle it, creatinine has a relatively high, constant clearance rate, making it an efficient indicator of kidney function.

Your body produces creatinine in proportion to your muscle mass and excretes it steadily in urine.

Why is this test done?

The test for creatinine is performed to help assess kidney function.

What should you know before the test?

- You won't need to restrict fluids, but you should not eat an excessive amount of meat before the test.
- You should avoid strenuous physical exercise during the collection period.
- The test usually requires urine collection over a 24-hour period.
- The nurse may ask you about medications that could interfere with the test. The doctor may restrict such drugs before the test.

What happens during the test?

- You're asked to urinate into a special container over a 24-hour period.
- Void and discard the urine, and then begin 24-hour collection with the next voiding.
- After you place the first specimen in the container, add the preservative given to you by the nurse or medical technician.
- Add each voiding to the container immediately. If any urine is lost, restart the test.

- Plan the start of your test so that collection ends at a time when the lab is open.
- Just before the end of the test period, make an effort to void and add that urine to the container.
- Be sure not to contaminate the specimen with toilet paper or stools.

What happens after the test?

- You can resume any medications withheld during the test.
- You may resume normal diet and activity.

What are the normal results?

Normally, urine creatinine levels range from 1 to 1.9 grams per 24 hours for men and from 0.8 to 1.7 grams per 24 hours for women.

What do abnormal results mean?

Decreased urine creatinine levels may be caused by impaired kidney activity (associated with shock, for example) or from kidney disease due to urinary tract obstruction or other diseases. Increased levels generally have little diagnostic significance.

CREATININE CLEARANCE BY THE KIDNEYS

This test evaluates kidney function by measuring how efficiently the kidneys are clearing a substance called *creatinine* from the blood. The rate of clearance is expressed in terms of the volume of blood (in milliliters) that can be cleared of creatinine in 1 minute. Creatinine levels become abnormal when the kidneys sustain substantial damage.

Why is this test done?

The creatinine clearance test may be performed for the following reasons:

- To check kidney function (primarily glomerular filtration)
- To monitor progression of kidney failure.

What should you know before the test?

- The test requires a timed urine specimen and at least one blood sample. A timed urine specimen can be taken over 2, 12, or 24 hours.
- You won't need to change your diet before the test, but you should not eat an excessive amount of meat before the test.
- You should avoid strenuous physical exercise during the urine collection period.
- The nurse will ask about any medications that may interfere with the test.

What happens during the test?

- You're asked to urinate into a special container over a prescribed period.
- Void and discard the urine, and then begin collection with the next voiding.
- After you place the first specimen in the container, add the preservative given to you by the nurse or medical technician.
- Add each voiding to the container immediately. If any urine is lost, restart the test.
- Plan the start of your test so that collection ends at a time when the lab is open.
- Just before the end of the test period, make an effort to void and add that urine to the container.
- Be sure not to contaminate the specimen with toilet paper or stools.
- For the blood sample, a nurse or medical technician inserts a needle into a vein, usually in your forearm. A blood sample is collected in a tube, which is then sent to a lab for testing.
- Although you may feel a sting from the needle and pressure from the tourniquet, collecting the sample takes only a few minutes.

What happens after the test?

- You may resume any medications withheld before the test.
- You may resume normal diet and activity.
- If swelling develops at the needle puncture site, apply warm soaks.

What are the normal results?

For men, normal creatinine clearance ranges from 85 to 125 milliliters per minute. For women, it ranges from 75 to 115 milliliters per minute. For older people, creatinine clearance normally decreases by 6 milliliters per minute for each decade.

What do abnormal results mean?

Low creatinine clearance may be caused by reduced kidney blood flow (associated with shock or kidney artery obstruction) or a long list of kidney disorders. It also may suggest congestive heart failure or severe dehydration.

High creatinine clearance rates generally have little diagnostic significance.

UREA CLEARANCE BY THE KIDNEYS

This test evaluates your kidney function by analyzing urine levels of urea, the main nitrogenous component in urine and the end product of protein metabolism. It's most useful for assessing overall kidney function. (See *Getting rid of urea,* page 592.)

Why is this test done?

The urea clearance test is performed to check your total kidney function.

What should you know before the test?

- The test requires two timed urine specimens and one blood sample.
- You must fast from midnight before the test and abstain from exercise before and during the test.
- The nurse will ask about any medications that might interfere with the test.

What happens during the test?

- For the blood test, a nurse or medical technician inserts a needle into a vein, usually in your forearm. A blood sample is collected in a tube, which is then sent to a lab for testing.
- Although you may feel a sting from the needle and pressure from the tourniquet, collecting the sample takes only a few minutes.
- For the urine sample, you first empty your bladder and discard the urine.
- You drink water to ensure adequate urine output.
- Collect two specimens 1 hour apart, and mark the collection time on the lab slip.

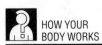

Getting rid of urea

When the body has taken everything useful out of the proteins it has received, all that's left is a toxic ammonia-containing waste called *urea*, which must be disposed of quickly.

It starts with the liver...

Amino acids absorbed from proteins by the intestine pass into the liver. Since the liver stores only small amounts of these amino acids — which are later returned to the blood to make enzymes, hormones, or new protoplasm — the liver converts the leftovers into other substances, such as glucose, glycogen, or fat. Before this conversion, the amino acids lose their nitrogen-containing amino groups. The amino groups are then converted to ammonia. The ammonia then combines with carbon dioxide to form urea, which is released into the blood and flows to the kidneys.

...And ends with the kidneys

The kidneys are the last station in urea's journey outside the body. Because the ammonia contained in urea is very toxic, especially to the brain, it must be removed as quickly as it's formed. (Serious liver disease causes elevated blood ammonia levels and eventually leads to coma.)

What happens after the test?

- You can resume any medications withheld before the test.
- You may resume normal diet and activity.

What are the normal results?

Normally, the urea clearance rate ranges from 64 to 99 milliliters per minute, with maximum clearance. If the flow rate is less than 2 milliliters per minute, normal clearance is 41 to 68 milliliters per minute.

What do abnormal results mean?

Low urea clearance values may indicate decreased kidney blood flow (due to shock or kidney artery obstruction), a long list of other kidney disorders, congestive heart failure, or dehydration. High urea clearance usually is not diagnostically significant.

URIC ACID

This test measures your body's production and excretion of a waste product known as *uric acid*. The analysis of uric acid levels in urine may supplement blood uric acid testing when the doctor is working to identify disorders that alter production or excretion of uric acid (such as leukemia, gout, and kidney dysfunction).

Why is this test done?

The uric acid test may be performed for the following reasons:
- To detect enzyme deficiencies and metabolic disturbances that affect uric acid production
- To help measure the efficiency of the kidney.

What should you know before the test?

- You won't need to change your diet before the test.
- The nurse will ask about any medications you take that may interfere with the test.

What happens during the test?

- You're asked to urinate into a special container over a 24-hour period.
- Void and discard the urine, and then begin 24-hour collection with the next voiding.
- After you place the first specimen in the container, add the preservative given to you by the nurse or medical technician.
- Add each voiding to the container immediately. If any urine is lost, restart the test.
- Plan the start of your test so that collection ends at a time when the lab is open.
- Just before the end of the test period, make an effort to void and add that urine to the container.
- Be sure not to contaminate the specimen with toilet paper or stools.

What happens after the test?

You can resume any medications withheld before the test.

What are the normal results?

Normal urine uric acid values vary with diet, but generally range from 250 to 750 milligrams per 24 hours.

What do abnormal results mean?

Elevated urine uric acid levels may be caused by such problems as blood disorders, multiple tumors or, in one case of good news, early remission in pernicious anemia.

Low urine uric acid levels show up in gout (when there's normal uric acid production but inadequate excretion) and in severe kidney damage.

HEMOGLOBIN

This test checks urine for hemoglobin, the protein that gives blood its color. Its presence in urine is an abnormal finding. It indicates excessive red blood cell destruction. It may be related to some kinds of anemia, infection, strenuous exercise, or severe effects of a transfusion reaction.

When red blood cell destruction occurs within the circulation, free hemoglobin enters the plasma and binds with a material called *haptoglobin*. If hemoglobin levels exceed haptoglobin levels, the excess of unbound hemoglobin is excreted in the urine.

Why is this test done?

The test for hemoglobin may be performed to aid the diagnosis of some anemias, infection, or severe effects of transfusion reaction.

What should you know before the test?

- You won't need to change your diet before the test.
- The test requires a random urine specimen.
- Because contamination of the specimen with menstrual blood alters results, a woman who's menstruating should reschedule her test.
- You should be careful not to contaminate the specimen with toilet paper or stools.
- The nurse will ask about any medications that might affect the test.

What happens during the test?

You're asked to urinate once into a special container.

What happens after the test?

You can resume any medications withheld during the test.

What are the normal results?

Normally, hemoglobin is not present in urine.

What do abnormal results mean?

Hemoglobin in the urine may be caused by severe blood breakdown in the veins, due to a blood transfusion reaction, burns, or a crushing injury. It may be caused by acquired anemias caused by chemical or drug intoxication or malaria. Other causes include inherited anemias, such as enzyme defects and, less commonly, it may signal cystitis or ureteral stones or infection. Hemoglobin and blood in the urine also show up in kidney damage, which may be caused by acute glomerulonephritis or pyelonephritis, kidney tumor, and tuberculosis.

MYOGLOBIN

This test helps evaluate muscle injury or disease by detecting a red pigment called *myoglobin* in the urine.

Myoglobin is normally found in muscle cells. When muscle cells are extensively damaged, myoglobin gets into the blood and then quickly into the urine. The damage may be due to disease or a severe crushing injury. For example, myoglobin appears in the urine within 24 hours after a heart attack.

Why is this test done?

The test for myoglobin may be performed for the following reasons:

- To help the doctor diagnose muscle disease
- To detect extensive injury to muscle tissue
- To measure the extent of muscle damage from crushing injuries.

What should you know before the test?

- You won't need to change your diet before the test.
- The test requires a random urine specimen.
- Test results are generally available in 1 day.

What happens during the test?

You're asked to urinate once into a special container.

What are the normal results?

Normally, myoglobin does not appear in urine.

What do abnormal results mean?

Myoglobin in the urine is a sign of acute or chronic muscle disease, alcoholic muscle damage, an extensive heart attack, or simply a family trait. Myoglobin can appear after such traumas as a crushing injury, extreme hyperthermia, or severe burns. It also appears after strenuous or prolonged exercise, but disappears after rest.

PORPHYRINS

This test detects abnormal hemoglobin formation by checking the urine for substances called *porphyrins*. The test counts specific porphyrins (uroporphyrins and coproporphyrins) and their precursors (such as porphobilinogen). Porphyrins are red-orange, fluorescent compounds that are produced when the body creates heme, which is part of hemoglobin.

Porphyrins are present in all of the body's protoplasm, take part in energy storage and utilization, and are normally excreted in urine in small amounts. Elevated urine levels of porphyrins or porphyrinogens reflect impaired heme creation. That problem may be caused by inherited enzyme deficiencies (congenital porphyrias) or by disorders such as hemolytic anemias and liver disease (acquired porphyrias).

Porphyrins are present in all of the body's protoplasm, helping with energy storage and utilization.

Why is this test done?

The test for porphyrins may be performed to aid diagnosis of inherited or acquired porphyrias.

What should you know before the test?

- You won't need to change your diet before the test.
- If you're a pregnant or menstruating woman, you may want to reschedule the test to avoid making it less accurate.
- The nurse will ask about any medications that might interfere with test results. The doctor may reschedule the test or restrict drugs before the test.

What happens during the test?

- You're asked to urinate into a special container over a 24-hour period.
- Void and discard that urine, and then begin 24-hour collection with the next voiding.
- After you place the first specimen in the container, add the preservative given to you by the nurse or medical technician.
- Add each voiding to the container immediately. If any urine is lost, restart the test.
- Plan the start of your test so that collection ends at a time when the lab is open.

- Just before the end of the test period, make an effort to void and add that urine to the container.

What happens after the test?

You may resume any medications withheld during the test.

What are the normal results?

Normal porphyrin and precursor values for urine occur in the following ranges:
- Uroporphyrins: in women, 1 to 22 micrograms per 24 hours; in men, undetectable to 42 micrograms per 24 hours
- Coproporphyrins: in women, 1 to 57 micrograms per 24 hours; in men, undetectable to 96 micrograms per 24 hours
- Porphobilinogen: in both sexes, up to 1.5 micrograms per 24 hours.

What do abnormal results mean?

Increased urine levels of porphyrins and porphyrin precursors are characteristic of porphyria. Infectious hepatitis, Hodgkin's disease, central nervous system disorders, cirrhosis, and heavy metal, benzene, or carbon tetrachloride poisoning may also increase porphyrin levels.

DELTA-AMINOLEVULINIC ACID

A test called the *delta-aminolevulinic acid test* may be performed to help diagnose porphyrias, liver disease, and lead poisoning.

Why is this test done?

The test may be performed for the following reasons:
- To screen for lead poisoning
- To help the doctor diagnose porphyrias and certain liver disorders, such as hepatitis and liver cancer.

What should you know before the test?

- If you or your child is having the test, you won't need to change your diet beforehand.

■ The nurse will ask about any medications that might interfere with test results. The doctor may reschedule the test or restrict drugs before the test.

Doctors can use this urine test to diagnose lead poisoning in children.

What happens during the test?

■ You're asked to urinate into a special container over a 24-hour period.

■ Void once and discard the urine, and then begin 24-hour collection with the next voiding.

■ After you collect the first specimen in the container, add the preservative given to you by the nurse or medical technician.

■ Add each urine specimen to the container immediately. If any urine is lost, restart the test.

■ Plan the start of your test so that collection ends at a time when the lab is open.

■ Just before the end of the test period, make an effort to void and add that urine to the container.

What happens after the test?

The doctor will resume administration of medications withheld during the test.

What are the normal results?

Normally, urine delta-aminolevulinic acid values range from 1.5 to 7.5 milligrams per deciliter per 24 hours.

What do abnormal results mean?

Elevated urine delta-aminolevulinic acid levels may occur in lead poisoning, acute porphyria, hepatic carcinoma, or hepatitis.

BILIRUBIN

This test helps determine the cause of jaundice. It's a screening test that detects water-soluble bilirubin in the urine. Detectable amounts of bilirubin may indicate liver disease caused by infections, bile-duct disease, or a toxic condition.

When combined with urobilinogen measurements, this test helps identify disorders that can cause jaundice. The analysis can be performed in the lab or at a person's bedside using a chemically treated strip.

Why is this test done?

The test for bilirubin may be performed to help the doctor identify the cause of jaundice.

What should you know before the test?

- You won't need to change your diet before the test.
- You'll be told that the test requires a random urine specimen.
- You'll be told that the specimen will be tested at bedside or in the lab. Bedside analysis can be performed immediately. Lab analysis is completed in 1 day.

What happens during the test?

You're asked to urinate once directly into a special container.

What are the normal results?

Normally, bilirubin is not found in urine in a routine screening test.

What do abnormal results mean?

High concentrations of direct bilirubin in urine may be evident from the specimen's appearance (dark, with a yellow foam). To diagnose jaundice, however, the doctor will correlate the bilirubin in urine with blood test results and with urine and fecal urobilinogen levels.

A nurse may quickly check out the cause of your jaundice with a bedside test, using a chemically treated strip.

UROBILINOGEN

This test helps check your liver and biliary tract function by measuring urine levels of urobilinogen. Urobilinogen is a colorless, water-soluble product that results from the reduction of bilirubin by intestinal bacteria. Absent or altered urobilinogen levels can indicate liver damage or dysfunction. Increased urine urobilinogen may indicate destruction of red blood cells. The urine sample is mixed with a chemical and the lab technician uses a microscope to watch a color reaction.

Why is this test done?

The test for urobilinogen may be performed for the following reasons:

- To aid the diagnosis of obstructions outside the liver such as blockage of the common bile duct
- To help diagnose liver and blood disorders.

What should you know before the test?

You won't need to change your diet except to avoid eating bananas for 48 hours before the test.

What happens during the test?

- You're asked to urinate into a special container over a 2-hour period.
- Void and discard the urine, and then begin 2-hour collection with the next voiding.
- After you place the first specimen in the container, add any preservative given to you by the nurse or medical technician.
- Add each voiding to the container immediately. If any urine is lost, restart the test.
- Plan the start of your test so that collection ends at a time when the lab is open.
- Just before the end of the test period, make an effort to void and add that urine to the container.

What happens after the test?

- You may resume your normal diet.
- You may resume any drugs withheld during the test.

What are the normal results?

Normally, urine urobilinogen values range from 0.1 to 1.1 Ehrlich units every 2 hours in women and 0.3 to 2.1 Ehrlich units every 2 hours in men.

What do abnormal results mean?

Absence of urine urobilinogen may be caused by complete obstructive jaundice or by broad-spectrum antibiotics, which destroy the intestinal bacterial flora. Low urine urobilinogen levels may be caused by congenital enzymatic jaundice (hyperbilirubinemia syndromes) or from treatment with drugs that acidify urine, such as ammonium chloride or ascorbic acid.

Elevated levels may indicate hemolytic jaundice, hepatitis, or cirrhosis.

COPPER REDUCTION TEST FOR SUGAR

The copper reduction test checks the urine for sugar levels, usually for the sake of diagnosing or monitoring people with diabetes.

The copper reduction test measures the concentration of substances in the urine through the reaction of these substances with a commercially prepared tablet called *Clinitest*. Clinitest reacts to glucose and to other sugars. The test is most valuable for providing diabetics with a simple, at-home method of monitoring urine glucose level. It's sometimes used as a rapid screening tool by labs.

Why is this test done?

The copper reduction test may be performed for the following reasons:
- To detect evidence of diabetes
- To monitor urine glucose levels during insulin therapy.

What should you know before the test?

- If you've been recently diagnosed as diabetic, the nurse or medical technician will teach you how to perform the Clinitest tablet test.
- The nurse will ask about any medications that might interfere with test results. The doctor may reschedule the test or restrict drugs before the test.

What happens during the test?

- First, you void, and then you drink water to ensure urine flow for the test.
- You're asked to void again after 30 to 45 minutes into a special container.
- Be sure not to contaminate the specimen with toilet tissue or stools.

The test is most valuable for helping diabetics monitor urine glucose levels at home.

The five-drop Clinitest tablet test

- Hold the medicine dropper vertically, and put five drops of urine from the specimen container into the test tube.
- Rinse the dropper with water, and add 10 drops of water to the test tube.
- Add one Clinitest tablet, and observe the color change, especially during effervescence or fizzing (the pass-through phase).
- Wait 15 seconds after effervescence subsides, and gently shake the test tube.
- If color develops at the 15-second interval, read the color against the Clinitest color chart and record the results.
- Ignore any changes that develop after 15 seconds.
- Rapid color changes (bright orange to dark brown or green-brown) in the pass-through phase in a five-drop Clinitest reaction indicate glucose in the urine of 2% or more. Record the results as over 2% without comparison to the color chart.

The two-drop Clinitest tablet test

- Hold the medicine dropper vertically, and put two drops of urine into the test tube.
- Flush urine residue from the dropper with water, and add 10 drops of water to the test tube.
- Add one Clinitest tablet, and observe the color change during the pass-through phase.
- Wait 15 seconds after effervescence stops, compare the color with the appropriate color reference chart, and record results.
- In a two-drop Clinitest reaction, rapid color changes (bright orange to dark brown or green-brown) in the pass-through phase indicate glucose in the urine of 5% or more.

What happens after the test?

- Store tablets in a well-marked, childproof bottle to prevent accidental ingestion.
- Don't use discolored tablets (dark blue). The normal color of fresh tablets is light blue, with darker blue flecks.
- During effervescence, hold the test tube near the top to avoid burning your hand; it becomes boiling hot.

Does the test have risks?

Make sure your hands are dry when handling Clinitest tablets and avoid contact with eyes, mucous membranes, gastrointestinal tract, and clothing because the sodium hydroxide and moisture produce caustic burns.

What are the normal results?

Normally, no glucose is present in urine.

What do abnormal results mean?

Glucose in the urine occurs in diabetes, adrenal and thyroid gland disorders, liver and central nervous system diseases, conditions involving low kidney function, toxic kidney tubular disease, heavy metal poisoning, pregnancy, and intravenous feeding. It also occurs with administration of large amounts of glucose and some drugs.

GLUCOSE TEST

The glucose oxidase test measures the concentration of glucose in your urine. It involves the use of commercial, plastic-coated, chemically-treated strips (Clinistix, Diastix) or Tes-Tape. The glucose oxidase test is used primarily to monitor urine glucose in people with diabetes. It's so simple and convenient that you can do it at home.

Why is this test done?

The glucose oxidase test may be performed for the following reasons:
- To detect glucose in the urine
- To monitor urine glucose levels during insulin therapy.

What should you know before the test?

- If you're newly diagnosed with diabetes, the nurse will teach you how to perform a chemical strip test.
- If you're receiving certain types of drug therapy, the nurse may recommend a Clinitest strip instead.

What happens during the test?

- First void, and then drink some water to ensure urine flow for the test.
- You urinate into a special container 30 to 45 minutes later.

The glucose oxidase test is so simple and convenient that you can do it at home.

The Clinistix test

- Dip the test area of the chemically treated strip into the specimen for 2 seconds.
- Remove excess urine by tapping the strip against a clean surface or the side of the container, and begin timing.
- Hold the strip in the air, and read the color exactly 10 seconds after taking the strip out of the urine. You read it by comparing it with the reference color blocks on the label of the container.
- Record the results.
- Ignore color changes that develop after 10 seconds.

The Diastix test

- Dip the reagent strip in the specimen for 2 seconds.
- Remove excess urine by tapping the strip against the container, and begin timing.
- Hold the strip in the air, and compare the color to the color chart exactly 30 seconds after taking the strip out of the urine.
- Record the results.
- Ignore color changes that develop after 30 seconds.

How to use Tes-Tape

- Withdraw about 1½ inches (3.8 centimeters) of the tape from the dispenser; dip 1¼ inches (3.1 centimeters) of it into the specimen for 2 seconds.
- Remove excess urine by tapping the strip against the side of the container, and begin timing.
- Hold the tape in the air, and compare the color of the darkest part of the tape to the color chart exactly 60 seconds after taking the strip out of the urine.
- If the tape indicates 0.5% or higher, wait an additional 60 seconds to make the final color comparison.
- Record the results.
- Be sure not to contaminate the urine specimen with toilet tissue or stools.

What happens after the test?

- Keep the test strip container tightly closed to prevent deterioration of strips by exposure to light or moisture.
- Store it in a cool place (under 86° F [30° C]) to avoid heat degradation.
- Don't use discolored or darkened Clinistix or Diastix or dark yellow or yellow-brown Tes-Tape.

What are the normal results?

Normally, no glucose is present in urine.

What do abnormal results mean?

Glucose in the urine occurs in diabetes, adrenal and thyroid disorders, liver and central nervous system diseases, conditions involving low kidney function, toxic kidney tubular disease, heavy metal poisoning, pregnancy, and intravenous feeding. It also shows up when people are given large amounts of glucose and certain drugs.

KETONE TEST

The ketone test evaluates your fat metabolism by measuring the level of ketone bodies in your urine. Ketone bodies are the by-products of fat metabolism; they include acetoacetic acid, acetone, and beta-hydroxybutyric acid. Excessive amounts may appear in people with carbohydrate dehydration, which may occur in starvation or diabetic ketoacidosis. Commercially available tests include the Acetest tablet, Chemstrip K, Ketostix, or Keto-Diastix. Each product measures a specific ketone body. For example, Acetest measures acetone, and Ketostix measures acetoacetic acid.

Why is this test done?

The ketone test may be performed for the following reasons:
- To screen for ketones in the urine
- To identify diabetic ketoacidosis and carbohydrate deprivation
- To distinguish between a diabetic and a nondiabetic coma
- To monitor control of diabetes, ketogenic weight reduction, and treatment of diabetic ketoacidosis.

What should you know before the test?

- If you're newly diagnosed with diabetes, the nurse will tell you how to perform the test.
- The nurse will ask about any medications that might interfere with test results. The doctor may reschedule the test or restrict drugs before the test.

What happens during the test?

- First, you void, and then you drink water to ensure urine flow for the test.
- You're asked to urinate into a special container about 30 minutes later using a method to get a midstream specimen. (See *How to catch a midstream specimen,* page 586.)

How to use Acetest

- Lay the tablet on a piece of white paper, and place one drop of urine on the tablet.
- Compare the tablet color (white, lavender, or purple) with the color chart after 30 seconds.

How to use Ketostix

- Dip the chemically treated stick into the specimen and remove it immediately.
- Compare the stick color (buff or purple) with the color chart after 15 seconds.
- Record the results as negative or positive for small, moderate, or large amounts of ketones.

How to use Keto-Diastix

- Dip the chemically treated strip into the specimen, and remove it immediately.
- Tap the edge of the strip against the container or a clean, dry surface to remove excess urine.
- Hold the strip horizontally to prevent mixing the chemicals from the two areas.
- Interpret each area of the strip separately. Compare the color of the ketone section (buff or purple) with the appropriate color chart after exactly 15 seconds; compare the color of the glucose section after 30 seconds.
- Ignore color changes that occur after the specified waiting periods.
- Record the results as negative or positive for small, moderate, or large amounts of ketones.

What happens after the test?

- Test the specimen within 60 minutes after it's obtained, or you must refrigerate it.
- Allow refrigerated specimens to return to room temperature before testing.
- Don't use tablets or strips that have become discolored or darkened.

The two-part strip is easy to use. Just hold it horizontally to prevent mixing the chemical from the two areas.

What are the normal results?

Normally, no ketones are present in urine.

What do abnormal results mean?

Ketones in the urine may show up in people with uncontrolled diabetes or starvation. It also occurs as a metabolic complication of intravenous or tube feeding.

VITAMINS & MINERALS

VITAMIN B$_6$

The tryptophan challenge test measures your body's stores of vitamin B$_6$ by measuring the level of xanthurenic acid in your urine after you receive a dose of a drug called *tryptophan*. This test can detect a deficiency of vitamin B$_6$ long before symptoms appear. The test is especially important because, so far, there's no way to directly measure your vitamin B$_6$ reserve.

Vitamin B$_6$ deficiency can cause a form of anemia without iron deficiency and central nervous system disturbances. In certain cases, vitamin B$_6$ deficiency may be associated with stones in the urinary tract.

Why is this test done?

The tryptophan challenge test may be performed to detect vitamin B$_6$ deficiency.

What happens before the test?

- You'll be given an oral dose of medication.
- The nurse will ask about any medications that might interfere with test results. The doctor may reschedule the test or restrict drugs before the test.

What happens during the test?

- You're asked to urinate into a special container over a 24-hour period.
- Void and discard the urine, and then begin 24-hour collection with the next voiding.
- After you place the first specimen in the container, add the preservative given to you by the nurse or medical technician.
- Add each voiding to the container immediately. If any urine is lost, restart the test.
- Plan the start of your test so that collection ends at a time when the lab is open.
- Just before the end of the test period, make an effort to void and add that urine to the container.

What are the normal results?

Normal excretion of xanthurenic acid after a tryptophan challenge dose is less than 50 milligrams per 24 hours.

What do abnormal results mean?

Urine levels of xanthurenic acid exceeding 100 milligrams per 24 hours indicate vitamin B_6 deficiency. This rare disorder may result from malnutrition, cancer, pregnancy, a family trait, or use of oral contraceptives or some drugs.

Note that if you have a vitamin B_6 deficiency, yeast, wheat, corn, liver, and kidneys are good sources of the vitamin.

VITAMIN C

This test measures levels of vitamin C (ascorbic acid) in the urine. It's particularly useful in diagnosing scurvy, an extreme deficiency of vitamin C marked by the degeneration of connective and bone--covering tissues and teeth. Although now uncommon in North America, scurvy may occur in alcoholics, people on low-fiber or low-citrus diets, and infants who've been weaned to cow's milk that doesn't contain a vitamin C supplement.

Why is this test done?

The test for vitamin C is performed to aid diagnosis of scurvy, scurvylike conditions, and metabolic disorders such as malnutrition.

What should you know before the test?

- You won't need to change your diet before the test.
- The nurse will ask about any medications that might interfere with test results. The doctor may reschedule the test or restrict drugs before the test.

What happens during the test?

- You're asked to urinate into a special container over a 24-hour period.
- Void and discard the urine, and then begin 24-hour collection with the next voiding.
- After you place the first specimen in the container, add the preservative given to you by the nurse or medical technician.
- Add each voiding to the container immediately. If any urine is lost, restart the test.
- Plan the start of your test so that collection ends at a time when the lab is open.
- Just before the end of the test period, make an effort to void and add that urine to the container.
- Note that if you have a vitamin C deficiency, citrus fruits, tomatoes, potatoes, cabbage, and strawberries are good dietary sources of vitamin C.

What are the normal results?

Normal urine vitamin C excretion is 30 milligrams per 24 hours.

What do abnormal results mean?

Low levels of vitamin C in the urine are common in people with infection, cancer, burns, or other stress-producing conditions. Decreased vitamin C levels may also indicate malnutrition, malabsorption, kidney deficiencies, or prolonged intravenous or tube feeding without vitamin C replacement. Severe vitamin C deficiency causes scurvy. (See *Scurvy: A brief history*.)

SODIUM AND CHLORIDE

This test helps determine the balance of salt and water in the body. Less significant than blood levels (and, consequently, performed less frequently), measurement of urine sodium and urine chloride con-

---

Scurvy: A brief history

Scurvy was probably the first disease to be recognized as a dietary deficiency. Although it rarely occurs now, scurvy once was common in places where fresh fruits and vegetables — major sources of vitamin C — weren't accessible in the winter.

A sailor's plague

Known as the "plague of the seas," scurvy was most prevalent in sailors because perishable foods couldn't be stored aboard ship. Famine or wartime food scarcity also caused scurvy.

When the Portuguese explorer Vasco da Gama first sailed around the Cape of Good Hope in 1497, more than half his crew died of the disease. Several centuries later, in 1747, Scottish naval surgeon James Lind found he could cure sailors of scurvy by giving them lemons and oranges.

The lime-juice cure

In an effort to duplicate Dr. Lind's success, lime juice was distributed in 1797 to the crews of British navy ships during long sea voyages, which explains the nickname "limeys," for British sailors.

centrations is used to evaluate kidney conservation of these two electrolytes and to confirm blood tests.

Why is this test done?

The tests for sodium and chloride may be given for the following reasons:

- To help evaluate fluid and electrolyte imbalance
- To monitor the effects of a low-salt diet
- To help evaluate kidney and adrenal gland disorders.

What should you know before the test?

- You won't need to change your diet before the test.
- If you're a pregnant or menstruating woman, you may want to reschedule the test to ensure more accurate results.
- The nurse will ask about any medications that might interfere with test results. The doctor may reschedule the test or restrict drugs before the test.

What happens during the test?

- You're asked to urinate into a special container over a 24-hour period.
- Void and discard the urine, and then begin 24-hour collection with the next voiding.
- After you place the first specimen in the container, add the preservative given to you by the nurse or medical technician.
- Add each voiding to the container immediately. If any urine is lost, restart the test.
- Plan the start of your test so that collection ends at a time when the lab is open.
- Just before the end of the test period, make an effort to void and add that urine to the container.
- Be sure not to contaminate the specimen with toilet paper or stools.

What are the normal results?

Normal ranges of sodium and chloride in the urine vary greatly with dietary salt intake and perspiration.

What do abnormal results mean?

Usually, levels of sodium and chloride in the urine are parallel, rising and falling together. Abnormal levels of both minerals may indicate the need for more specific testing. Elevated levels of sodium in the urine may reflect increased salt intake, adrenal failure, a diabetic condition, salt-losing tissue damage, and dehydration.

Decreased levels of sodium in the urine suggest decreased salt intake, primary aldosteronism (which causes high blood pressure), acute kidney failure, and congestive heart failure.

POTASSIUM

This test evaluates your kidney function. It measures urine levels of potassium, a major electrolyte that helps regulate acid-base balance and neuromuscular function. Potassium imbalance may cause the person to have muscle weakness, nausea, diarrhea, confusion, low blood pressure, and electrocardiogram changes. A severe imbalance may lead to cardiac arrest.

Most commonly, a blood test is performed to detect abnormally high or abnormally low potassium levels. A test of the level of potassium in the urine may be performed if doctors cannot uncover the cause of this condition through other means. If results suggest a kidney disorder, additional tests may be ordered.

Potassium imbalance may cause muscle weakness, nausea, diarrhea, confusion, low blood pressure, and electrocardiogram changes.

Why is this test done?
The test for potassium may be done to determine whether hypokalemia is caused by kidney or other disorders.

What should you know before the test?
- You won't need to change your diet before the test.
- If you're a pregnant or menstruating woman, you may want to reschedule the test to avoid making it less accurate.
- The nurse will ask about any medications that might interfere with test results. The doctor may reschedule the test or restrict drugs before the test.

What happens during the test?
- You're asked to urinate into a special container over a 24-hour period.
- Void and discard the urine, and then begin 24-hour collection with the next voiding.

- After you place the first specimen in the container, add the preservative given to you by the nurse or medical technician.
- Add each voiding to the container immediately. If any urine is lost, restart the test.
- Plan the start of your test so that collection ends at a time when the lab is open.
- Just before the end of the test period, make an effort to void and add that urine to the container.
- Refrigerate the specimen or place it on ice during the collection period.

What happens after the test?

- You may be given potassium supplements and you may have a blood test to monitor your potassium levels.
- You may need dietary supplements and nutritional counseling.
- You may be given intravenous or oral fluids to replace lost potassium.
- You may resume drugs withheld during the test.

What are the normal results?

Normal potassium excretion is 25 to 125 milliequivalents per 24 hours, with an average potassium concentration of 25 to 100 milliequivalents per liter.

What do abnormal results mean?

In a person with potassium deficiency, urine potassium concentration less than 10 milliequivalents per liter suggests normal kidney function, indicating that potassium loss is most likely caused by a gastrointestinal disorder.

In a person with potassium deficiency lasting more than 3 days, urine potassium concentration above 10 milliequivalents per liter indicates kidney loss of potassium. These losses may be caused by such disorders as aldosteronism or kidney problems or failure. However, disorders that don't involve the kidney, such as dehydration, starvation, Cushing's disease, or salicylate intoxication, may also elevate urine potassium levels.

CALCIUM AND PHOSPHATES

This test measures the levels of calcium and phosphates in the urine. They're essential for the formation and resorption of bone. Urine calcium and phosphate levels generally parallel levels of these minerals in the blood.

Normally absorbed in the upper intestine and excreted in feces and urine, calcium and phosphates help maintain tissue and fluid pH, electrolyte balance in cells and extracellular fluids, and permeability of cell membranes. Calcium promotes enzymatic processes, aids blood coagulation, and lowers neuromuscular irritability. Phosphates aid carbohydrate metabolism.

Why is this test done?

The test for calcium and phosphates may be performed for the following reasons:
- To evaluate calcium and phosphate metabolism and excretion
- To monitor treatment of calcium or phosphate deficiency.

What should you know before the test?

- You should be as active as possible before the test.
- The doctor may suggest you go on a diet called the *Albright-Reifenstein diet* (which contains about 130 milligrams of calcium per 24 hours) for 3 days before the test.
- If you're a pregnant or menstruating woman, you may want to reschedule the test to avoid making it less accurate.
- The nurse will ask about any medications that might interfere with test results. The doctor may reschedule the test or restrict drugs before the test.

What happens during the test?

- You're asked to urinate into a special container over a 24-hour period.
- Void and discard the urine, and then begin 24-hour collection with the next voiding.
- After you place the first specimen in the container, add the preservative given to you by the nurse or medical technician.
- Add each voiding to the container immediately. If any urine is lost, restart the test.

Before the test, you should be as active as possible and you may be asked to follow a diet that regulates your calcium intake.

- Plan the start of your test so that collection ends at a time when the lab is open.
- Just before the end of the test period, make an effort to void and add that urine to the container.

What are the normal results?

Normal values depend on dietary intake. Men excrete less than 275 milligrams of calcium per 24 hours. Women excrete less than 250 milligrams per 24 hours. Normal excretion of phosphate in both sexes is less than 1,000 milligrams per 24 hours.

What do abnormal results mean?

A variety of disorders may affect calcium and phosphorus levels. The doctor will probably do more testing.

MAGNESIUM

This test determines urine magnesium levels. Measurement of urine magnesium is especially useful because magnesium deficiency is detectable in the person's urine before it shows up in the blood. This test may be used to rule out magnesium deficiency as the cause of neurologic symptoms and to help evaluate glomerular function in suspected kidney disease.

Magnesium is found primarily in the bones and in intracellular fluid. An imbalance of this element in the body may cause a variety of symptoms, such as excessive perspiration, muscle weakness, visual disturbances, lethargy, confusion, hallucinations, or nausea and vomiting.

The test is especially useful because magnesium deficiency is detectable in the person's urine before it shows up in the blood.

Why is this test done?

The test for magnesium may be performed for the following reasons:
- To rule out magnesium deficiency in people with symptoms of central nervous system irritation
- To detect excessive urinary excretion of magnesium
- To help evaluate glomerular function in kidney disease.

What should you know before the test?

- You won't need to change your diet before the test.
- If you're a pregnant or menstruating woman, you may want to reschedule the test to avoid making it less accurate.
- The nurse will ask about any medications that might interfere with test results. The doctor may reschedule the test or restrict drugs before the test.

What happens during the test?

- You're asked to urinate into a special container over a 24-hour period.
- Void and discard the urine, and then begin 24-hour collection with the next voiding.
- After you place the first specimen in the container, add the preservative given to you by the nurse or medical technician.
- Add each voiding to the container immediately. If any urine is lost, restart the test.
- Plan the start of your test so that collection ends at a time when the lab is open.
- Just before the end of the test period, make an effort to void and add that urine to the container.

What are the normal results?

Normal urinary excretion of magnesium is less than 150 milligrams per 24 hours.

What do abnormal results mean?

Low urine magnesium levels may be caused by poor absorption, acute or chronic diarrhea, a diabetic condition, dehydration, pancreatitis, advanced kidney failure, and primary aldosteronism. They also may be caused by decreased dietary intake of magnesium.

Elevated urine magnesium levels may be caused by early chronic kidney disease, an adrenal gland problem, chronic alcoholism, or chronic ingestion of magnesium-containing antacids.

IRON

The hemosiderin test helps determine if the body is accumulating excessive amounts of iron. The test measures the urine level of hemosiderin — one of the two forms of storage iron deposited in body tissue.

When iron storage mechanisms fail to manage iron overload, excess iron may escape to cells unaccustomed to high iron concentrations and may produce toxic effects. Toxicity may affect the liver, the heart lining, bone marrow, pancreas, kidneys, and skin. Subsequent tissue damage is referred to as *hemochromatosis*. Hemochromatosis may occur in a rare hereditary form (primary hemochromatosis) as well as forms caused by outside influences.

When iron storage mechanisms fail, iron overload may produce toxic effects.

Why is this test done?

The test for hemosiderin may be performed to aid the diagnosis of hemochromatosis.

What should you know before the test?

You'll be told that no restrictions are necessary and that the test requires a urine specimen.

What happens during the test?

You're asked to urinate once into a special container.

What are the normal results?

Normally, hemosiderin is not found in urine.

What do abnormal results mean?

The presence of hemosiderin, appearing as yellow-brown granules in urinary sediment, indicates hemochromatosis. A liver or bone marrow biopsy is necessary to confirm the condition. Hemosiderin may also suggest some forms of anemia, multiple blood transfusions, and a reaction to excessive iron injections or dietary intake of iron.

15

CULTURES:
Pinpointing the Cause of Infection

GENERAL CULTURES

URINE CULTURE

This test detects urinary tract infections, especially bladder infections. Urine in the kidneys and bladder is normally sterile, but a urine specimen may still contain various organisms because it has passed through the nonsterile urethra and external genitalia.

Why is this test done?
The urine culture may be performed for the following reasons:
- To diagnose urinary tract infection in an adult or a child
- To check for the growth of bacteria after the doctor inserts a urinary catheter.

What should you know before the test?
- You won't need to change your diet before the test.
- The doctor or nurse will ask whether you're taking an antibiotic. He or she may discontinue the medication before the test.

What happens during the test?
- You're asked to collect a clean-voided midstream urine specimen. (If you'll be collecting a urine specimen from a baby, see *How to put a urine collector on your baby*.)
- Make sure you don't contaminate the specimen with toilet paper or feces.
- For the person with suspected tuberculosis, specimen collection may be required on three consecutive mornings.

What happens after the test?
You can resume any medications discontinued for the test.

What are the normal results?
Culture results of sterile urine are normally reported as "no growth," which usually indicates the absence of a urinary tract infection. However, a single negative culture doesn't always rule out an infection.

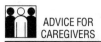

ADVICE FOR CAREGIVERS

How to put a urine collector on your baby

If the doctor needs samples of your baby's urine to diagnose or treat an illness, you'll be given some special equipment to collect the urine. The same plastic disposable collection bags with adhesive rings around their openings are used for boys and girls, but the methods used to attach the bags are different.

For a girl
Stretch the perineum (the skin between the anus and the labia) to smooth the skin around the vagina. Working upward from the perineum, press the bag's adhesive ring inside the labia.

For a boy
Make sure the adhesive seal attaches firmly to the skin around the scrotum and penis and doesn't pucker.

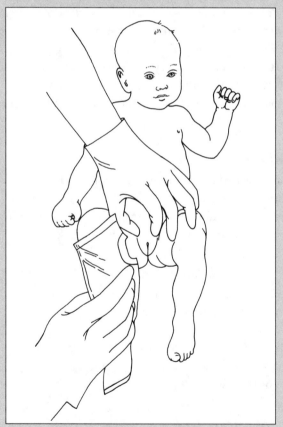

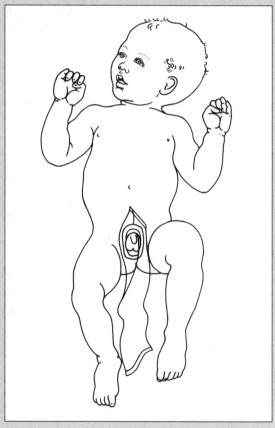

What do abnormal results mean?

Bacterial counts of 100,000 or more organisms of a single microbe species per milliliter indicate a probable urinary tract infection. Counts under 100,000 may be significant, depending on your age, sex, history, and other individual factors. A special test isolates bacteria that indicate tuberculosis of the urinary tract.

STOOL CULTURE

This test is used to determine the cause of gastrointestinal distress or to see if you're a carrier of infectious organisms. Normal bacteria in feces include several potentially harmful organisms. A bacteriologic exam is valuable for identifying organisms that cause digestive tract diseases, such as typhoid and dysentery. A sensitivity test may follow isolation of the causative organism. A stool culture may also be used to detect certain viruses, such as enterovirus, which can cause meningitis.

Why is this test done?

A stool culture may be performed for the following reasons:
- To identify harmful bacteria, especially in a debilitated person
- To help the doctor treat disease, prevent possibly life-threatening complications, and confine highly infectious diseases.

What should you know before the test?

- You won't need to change your diet before the test.
- The test may require collection of a stool specimen on 3 consecutive days.
- The nurse will ask about dietary patterns, recent antibiotic therapy that might affect the test, and recent travel that might suggest endemic infections or infestations.

What happens during the test?

You're asked to place a stool specimen directly into a special container. The specimen must represent the first, middle, and last portion of the feces passed.

What are the normal results?

Approximately 96% to 99% of normal fecal bacteria species can't survive in the open air. The remaining 1% to 4% of species include gram-negative bacilli (predominantly *Escherichia coli* and other Enterobacteriaceae), *Pseudomonas*, gram-positive cocci (mostly enterococci), and a few yeasts.

What do abnormal results mean?

The most common harmful organisms of the digestive tract are called *Shigella*, *Salmonella*, and *Campylobacter jejuni*. Isolation of these organisms in people with acute diarrhea indicates bacterial infection and may require special tests. The doctor will also look for evidence of such problems as food poisoning, staphylococcal infection, yeast infection, and aseptic meningitis.

THROAT CULTURE

A throat culture can isolate and identify harmful organisms. Culture results are considered in relation to your health status, recent antibiotic therapy, and amount of normal organisms.

Why is this test done?

A throat culture may be performed for the following reasons:
- To isolate and identify group A beta-hemolytic streptococci, a type of microorganism; this allows for early treatment of pharyngitis and may help to prevent such complications as rheumatic heart disease or glomerulonephritis
- To check a person who has no symptoms but who may actually have a harmful infection
- To identify *Candida albicans* (which may cause thrush).

What should you know before the test?

- You won't need to change your diet before the test.
- A nurse or medical technician will use a sterile swab to collect material from your throat. You may gag during the swabbing.
- The test takes less than 30 seconds, and test results should be available in 2 or 3 days.

The doctor may use a throat culture to check a person who has no symptoms but who may actually have a harmful infection.

- The nurse will ask about any recent antibiotic therapy and may want to know your immunization history.

What happens during the test?
- The nurse asks you to tilt your head back and close your eyes.
- With your throat well illuminated, the nurse checks for inflamed areas using a tongue depressor, and then swabs the tonsil area.

What are the normal results?
Normally, the throat contains some forms of staphylococci and *Haemophilus,* diphtheroids, pneumococci, yeasts, and enteric gram-negative bacteria.

What do abnormal results mean?
Organisms that may be harmful include the ones that can cause scarlet fever, pharyngitis, thrush, diphtheria, and whooping cough. The lab report should indicate the prevalent organisms and the quantity of pathogens cultured.

NASOPHARYNGEAL CULTURE

This test is used to isolate the cause of a nose and throat infection. It checks secretions for the presence of harmful organisms. To obtain results, a specimen is stained and then examined under a microscope. The doctor uses the information to determine the need for additional testing and to choose an effective antibiotic.

Why is this test done?
A nasopharyngeal culture may be performed for any of the following reasons:
- To identify harmful organisms causing upper respiratory tract symptoms
- To identify growth of normal nasopharyngeal organisms, which may be harmful to debilitated people or to those who have a damaged immune system

- To identify microorganisms that may cause whooping cough or meningitis (may be especially important in very young, elderly, or debilitated people and in people who don't have symptoms of illness but are nevertheless suspected of having an infection)
- Less frequently, to isolate viruses, especially to identify people who may be carrying influenza virus A or B.

What should you know before the test?

- A nurse or medical technician will collect secretions from the back of your nose and your throat using a cotton-tipped swab.
- Obtaining the specimen takes less than 15 seconds. You may feel slight discomfort and may gag.
- Initial test results are available in 48 to 72 hours. It may take longer to obtain viral test results.

What happens during the test?

- You're asked to cough before collection of the specimen. Next, you're positioned with your head tilted back.
- Using a penlight and tongue depressor, the examiner inspects your throat and the back of your nose.
- The nurse or medical technician gently passes a swab through the nostril into the nasopharynx (the upper part of the pharynx that connects with the nasal passages). Alternatively, the examiner may place a pyrex tube into your nostril and then pass the swab through this tube.

What are the normal results?

Organisms commonly found in the nasopharynx include some types of streptococci and other bacteria.

What do abnormal results mean?

Harmful organisms include some forms of streptococci (organisms that cause whooping cough and diphtheria) and excessive amounts of organisms that may cause flu, pneumonia, or candidiasis.

A nose and throat culture may be performed to detect microorganisms that can cause whooping cough or meningitis.

SPUTUM CULTURE

This test is used to identify the organism causing a respiratory tract infection. Checking the bacteria in sputum — material raised from the lungs and bronchi — is an important aid for the doctor in the management of lung disease.

The usual method of specimen collection is to have the person cough deeply and spit out a specimen. Other methods include tracheal (windpipe) suctioning and bronchoscopy.

Why is this test done?

A sputum culture is performed to identify the cause of a lung infection. The results help the doctor diagnose bronchitis, tuberculosis, lung abscess, and pneumonia.

What should you know before the test?

- The test requires a sputum specimen, which a nurse or medical technician will help you produce.
- If the specimen is to be collected by expectoration (spitting out), the nurse will tell you to drink fluids the night before collection to help increase sputum production.
- The nurse will teach you how to expectorate by taking three deep breaths and forcing a deep cough. It's important to remember that sputum is not the same as saliva, which is unacceptable for culturing.
- Don't brush your teeth or use mouthwash before the test. (If you do, the tests results will be unreliable.) You may rinse your mouth with water.
- If the specimen is to be collected by tracheal suctioning, you'll experience discomfort as the catheter passes into your trachea.
- If the specimen is to be collected by bronchoscopy, you'll fast for 6 hours before the procedure. You'll receive a local anesthetic just before the test to minimize discomfort during passage of the tube.
- Because the bronchoscopy requires an anesthetic, the nurse will ask you to sign a consent form.
- If the doctor suspects that you have tuberculosis, at least three morning specimens may be required.
- Test results are usually available in 48 to 72 hours. However, because cultures for tuberculosis take up to 2 months, the diagnosis of this disorder is generally based on the person's symptoms and on results of an acid-fast bacilli test, a chest X-ray, and a skin test.

Don't brush your teeth or use mouthwash before the test. (If you do, the test results will be unreliable.)

What happens during the test?

- For expectoration, the nurse asks you to cough deeply and spit into the container. If the cough doesn't produce sputum, the nurse may use chest physiotherapy or nebulization (a heated aerosol spray) to induce it.
- For tracheal suctioning, the nurse slips a lubricated tube through your nostril and into the trachea, then suctions for up to 15 seconds. This method makes you cough.
- For bronchoscopy, a local anesthetic is sprayed into your throat (or you gargle with a local anesthetic); then the doctor inserts the bronchoscope through your throat and into the bronchus. Secretions are collected with a bronchial brush or aspirated through the inner channel of the scope.
- Tracheal suctioning is not used if you have abnormalities in your esophagus or if you have heart disease.

What are the normal results?

Normally, sputum is contaminated with harmless organisms, such as some types of streptococci and yeasts. These organisms are not worrisome if your overall condition is healthy.

What do abnormal results mean?

Harmful organisms most often found in sputum include the bacteria that cause pneumonia, tuberculosis, and other diseases. Isolation of the bacterium that causes tuberculosis is always a significant finding.

Diagnosis of respiratory viruses usually requires blood tests rather than a sputum culture.

BLOOD CULTURE

This test helps the doctor identify the organism causing your symptoms. A blood culture can isolate the harmful organisms that cause bacteremia (bacterial invasion of the bloodstream) and septicemia (systemic spread of such infection). The lab takes a sample of your blood, inoculates a culture medium where it can grow, and incubates it.

Why is this test done?

A blood culture may be performed for the following reasons:

- To confirm bacteremia
- To identify the causative organism in bacteremia and septicemia.

What should you know before the test?

- You won't need to change your diet before the test.
- You may be told to expect slight discomfort from the tourniquet pressure and the needle puncture.
- Drawing a blood sample takes less than 3 minutes.

What happens during the test?

A nurse or medical technician inserts a needle into a vein, usually in your forearm. A blood sample is collected in a tube, which is then sent to the lab for testing.

What happens after the test?

If swelling develops at the needle puncture site, warm soaks are applied to the area to ease discomfort.

What are the normal results?

Normally, blood cultures are sterile.

What do abnormal results mean?

Positive blood cultures do not necessarily confirm a spreading bacterial infection. Mild, short-term invasions of bacteria may occur during many infectious diseases and other disorders. Persistent, continuous, or recurrent bacteremia reliably confirms the presence of serious infection. To detect the cause, blood samples are ideally drawn on 2 consecutive days. Isolation of most organisms takes about 72 hours; however, negative cultures are held for 1 week or more before being reported negative.

WOUND CULTURE

Performed to confirm infection, a wound culture is a microscopic analysis of a specimen from a laceration or lesion. Wound cultures may be aerobic (to detect organisms that can live in the open air and usually appear in a superficial wound) or anaerobic (to detect organisms that cannot live in the presence of oxygen and that appear in postoperative wounds, ulcers, or compound fractures).

The doctor may perform this culture when a person has a fever and an inflamed, draining wound.

Why is this test done?

A wound culture may be performed to identify an infection.

What should you know before the test?

- A drainage specimen from the wound will be withdrawn by a syringe or removed on cotton swabs.
- Collecting the drainage specimen takes less than 3 minutes.

What happens during the test?

The nurse first cleans the area around the wound with an antiseptic solution.

Collecting an aerobic culture

The nurse will press the wound and swab as much discharge as possible or insert the swab deeply into the wound and gently rotate it.

Collecting an anaerobic culture

- The nurse will insert the swab deeply into the wound, gently rotate it, and immediately place it in a special container.
- Alternatively, the nurse may insert a needle into the wound, withdraw 1 to 5 milliliters of discharge into the syringe, and inject the discharge into a tube.
- The wound is then dressed.

What are the normal results?

Normally, no harmful organisms are present in a clean wound.

The doctor may perform this culture when a person has a fever and an inflamed, draining wound.

What do abnormal results mean?

The most common aerobic organisms in a wound infection include *Staphylococcus aureus*, group A beta-hemolytic streptococci, *Proteus*, *Escherichia coli*, and other such bacteria. The most common anaerobic organisms are certain species of *Clostridium* and *Bacteroides*.

STOMACH CULTURE

Used to diagnose tuberculosis, this test requires removal of a small amount of the stomach's contents and cultivation of any microbes present. It's performed in conjunction with a chest X-ray and a skin test. This test is especially useful when a sputum specimen can't be obtained.

In an infant with an infection, gastric aspiration also provides a specimen for rapid identification of bacteria.

The microbes in your stomach can be cultured to show whether you have tuberculosis. In infants, they can reveal the cause of an infection.

Why is this test done?

A stomach culture may be performed for the following reasons:
- To help the doctor diagnose tuberculosis
- To identify the causative agent in an infant with an infection.

What should you know before the test?

- You or your infant will fast for 8 hours before the test.
- The same procedure may be performed on three consecutive mornings.
- The doctor or nurse will ask about any recent medications you've taken that could affect test results. Use of such medications may be discontinued.
- You or your infant should remain in bed each morning until the specimen is collected, to prevent premature emptying of stomach contents.
- The examiner will insert a tube through your nostril and into your stomach to withdraw the specimen. The tube may make you gag, but it will pass more easily if you relax and follow instructions about breathing and swallowing.
- Just before the procedure, the nurse will check your heart rate.
- It may take as long as 2 months to obtain test results.

What happens during the test?

As soon as you awaken in the morning, the examiner inserts the tube through your nose and collects stomach contents.

What happens after the test?

- You can resume your normal diet and any medications discontinued before the test.
- You'll be told not to blow your nose for at least 4 hours to prevent bleeding.

Does the test have risks?

You won't be given the test if you're pregnant or have a condition such as an esophageal disorder, cancer, recent severe gastric hemorrhage, aortic aneurysm, or heart failure.

What are the normal results?

Normally, the culture specimen shows no harmful organisms.

What do abnormal results mean?

Isolation and identification of the organism *Mycobacterium tuberculosis* indicates active tuberculosis. Other species of *Mycobacterium* may cause lung disease that produces the same symptoms as tuberculosis. Treatment of these diseases may be difficult and commonly requires further studies to help the doctor find an effective antibiotic.

Harmful bacteria causing an infant's infection may also be identified through culture.

INTESTINAL CULTURE

This test requires putting a tube into the duodenum (the top part of the intestine), withdrawing some contents, and cultivating the microbes found there. The culture will help the doctor identify harmful organisms that may cause intestinal diseases, such as duodenitis, cholecystitis, or cholangitis. Occasionally, a specimen may be obtained during surgery.

Why is this test done?

An intestine culture may be performed for the following reasons:
- To detect bacterial infection of the bile ducts and duodenum
- To differentiate between infection and gallstones
- To rule out bacterial infection as the cause of persistent stomach pain, nausea, vomiting, and diarrhea.

What should you know before the test?

- You'll have to restrict food and fluids for 12 hours before the test.
- A tube will be inserted through your nostril and into your stomach. Although this procedure is uncomfortable, it isn't dangerous.
- The passage of the tube may cause gagging, but following the examiner's instructions about proper positioning, breathing, swallowing, and relaxing will minimize discomfort.
- To increase your comfort level, you should empty your bladder before the procedure.

Normally, an intestine culture reveals no harmful organisms. The bacterial count is relatively low.

What happens during the test?

- After the tube is inserted, you lie on your left side with your feet elevated.
- The examiner may use a fluoroscope to confirm the correct position of the tube.
- The examiner withdraws duodenal contents.

What happens after the test?

- You'll be kept in bed until you feel stronger.
- You can resume your normal diet.

Does the test have risks?

You shouldn't undergo this test if you're pregnant, have had a heart attack or a recent severe stomach hemorrhage, or have acute pancreatitis or cholecystitis, abnormalities of the esophagus, an aortic aneurysm, or congestive heart failure.

What are the normal results?

Normally, an intestine culture contains small amounts of white blood cells and tissue cells with no harmful organisms. The bacterial count is usually relatively low: less than 100,000 per milliliter of body fluid.

What do abnormal results mean?

Generally, bacterial counts of 100,000 or more per milliliter of body fluid or the presence of harmful organisms, such as *Escherichia coli*, *Staphylococcus aureus*, and *Salmonella*, in any number indicates infection.

Numerous white blood cells, copious mucous debris, and bile-stained cells in the bile fluid suggest inflammation of the bile ducts. Other findings can suggest inflammation of the pancreas, the duodenum, or bile ducts. To make a definitive diagnosis, the doctor may require more testing.

GENITAL CULTURES

CULTURE FOR GONORRHEA

This test confirms gonorrhea, a disease that's almost always caused by sexual transmission of the organism *Neisseria gonorrhoeae*. A stained smear of genital discharge can confirm gonorrhea in 90% of men with characteristic symptoms, but a culture is often necessary, especially in women with no symptoms. Specimens may be taken from the urethra (the usual site in men), endocervix (the usual site in women), anal canal, or throat.

Why is this test done?

This culture is performed to confirm gonorrhea.

What should you know before the test?

Test results are usually available within 24 to 72 hours.

For women

You'll be told not to douche for 24 hours before the test.

For men

- You'll be told not to urinate during the hour preceding the test.
- Men sometimes experience nausea, sweating, weakness, and fainting due to stress or discomfort when the cotton swab or wire loop is introduced into the urethra.

What happens during the test?

Endocervical culture

- You lie on the examining table with your feet in stirrups (much like when you have a Pap test). You're draped, and the examiner instructs you to take deep breaths.
- The examiner inserts a vaginal speculum that's lubricated with warm water and wipes mucus from the cervix with cotton balls.
- The examiner inserts a dry, sterile cotton swab into the endocervical canal to collect the specimen.

Urethral culture

- You lie on the examining table, covered with a drape.
- The examiner cleans around the urethral opening with a sterile gauze pad or a cotton ball, then inserts a thin swab or a wire loop into the urethra, and rotates the swab or loop from side to side.
- In another method, the urethra may be milked, bringing urethral secretions to the opening for collection on a cotton swab.

Rectal culture

After the examiner has obtained an endocervical or urethral specimen (while you're still on the examining table), a sterile cotton swab is inserted into the anal canal to obtain another specimen.

Throat culture

- You sit with your head tilted back.
- The nurse checks your throat for inflamed areas using a tongue depressor, then rubs a sterile swab from side to side over the tonsil area to collect the specimen.

What happens after the test?

- You'll be told to avoid all sexual contact until test results are available.
- If the test confirms gonorrhea, this finding must be reported to the local health department.
- The nurse will explain that treatment usually begins after confirmation of positive culture, except in a person who has symptoms of gonorrhea or a person who's had intercourse with someone known to have gonorrhea.
- A repeat culture is required 1 week after completion of treatment to evaluate therapy.

If the test confirms gonorrhea, this finding must be reported to the local health department.

What are the normal results?

Normally, *Neisseria gonorrhoea* does not appear in the culture.

What do abnormal results mean?

A positive culture confirms gonorrhea.

CULTURE FOR HERPES

This test detects infection by the herpes simplex virus. About 85% of the people with this common infection don't experience noticeable symptoms at first. The rest have local lesions. After the initial infection, the person becomes a carrier who's subject to recurrent attacks. Symptoms depend on the location of the infection.

Herpes simplex type 1 is transmitted primarily by contact with oral secretions and occurs primarily in children. Herpes simplex type 2 is transmitted primarily by contact with genital secretions, mainly affects the genitalia, and usually occurs in adolescents and young adults. (See *The genital herpes cycle*, page 634.) In a person with a damaged immune system, infection with herpes simplex may lead to numerous illnesses.

Approximately 50% of the strains of herpes simplex virus can be detected within 24 hours after the lab receives the specimen. Five to 7 days are required to detect the remaining strains of herpes simplex.

About 85% of the people with this common infection don't have noticeable symptoms at first.

Why is this test done?

This culture may be performed to confirm a diagnosis of herpes simplex virus infection.

What should you know before the test?

The nurse will explain that specimens will be collected from suspected lesions.

What happens during the test?

The examiner collects a specimen for culture in a special collection device. For the throat, skin, eye, or genital area, the examiner uses a special swab.

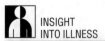

INSIGHT
INTO ILLNESS

The genital herpes cycle

After the initial genital herpes infection, a latent (inactive) period follows. During this time, the virus enters the nerves surrounding the lesions and remains there permanently.

Repeated outbreaks of herpes may develop at any time, again followed by a latent stage when healing is complete. These outbreaks may recur as often as three to eight times yearly. Although the cycle continues indefinitely, some people remain symptom-free for years.

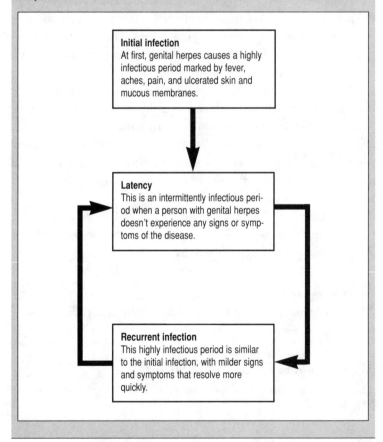

Initial infection
At first, genital herpes causes a highly infectious period marked by fever, aches, pain, and ulcerated skin and mucous membranes.

Latency
This is an intermittently infectious period when a person with genital herpes doesn't experience any signs or symptoms of the disease.

Recurrent infection
This highly infectious period is similar to the initial infection, with milder signs and symptoms that resolve more quickly.

SELF-HELP

How to prevent genital herpes from destroying your relationship

Genital herpes can cause long-term problems in a sexual relationship. Your herpes-free partner always runs the risk of acquiring the disease through sexual intercourse. You may feel like hiding your condition from your partner or hesitate to initiate a relationship.

Guidelines for decreasing the risk of transmission

Avoid having sexual intercourse from the time symptoms first occur until 10 days after the lesions heal. Although herpes can be transmitted at any time, transmission occurs less frequently during symptom-free periods.

Understand that the use of condoms doesn't guarantee protection against herpes, but it does decrease the risk.

A tough topic: Talking about herpes

If you're in a relationship, approach your partner with honesty, but avoid shocking revelations like "I have something terrible to tell you." Instead, broach the subject of herpes with discretion at a convenient time. Use neutral words and terms. For instance, think of herpes as "an infection that comes and goes" rather than "incurable."

What are the normal results?

Normally, herpes simplex virus doesn't appear in specimens from people with healthy immune systems who show no outward signs of the disease.

What do abnormal results mean?

Isolation of the virus from local lesions helps to confirm a diagnosis of herpes virus infection.

If you're diagnosed with genital herpes, you should seek medical advice about treatment and informing sexual partners. (See *How to prevent genital herpes from destroying your relationship*.)

CULTURE FOR CHLAMYDIA

The most common sexually transmitted disease in North America is caused by a protozoan called *Chlamydia trachomatis*. This parasite is identified in the lab by culturing in cells susceptible to the infection. After the culture's incubated, the lab can detect *Chlamydia*-infected cells by looking for antibodies or by iodine staining.

Why is this test done?

This culture is performed to confirm infections caused by the organism *Chlamydia trachomatis.*

What should you know before the test?

- The nurse will describe the procedure for collecting a specimen for culture, which varies depending on the site of infection.
- If the specimen is to be collected from your genital tract, you'll be instructed not to urinate for 3 to 4 hours before the specimen is taken.

What happens during the test?

- The examiner obtains a specimen from the infected site. In adults, these sites may include the eye, urethra (not the pus-filled discharge), endocervix, or rectum.
- For a man, the examiner may obtain a urethral specimen with a cotton-tipped applicator. For a woman, the examiner may collect a specimen from the endocervix using a swab or brush.
- You're advised to avoid all sexual contact until after test results are available.

What are the normal results?

Normally, *Chlamydia trachomatis* does not appear in the culture.

What do abnormal results mean?

A positive culture confirms *Chlamydia trachomatis* infection. If you're diagnosed with chlamydia, you should seek medical advice about treatment and inform any sexual partners about your infection.

16

FLUID ANALYSIS:
Evaluating the Body's Other Liquids

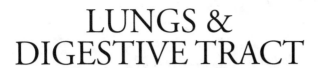

LUNGS & DIGESTIVE TRACT

LUNG PARASITES

This test is used to check your sputum or phlegm for parasites or their eggs that might be living in your lungs. Lung parasite infestation is rare in North America, but if the doctor suspects you've been exposed, he or she will look for parasites such as hookworms. The specimen is obtained by coughing and spitting or by suctioning of the windpipe.

Why is this test done?
The sputum may be examined to identify parasites in your lungs.

What should you know before the test?
- The test requires a sputum specimen or, if necessary, suctioning of the windpipe.
- Early morning collection is preferred because secretions accumulate overnight.
- You can help sputum production by drinking fluids the night before collection.

What happens during the test?
You're asked to spit by taking three deep breaths and forcing a deep cough. The sputum you produce is put into a container and sent to a lab.

If you have suctioning
- If suctioning of your windpipe is required to provide a sample, you'll feel some short-term discomfort from the catheter.
- The doctor or nurse passes a catheter through your nostril, without using suction. You cough when the catheter passes into your voice box.
- The nurse applies suction for 5 or 10 seconds — no longer than 15 seconds — and then removes the catheter and sends the sample to the lab.

What are the normal results?

Normally, no parasites or eggs are found.

What do abnormal results mean?

The doctor can match the parasite to the type of lung infection you have. The parasite, in its adult state, may also cause an intestinal infection. Examples of parasites that may be found include *Entamoeba histolytica* (amebiasis), *Ascaris lumbricoides* (roundworm), *Echinococcus granulosus, Strongyloides stercoralis* (threadworm), *Paragonimus westermani* (lung fluke), or *Necator americanus* (hookworm).

LUNG FLUID

This test, which doctors call *pleural fluid analysis*, is used to check the space around your lungs for excess fluid. The pleura, a two-layer membrane that covers the lungs and lines the chest cavity, keeps a little lubricating fluid between its layers to minimize friction when you breathe. Increased fluid in this space may be caused by diseases such as cancer or tuberculosis or from blood or lymphatic disorders. Too much of it can cause difficult breathing. (See *The pleura: Protecting your lungs*.)

Why is this test done?

Pleural fluid analysis may be performed to find the cause and nature of excess liquid around the lungs.

What should you know before the test?

- You won't need to change your diet before the test.
- The doctor may use chest X-rays or ultrasound before the test to help locate the fluid.
- You'll be given a local anesthetic before the test; you may feel a stinging sensation when it's injected.
- You'll be asked not to cough, breathe deeply, or move during the test to minimize the risk of injury to the lung.
- The nurse may shave the area around the needle insertion site.

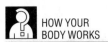

HOW YOUR
BODY WORKS

The pleura: Protecting your lungs

If your doctor has ordered a pleural fluid analysis, understanding the function of pleura (the sacs that surround the lungs) may help you prepare for this test.

The pleural layers protect your lungs. The outer *parietal pleura* lines the inside of the chest. The inner *visceral pleura* envelops the lung itself. Between the parietal pleura and the visceral pleura, the *pleural space* contains a thin film of fluid. This lubricates the pleural surfaces and prevents friction between the layers when they expand as you inhale.

Where the breath goes

You breathe through hollow tubes in the lungs. Beginning at your mouth, the largest tube, called the *trachea* (windpipe) leads to hollow tubes called *bronchi*, which resemble tree branches. These gradually become smaller, until each bronchus eventually branches into *bronchioles* and finally terminates in clusters of air sacs. In these tiny air sacs, called alveoli, the exchange of oxygen and carbon dioxide takes place.

Any disorder of the pleura interferes with smooth and efficient gas exchange, thus hindering respiration.

LEFT LUNG

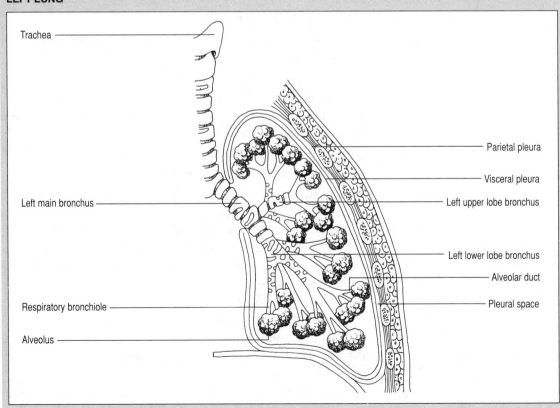

Trachea

Left main bronchus

Respiratory bronchiole

Alveolus

Parietal pleura

Visceral pleura

Left upper lobe bronchus

Left lower lobe bronchus

Alveolar duct

Pleural space

What happens during the test?

- A nurse or medical technician asks you to sit at the edge of the bed with a chair or stool supporting your feet and your head and arms resting on a padded overbed table. If you can't sit up, you may be positioned on your side with your arm above your head.
- The nurse reminds you not to cough, breathe deeply, or move suddenly during the procedure.
- During thoracentesis (pleural fluid aspiration), the doctor punctures the chest wall with a large needle and withdraws a specimen of pleural fluid for analysis or draws off liquid through the needle to relieve lung compression and breathing problems.
- You may feel some pressure during withdrawal of the fluid.
- After the needle is removed, the nurse applies light pressure and a small adhesive bandage to the puncture site.
- You must remain on your side for at least 1 hour to seal the puncture site; notify the nurse if you have trouble breathing.

The doctor draws off lung fluid for analysis or to relieve lung compression and breathing problems.

Does the test have risks?

This procedure isn't used for people who have histories of bleeding disorders.

What are the normal results?

Normally, the pleural cavity maintains negative pressure and contains less than 20 milliliters of fluid.

What do abnormal results mean?

Too much fluid is caused by the abnormal formation or reabsorption of pleural fluid. Certain characteristics classify pleural fluid as either a transudate (a low-protein fluid that's leaked from normal blood vessels) or an exudate (a protein-rich fluid that's leaked from blood vessels with increased permeability). Pleural fluid may contain blood, chyle, or pus and dead tissue.

The doctor will analyze the fluids to determine the cause, which may include high blood pressure, congestive heart failure, cirrhosis of the liver, nephritis, lymphatic drainage interference, infections, lung damage, rheumatoid arthritis, complications of pneumonia, cancer, and a variety of infections.

Cultures of pleural fluid may reveal bacteria or other pathogens.

STOMACH ACID SECRETION TEST

This procedure, which doctors call the *basal gastric secretion test*, is used to measure your stomach's secretion of acid. The test is done while you fast by withdrawing some stomach contents through a tube running from your nose to your stomach.

The doctor may perform this test if you have obscure stomach pain, loss of appetite, and weight loss. Because certain factors around you — such as the sight or odor of food — and psychological stress stimulate stomach acid secretion, accurate testing requires that you be relaxed and isolated from all sources of sensory stimulation. Although abnormal stomach acid secretion can suggest various stomach and duodenal disorders, the doctor may follow this test with the stomach acid stimulation test to obtain a complete evaluation.

Why is this test done?

The stomach acid secretion test may be performed to determine the output of stomach acid that occurs while you're fasting.

What should you know before the test?

- You'll fast for 12 hours and restrict fluids and smoking for 8 hours before the test.
- The procedure takes approximately 1½ hours (or 2½ hours, if followed by the stomach acid stimulation test).
- If you're using antacids or other medications, they may be stopped for 24 hours before the test.
- The nurse will check your pulse rate and blood pressure just before the test. Then you'll be encouraged to relax.

What happens during the test?

- While you're seated, a nurse inserts a tube through your nose and into your stomach. You may initially feel discomfort and may cough or gag.
- The tube is attached to a large syringe used to withdraw your stomach contents.
- To ensure complete emptying of the stomach, you assume three positions in sequence — on your back, and then on your right and left sides — while the stomach contents are withdrawn.

- The tube from your nose to your stomach is connected to a suction machine that applies continuous low suction. The suction can also be performed manually with a syringe.

What happens after the test?

You can resume your usual diet and any medications that were withheld before the test, unless the stomach acid stimulation test will also be performed.

What are the normal results?

Normally, basal secretion ranges from 0.2 to 3.8 milliequivalents per hour in women and 1 to 5 milliequivalents per hour in men.

What do abnormal results mean?

Abnormal results don't provide specific enough information to make a diagnosis and the doctor will consider them with the results of the stomach acid stimulation test. A high rate of secretion may suggest an intestinal ulcer or, if it's very high, a condition called *Zollinger-Ellison syndrome*. A low amount of secretion may indicate stomach cancer or a benign stomach ulcer. Absence of secretion may indicate pernicious anemia.

The stomach acid secretion test goes hand-in-hand with the stomach acid stimulation test.

STOMACH ACID STIMULATION TEST

This test, which doctors call the *gastric acid stimulation test*, is used to find out if the stomach is secreting acid properly. It measures the secretion of stomach acid for 1 hour after you receive an injection of pentagastrin or a similar drug that stimulates stomach acid output. The doctor uses this test when the stomach acid secretion test suggests a problem. The stomach acid stimulation test is commonly performed immediately afterward. Although this test can detect abnormal stomach acid secretion, X-ray studies and endoscopy are necessary to determine the cause of such secretions.

Why is this test done?

The stomach acid stimulation test may be performed to help the doctor diagnose a duodenal ulcer, Zollinger-Ellison syndrome, pernicious anemia, and stomach cancer.

What should you know before the test?

- You'll be told not to eat, drink, or smoke after midnight before the test.
- If you're taking antacids or some other drugs, they may be stopped.

What happens during the test?

- The test takes 1 hour.
- The test may cause discomfort, such as abdominal pain, nausea, vomiting, flushing, transitory dizziness, faintness, and numbness of extremities. You should report symptoms immediately.
- After stomach acid secretions are collected for the stomach acid secretion test, the tube from your nose to your stomach remains in place.
- You'll receive an injection of pentagastrin. After 15 minutes, the examiner collects a specimen of stomach acid secretions from the tube every 15 minutes for 1 hour.

What happens after the test?

You may resume your usual diet and any medications withheld for the test.

What are the normal results?

Following stimulation, stomach acid secretion ranges from 11 to 21 milliequivalents per hour for women and 18 to 28 milliequivalents per hour for men.

What do abnormal results mean?

A high level of stomach acid secretion may indicate a duodenal ulcer; an extremely high level suggests Zollinger-Ellison syndrome. A low level of secretion may indicate stomach cancer; an absence of hydrochloric acid, which is normally found in secretions, may indicate pernicious anemia.

ABDOMINAL FLUID

This procedure, which doctors call *peritoneal fluid analysis*, is used to determine the cause of excess fluids in the abdomen or to detect abdominal injury. A sample of peritoneal fluid is withdrawn by a procedure called *paracentesis*. Peritoneal fluid is drawn from the peritoneum, a membrane sac that lines the abdominal and pelvic wall.

Why is this test done?

The analysis of peritoneal fluid may be performed for the following reasons:
- To determine the cause of fluid-filled sacs in the abdomen
- To detect abdominal injury.

What should you know before the test?

- You won't need to change your diet before the test.
- The test requires a peritoneal fluid sample. You'll receive a local anesthetic to make you comfortable; the procedure takes about 45 minutes.
- If you have severe pressure in your abdomen, the procedure will relieve your discomfort and allow you to breathe more easily.
- You should void any urine just before the test. This helps prevent accidental bladder injury during needle insertion.

What happens during the test?

- You sit on a bed or in a chair with your feet flat on the floor and your back well supported.
- You're draped to keep you from chilling.
- You're given a local anesthetic; you may feel a stinging sensation when it's injected.
- This procedure requires inserting a trocar (a sharp stylet inside a tube) through the abdominal wall after administration of the local anesthetic. If the fluid is being removed to provide relief, the trocar may be connected to a drainage system. However, if only a small amount of fluid is needed for a diagnosis, the test may be done with a needle.
- You may feel some pressure during withdrawal of the fluid.

This procedure is sometimes used to remove excess fluid from the abdominal cavity.

Does the test have risks?

The test must be performed very cautiously with pregnant women and people with bleeding tendencies or unstable vital signs.

What are the normal results?

Normally, the peritoneal fluid is sterile, odorless, and clear to pale yellow in color.

What do abnormal results mean?

The following are some of the abnormalities and the disorders they suggest:

- Milk-colored peritoneal fluid may be caused by fluid from a damaged thoracic duct, suggesting cancers, tuberculosis, parasitic infection, or liver cirrhosis.
- Cloudy or turbid fluid may indicate peritonitis due to primary bacterial infection, ruptured bowel (after injury), pancreatitis, strangulated intestine, or appendicitis.
- Bloody fluid may result from a benign or malignant tumor, hemorrhagic pancreatitis, or damage incurred during the test.
- Bile-stained, green fluid may indicate a ruptured gallbladder, acute pancreatitis, or perforated intestine or duodenal ulcer.

Lab tests on any red blood cells, protein, hormones, or even fungi found in the fluid will point to other possible disorders.

PARASITES IN THE DIGESTIVE TRACT

This procedure, which doctors call the *test for duodenal parasites*, is used to diagnose parasitic infection of the digestive tract by investigating duodenal contents. It's performed by passing a tube from the person's nose into the duodenum (top of the small intestine) or by using an Entero capsule to withdraw a specimen.

Why is this test done?

The test for duodenal parasites may be performed when the person has symptoms of parasitic infection but stool examinations are negative.

Intestinal parasites may include viruses, bacteria, fungi, single-celled amoeba, or several types of worms.

What should you know before the test?

- You'll restrict food and fluids for 12 hours before the test.
- A doctor or nurse will collect the specimen by putting a tube into your nose and stomach or by using a weighted gelatine capsule with a string attached.
- If the test is to be done with a tube through your nose, be aware that you may gag during the tube's passage. Following the examiner's instructions about positioning, breathing, and swallowing will minimize discomfort.
- You'll be told to empty your bladder just before the procedure.

What happens during the test?

Tube insertion

- After the tube is inserted, you lie on your left side, with your feet elevated, to allow your stomach's action to move the tube into the duodenum.
- Fluoroscopy may be used to confirm that the tube is in position and suction can start.

Entero capsule and string

- The doctor tapes the free end of the string to your cheek.
- You swallow the gelatin capsule with water.
- The string remains in place for 4 hours and then is pulled out gently and placed in a sterile container.

What happens after the test?

You can resume your normal diet.

Does the test have risks?

The test won't be given if you're a pregnant woman or have any of the following conditions: acute cholecystitis; acute pancreatitis; esophageal varices, stenosis, diverticula, or malignant cancers; recent, severe stomach hemorrhage; aortic aneurysm; or congestive heart failure.

What are the normal results?

Normally, no eggs or parasites appear.

What do abnormal results mean?

Diagnosis depends upon the type of parasite found. Finding *Giardia lamblia* indicates giardiasis, possibly causing malabsorption syndrome; *Strongyloides stercoralis* suggests strongyloidiasis; *Ancylostoma duodenale* and *Necator americanus* imply hookworm disease. Infestation of the bile ducts by liver flukes, such as *Clonorchis sinensis* and *Fasciola hepatica,* are rare in North America.

BLOOD IN FECES

This test, which doctors call the *fecal occult blood test,* is used to detect abnormal gastrointestinal bleeding. Fecal occult blood is detected by microscopic analysis or by chemical tests for hemoglobin. Normally, feces contain small amounts of blood (2 to 2.5 milliliters per day), so the test is for larger quantities. Additional tests are required to pinpoint the origin of the bleeding. (See *Common sites and causes of gastrointestinal blood loss,* page 650.)

Why is this test done?

The fecal occult blood test may be performed for the following reasons:
- To detect gastrointestinal bleeding
- To aid an early diagnosis of colorectal cancer.

What should you know before the test?

- You'll be told to maintain a high-fiber diet and to refrain from eating red meats, poultry, fish, turnips, and horseradish for 48 to 72 hours before the test as well as throughout the collection period.
- The test requires collection of three stool specimens. Occasionally, only a random specimen is collected.
- If you're taking certain medications, they may be stopped for 48 hours before and during the test.

What happens during the test?

- You collect three stool specimens or a random specimen, using a tongue depressor or a small applicator.
- You should be careful not to contaminate the specimen with urine or toilet paper.
- A lab technician or the nurse tests the specimen.

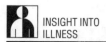

INSIGHT INTO
ILLNESS

Common sites and causes of gastrointestinal blood loss

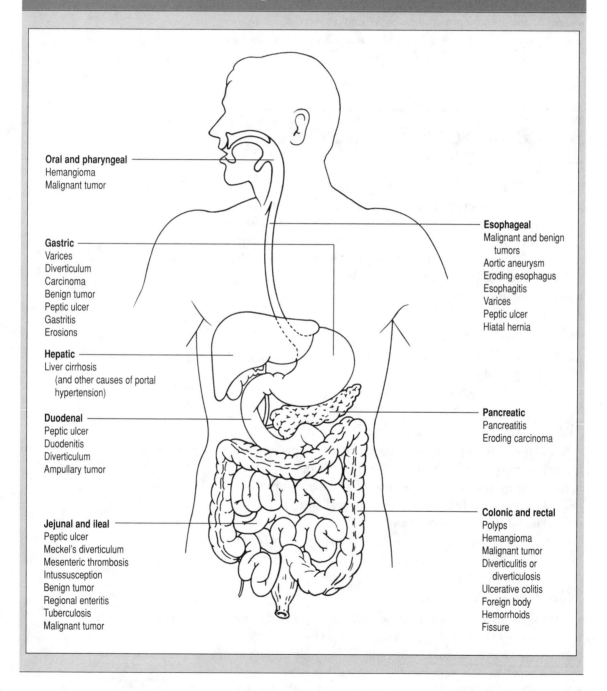

Oral and pharyngeal
Hemangioma
Malignant tumor

Esophageal
Malignant and benign
    tumors
Aortic aneurysm
Eroding esophagus
Esophagitis
Varices
Peptic ulcer
Hiatal hernia

Gastric
Varices
Diverticulum
Carcinoma
Benign tumor
Peptic ulcer
Gastritis
Erosions

Hepatic
Liver cirrhosis
    (and other causes of portal
    hypertension)

Pancreatic
Pancreatitis
Eroding carcinoma

Duodenal
Peptic ulcer
Duodenitis
Diverticulum
Ampullary tumor

Colonic and rectal
Polyps
Hemangioma
Malignant tumor
Diverticulitis or
    diverticulosis
Ulcerative colitis
Foreign body
Hemorrhoids
Fissure

Jejunal and ileal
Peptic ulcer
Meckel's diverticulum
Mesenteric thrombosis
Intussusception
Benign tumor
Regional enteritis
Tuberculosis
Malignant tumor

What happens after the test?

After the test you can resume your usual diet and medication schedule.

What are the normal results?

Normally, less than 2.5 milliliters of blood are found.

What do abnormal results mean?

Too much blood in the feces indicates gastrointestinal bleeding, which may be caused by many disorders, such as varices, peptic ulcer, cancer, ulcerative colitis, dysentery, or hemorrhagic disease. This test is particularly important for early diagnosis of colorectal cancer. Further tests, such as barium swallow, analyses of stomach contents, and endoscopic procedures, are necessary to define the site and extent of bleeding.

FATS IN FECES

This test, which doctors call the *fecal lipids test*, is used to evaluate your digestion of fats. When bile and pancreas secretions are adequate, dietary fats are almost completely absorbed in the small intestine. When they aren't, this procedure is used to extract unabsorbed fat from the feces and weigh it to evaluate the problem.

Why is this test done?

The fecal lipids test may be performed to confirm steatorrhea (excessive fat in the feces) and to investigate signs of poor absorption in the digestive tract, such as weight loss, abdominal distention, and scaly skin.

What should you know before the test?

- You'll be told not to drink alcohol and to maintain a high-fat diet (3.5 ounces [100 grams] per day) for 3 days before the test and during the collection period.
- The test requires a 72-hour stool collection.
- If you're taking medications that could affect the test results, they may be stopped.
- The nurse will teach you how to do a timed, 72-hour stool collection.
- The lab requires 1 or 2 days to complete the analysis.

What happens during the test?

- You collect stool specimens over a 72-hour period, using depressors or a commercially available kit with instructions.
- Be sure to avoid contaminating the stool specimens with toilet tissue or urine.

What happens after the test?

You may resume your usual diet and any medications withheld before the test.

What are the normal results?

Fecal fats normally comprise less than 20% of excreted solids, with excretion of less than 7 grams per 24 hours.

What do abnormal results mean?

Both digestive and absorptive disorders cause excessive fat in the feces. Digestive disorders may affect the production and release of pancreatic lipase or bile. Absorptive disorders may affect the integrity of the intestine. Investigating these disorders may lead the doctor to consider a long list of potential problems with the pancreas, liver, intestines, and lymph glands.

Symptoms that may prompt a doctor to order this test include weight loss, abdominal distention, and scaly skin.

STOOL TEST FOR INTESTINAL PARASITES

This test is used to look for intestinal parasitic infection. Examination of a stool specimen can reveal several types of intestinal parasites or their eggs. Some of these parasites are harmless. Others cause intestinal disease.

In North America, the most common parasites include the roundworms *Ascaris lumbricoides* and *Necator americanus* (hookworms); the pinworm *Enterobius follicularis;* the tapeworms *Diphyllobothrium latum, Taenia saginata*, and *T. solium* (rare); the amoeba *Entamoeba histolytica;* and the flagellate *Giardia lamblia.*

Why is this test done?

The examination of stool specimens is done to confirm or rule out intestinal parasitic infection and disease.

What should you know before the test?

- You'll be told to avoid treatments with castor or mineral oil, bismuth, magnesium or antidiarrheal compounds, barium enemas, and antibiotics for 7 to 10 days before the test.
- The test requires three stool specimens — one every other day or every third day. Up to six specimens may be required to confirm the presence of *Entamoeba histolytica*.
- If you have diarrhea, the nurse will ask about your recent dietary and travel history. The nurse will also ask about other drugs that might influence the test and whether you've taken them within the past 2 weeks.
- The nurse will teach you how to collect and store the specimens.

What happens during the test?

- Collect the specimen with a tongue depressor or a commercially available kit.
- Be careful not to contaminate the specimen with toilet paper or urine. Don't collect a specimen from the toilet bowl. Any contamination can kill the parasites and invalidate the test.
- If you're bedridden, the nurse collects the specimen in a bedpan and transfers it to a special container. (See *Checking for pinworms*.)

What are the normal results?

Normally, no parasites or eggs appear in stools.

What do abnormal results mean?

The presence of parasites confirms the suspected disorders and may lead to more tests.

Since injury to the person is difficult to detect — even when a worm's eggs or larvae appear — the number of worms usually correlates with the person's clinical symptoms. The information is used to distinguish between worm infestation and worm-caused diseases.

Parasites may be causing damage in other parts of the body. For example, the roundworm *Ascaris* may perforate the bowel wall, causing peritonitis, or may migrate to the lungs, causing pneumonia. Hookworms can cause a form of anemia due to bloodsucking and hemorrhage, especially in people with iron-deficient diets. The tapeworm *D. latum* may cause a form of anemia by removing vitamin B_{12}.

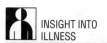 INSIGHT INTO ILLNESS

Checking for pinworms

The eggs of the pinworm seldom appear in feces because the female migrates to the person's anus and deposits her eggs there. To collect the eggs, the nurse places a piece of cellophane tape, sticky side out, on the end of a tongue depressor and presses it firmly to the anal area.

When eggs are found

The tape is transferred, sticky side down, to a slide. Since the female pinworm usually deposits her eggs at night, the best time to collect the specimen is early in the morning, before the person bathes or defecates.

INFECTIOUS DIARRHEA VIRUS

This procedure involves the examination of a stool sample for antigens to the rotavirus. This virus is the most frequent cause of infectious diarrhea in infants and young children. They're most prevalent in children ages 3 months to 2 years during the winter. Rotavirus causes diarrhea, vomiting, fever, and abdominal pain. Symptoms of infection may range from mild in adults to severe in young children, especially hospitalized infants.

Because human rotaviruses do not multiply well in lab cell cultures, a quick test with a sensitive, specific enzyme may be needed to catch them.

Why is this test done?
This stool examination is done to obtain a lab diagnosis of rotavirus gastroenteritis.

What should you know before the test?
- The test requires a stool specimen.
- If possible, collect the specimens when the disease is first suspected or during the acute stage of the infection to ensure detection of the viral antigens.

What happens during the test?
- Usually, a nurse or medical technician collects a 1-gram stool specimen in a screw-capped tube or vial. If a microbiological transport swab is used, it must be heavily stained with feces to detect the rotavirus.
- The child or adult being tested should be given extra fluids to avoid dehydration caused by vomiting and diarrhea.

What are the normal results?
Normally, there are no rotaviruses in stools.

What do abnormal results mean?
The detection of rotavirus by enzyme immunoassay indicates a current infection with the organism. The severity of disease is generally

greater in young children than in adults. Rotavirus infections are easily transmitted in group settings such as nursing homes, preschools, and day-care centers. Transmission is presumed to occur from person-to-person by the fecal-oral route — making hand washing the best defense.

REPRODUCTIVE SYSTEM

CHROMOSOME ANALYSIS

Chromosome analysis is done to study the relationship between the microscopic appearance of chromosomes and an individual's phenotype — the expression of the genes in physical, biochemical, or physiologic traits.

Ideally, chromosomes are studied during the middle phase of mitosis (cell division). Cells are harvested, stained, and then examined under a microscope. These cells are then photographed to record the karyotype — the systematic arrangement of chromosomes in groupings according to size and shape.

Only rapidly dividing cells, such as bone marrow or neoplastic cells, permit direct, immediate study. In other cells, mitosis is stimulated by the addition of phytohemagglutinin. Indications for the test determine the specimen required (blood, bone marrow, amniotic fluid, skin, or placental tissue) and the specific analytic procedure.

Why is this test done?

The chromosome analysis may be performed to identify chromosomal abnormalities as the underlying cause of malformation, irregular development, or disease.

What should you know before the test?

- The test will require a sample of your blood or a specimen of tissue, bone marrow, or amniotic fluid (to test a fetus).
- The length of time before results will be available varies according to the specimen required. For example, test results on a blood sample

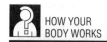

HOW YOUR BODY WORKS

Chromosomes and sex characteristics

A mammal's eggs fertilized by sperm bearing an X chromosome become females (XX), while those fertilized by sperm bearing a Y chromosome become males (XY).

The Y chromosome causes the indifferent gonad to organize testes. The testes then secrete testosterone, causing the male body type. In the absence of the Y chromosome and testosterone secretion, ovaries form, and the embryo becomes a female.

How people with female chromosomes develop testes

Occasionally, female XX embryos develop testes and become males, or male XY embryos develop ovaries and become females. Also, either type of embryo may have a combination of testicular and ovarian tissue (true hermaphroditism). It's believed that only a small portion of the Y chromosome causes testes to form. Therefore, XX persons with testes have probably conserved this critical portion of the Y chromosome, which remains active.

Reasons for chromosome studies

Listed below are common specimens used in chromosome analysis and the reasons for their use.

Blood
- To evaluate abnormal appearance or development suggesting chromosomal irregularity
- To evaluate couples with a history of miscarriages or to identify balanced translocation carriers having unbalanced offspring
- To detect chromosomal rearrangements in rare genetic diseases predisposing patient to malignant neoplasms

Blood or bone marrow
To identify Philadelphia chromosome and confirm chronic myelogenous leukemia

Skin
To evaluate abnormal appearance or development suggesting chromosomal irregularity

Amniotic fluid
To evaluate a developing fetus with possible chromosomal abnormality

Placental tissue
To evaluate products of conception after a miscarriage to determine if abnormality is fetal or placental in origin

are generally available in 72 to 96 hours. Analysis of skin biopsy specimens or amniotic fluid cells may take several weeks.

What happens during the test?
- A nurse or medical technician collects the sample, depending on the doctor's preferred method.
- If it's a blood sample, a nurse or medical technician inserts a needle into a vein, usually in your forearm. The blood sample is collected in a tube, which is then sent to a lab for testing.
- Although you may feel a sting from the needle and pressure from the tourniquet, collecting the sample takes only a few minutes.

What happens after the test?
If swelling develops at the needle puncture site, apply warm soaks.

What are the normal results?
The normal cell contains 46 chromosomes: 22 pairs of autosomes (nonsex chromosomes) and 1 pair of sex chromosomes (Y for the male-determining chromosome, X for the female-determining chromosome).

What do abnormal results mean?
Chromosome abnormalities may be in their numbers or their structures. The chromosome pairs may not have separated properly during cell division, or part of a chromosome may have broken off or traded parts to produce an unbalanced chromosome. The significance of chromosome analysis results depends on the specimen and indications for the test. (See *Chromosomes and sex characteristics*, page 655, and *Reasons for chromosome studies*.)

AMNIOCENTESIS

Amniocentesis, which doctors sometimes call *amniotic fluid analysis*, is used to detect fetal abnormalities. In this procedure, a doctor uses a needle to withdraw 10 to 20 milliliters of amniotic fluid from a pregnant woman for lab analysis.

This analysis may be used to detect certain birth defects, such as Down's syndrome or spina bifida. It can be used to find out the baby's due date and its sex and to detect diseases in the womb. It requires a level of amniotic fluid usually reached after the 16th week of pregnancy. The doctor may recommend amniocentesis if the mother is over age 35, if she's had a miscarriage, or if there's a family history of genetic, chromosomal, or neural tube defects.

Why is this test done?

Aspirating amniotic fluid may be performed for the following reasons:

- To detect fetal abnormalities, particularly chromosomal and neural tube defects
- To detect hemolytic disease of the newborn
- To diagnose metabolic disorders, amino acid disorders, and mucopolysaccharidoses
- To determine fetal age and maturity, especially lung maturity
- To assess fetal health by detecting the presence of meconium or blood or measuring amniotic levels of estriol and fetal thyroid hormone
- To identify fetal gender when one or both parents are carriers of a sex-linked disorder.

What should you know before the test?

- You won't need to change your diet before the test.
- The test requires a specimen of amniotic fluid; a nurse or doctor will perform the test.
- Normal test results can't guarantee a normal fetus because some fetal disorders are undetectable.
- You'll be asked to sign a consent form.
- You'll feel a stinging sensation when the local anesthetic is injected.
- You should empty your bladder just before the test to minimize the risk of puncturing the bladder and aspirating urine instead of amniotic fluid.

What happens during the test?

- The doctor locates a pool of amniotic fluid after finding the fetus and placental position, usually through palpation and ultrasound.
- Your skin is prepared with antiseptic and alcohol; then the anesthetic is injected.
- The doctor inserts a needle with a stylet into the amniotic cavity.

How the doctor aspirates amniotic fluid

After the doctor knows the position of the placenta and fetus, the aspirating needle is inserted through the abdominal wall at a right angle.

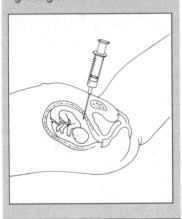

- A 10-milliliter syringe is attached to the needle; then the fluid is aspirated and placed in a test tube.
- The needle is withdrawn, and an adhesive bandage is placed over the needle insertion site.

What happens after the test?
- The doctor will monitor the fetal heart rate and your vital signs.
- The doctor will tell you to report any abdominal pain or cramping, chills, fever, vaginal bleeding or leakage of vaginal fluid, or unusually high or low fetal activity immediately.

Does the test have risks?
Although side effects are rare, there's a small chance of miscarriage, injury to the fetus or placenta, bleeding, premature labor, infection, and Rh sensitization from fetal bleeding into the mother's circulation. Due to the severity of possible complications, amniocentesis isn't used as a general screening test. (See *How the doctor aspirates amniotic fluid.*)

Another method of detecting fetal chromosomal and biochemical disorders in early pregnancy is chorionic villi sampling. (See *Answers to questions about chorionic villi sampling.*)

What are the normal results?
Normal amniotic fluid is clear, but may contain white flecks of a material called *vernix caseosa* when the fetus is near term.

What do abnormal results mean?
Blood in amniotic fluid is usually the mother's and doesn't indicate an abnormality. However, it does inhibit cell growth and crowd out other constituents. The other matter that's found in the fluid includes the following, along with their indications:
- Large amounts of bilirubin, a byproduct of red blood cell breakdown, may indicate hemolytic disease of the newborn.
- Meconium, found in the fetal gastrointestinal tract, passes into the amniotic fluid when low oxygen causes fetal distress and relaxation of the anal sphincter.
- Creatinine, a product of fetal urine, increases in the amniotic fluid as the fetal kidneys mature.
- Alpha-fetoprotein is produced first in the yolk sac and later in the liver and gastrointestinal tract. High levels indicate neural tube defects, but the alpha-fetoprotein levels may remain normal if the de-

STRAIGHT
TALK

Answers to questions about chorionic villi sampling

What is chorionic villi sampling?
Chorionic villi sampling, or biopsy, is a prenatal test for quick detection of fetal disorders that's done in the first trimester (3 months) of pregnancy.

What are chorionic villi?
The chorionic villi are fingerlike projections that surround the embryonic membrane and eventually form the placenta. Cells are fetal rather than maternal, so they can be checked for fetal abnormalities.

What are the benefits of this test?
Preliminary results may be available within hours; complete results within a few days. In contrast, amniocentesis cannot be performed before the 16th week of pregnancy, and the results aren't available for at least 2 weeks. Thus, chorionic villi sampling can detect fetal abnormalities as much as 10 weeks sooner than amniocentesis.

Chorionic villi sampling can be used to detect about 200 diseases prenatally. For example, direct analysis of rapidly dividing fetal cells can detect chromosome disorders. DNA analysis can detect blood disorders and lysomal enzyme assays can screen for lysosomal storage disorders such as Tay-Sachs disease.

When should it be performed?
Samples are best obtained between the 8th and 10th weeks of pregnancy — when the fetus has grown large enough to make the procedure less difficult. After the 10th week, it may be more dangerous.

What is the downside?
The test is reliable unless the sample contains too few cells or the cells fail to grow in the culture. The mother's risks for this procedure appear to be similar to those for amniocentesis — a small chance of miscarriage, cramps, infection, and bleeding. However, recent research reports an incidence of limb malformations in newborns when chorionic villi sampling has been performed.

Unlike amniocentesis, chorionic villi sampling can't detect complications in cases of Rh sensitization, uncover neural tube defects, or determine pulmonary maturity. However, it may prove to be the best way to detect other serious fetal abnormalities early in pregnancy.

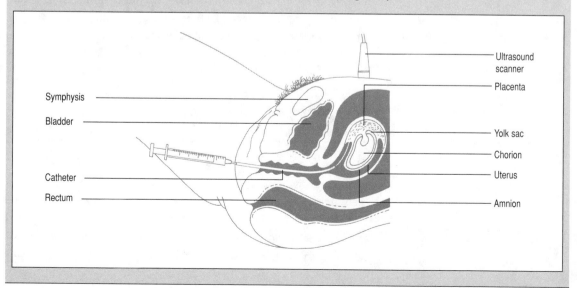

fect is small and closed. Elevated alpha-fetoprotein levels may occur in multiple pregnancy and in a number of serious disorders.

■ The amount of uric acid in the amniotic fluid increases as the fetus matures, but these levels fluctuate widely and can't accurately predict maturity.

■ Estrone, estradiol, estriol, and estriol conjugates appear in amniotic fluid in varying amounts. Severe erythroblastosis fetalis decreases the estriol level.

■ Blood in the amniotic fluid (in about 10% of people tested) is caused by a faulty tap. If the origin is the mother's, the blood generally has no special significance. However, "portwine" fluid may be a sign of a damaged placenta, while blood of fetal origin may indicate damage to the fetal, placental, or umbilical cord vessels by the amniocentesis needle.

■ The Type II cells lining the fetal alveoli (air sacs) in the lungs produce lecithin slowly in early pregnancy and then markedly increase production around the 35th week.

■ The sphingomyelin level helps confirm fetal pulmonary maturity or suggests a risk of respiratory distress.

■ Measuring sugar levels in the fluid can aid in assessing blood sugar control in the diabetic person.

■ Insulin levels increase sharply (up to 27 times normal) in a person with poorly controlled diabetes.

■ Lab analysis can identify at least 25 different enzymes (usually in low concentrations) in amniotic fluid, but they don't explain much.

■ When the mother carries an X-linked disorder, determination of fetal sex is important. If chromosome karyotyping identifies a male fetus, there's a 50% chance he'll be affected; a female fetus won't be affected but has a 50% chance of being a carrier.

If blood in amniotic fluid is the mother's, it doesn't usually indicate an abnormality.

PAP TEST

The Papanicolaou (Pap) test allows for the study of cervical cells. It's a widely known test for early detection of cervical cancer. A doctor or specially trained nurse scrapes secretions from the patient's cervix and spreads them on a slide, which is sent to the lab for analysis. The test relies on the shedding of malignant cells from the cervix and shows cell maturity, metabolic activity, and structure variations.

If a Pap test is positive or suggests malignancy, a cervical biopsy (removal and analysis of tissue) can confirm the diagnosis. The test is an important aid to the detection of cancer at a stage when the disease is often without symptoms and still curable. (See *How a Pap test is done,* page 662.)

Why is this test done?

The Pap test may be done for the following reasons:
- To detect malignant cells
- To detect inflammatory tissue changes
- To assess response to chemotherapy and radiation therapy
- To detect viral, fungal and, occasionally, parasitic invasion.

What should you know before the test?

- If you're menstruating, the test will be rescheduled. The best time to have it done is midcycle.
- You'll be told not to douche or insert vaginal medications for 24 hours before the test because doing so can wash away cellular deposits and change the vaginal pH.
- The procedure takes 5 to 10 minutes or slightly longer if the vagina, pelvic cavity, and rectum are examined too.
- The nurse or doctor will ask about your most recent Pap test, your menstrual periods, what sort of birth control you might be using, and other questions that might influence interpretation of the test results.
- The test results should be available within a few days.
- You'll be asked to empty your bladder just before the test.

What happens during the test?

- You undress from the waist down and drape yourself.
- You lie on the examining table and place your heels in the stirrups. (You may be more comfortable if you keep your shoes on.) You slide your buttocks to the edge of the table.
- The examiner puts on gloves and inserts an unlubricated speculum into your vagina. To make insertion easier, the speculum may be moistened with saline solution or warm water.
- After the cervix is located, the examiner collects secretions from the cervix and material from the endocervical canal with a saline-moistened cotton-tipped swab or wooden spatula.

How a Pap test is done

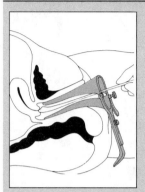 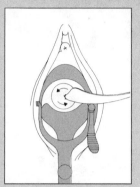 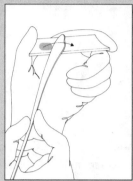 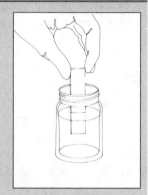

1 An unlubricated speculum is inserted into the vagina. To make insertion easier and more comfortable, the speculum is held under warm running water before insertion.

2 The cervix is exposed by opening the speculum blades. A saline-moistened Pap stick is inserted through the speculum and secretions are scraped from the cervical canal.

3 The specimen is spread on a slide.

4 Immediately, the slide is placed in a fixative solution, or sprayed with a commercial fixative.

What are the normal results?

Normally, no malignant cells or other abnormalities are present.

What do abnormal results mean?

Usually, malignant cells have relatively large nuclei and only small amounts of cytoplasm. They show abnormal nuclear chromatin patterns and marked variation in size, shape, and staining properties and may have prominent nucleoli. The results are reported in four grades of cells from normal to conclusively malignant. To confirm a suggestive or positive cytology report, the test may be repeated or followed by a biopsy.

SEMEN ANALYSIS

Semen analysis is a simple, inexpensive, and reasonably definitive test that's used in a broad range of applications. Analysis can check a man's fertility by measuring the volume of his semen, counting sperm, and examining sperm cells under a microscope. Motility and appearance are studied microscopically after staining a drop of semen.

If analysis detects an abnormality, additional tests (for example, liver, thyroid, pituitary, or adrenal function tests) may be performed. Significant abnormalities — such as greatly decreased sperm count or motility, or marked increase in abnormal forms — may require a testicular biopsy (removal and analysis of tissue).

Why is this test done?

Semen analysis may be performed for the following reasons:

- To evaluate male fertility in an infertile couple
- To prove the effectiveness of vasectomy
- To detect semen on the body or clothing of a suspected rape victim or elsewhere at the crime scene. (See *Semen identification: A tool for investigating crime*, page 664)
- To identify blood group substances to exonerate or incriminate a criminal suspect
- To rule out paternity on grounds of complete sterility.

What happens before and during the test?

Evaluation of fertility in men

- The doctor or nurse will give you written instructions and suggest that the most useful semen specimen requires masturbation, ideally in a doctor's office or a lab.
- You'll need to follow the instructions given you about avoiding sex before the test because this may increase your sperm count. Some doctors specify a fixed number of days, usually between 2 and 5. Others advise a period of continence equal to the usual interval between episodes of sexual intercourse.
- If you prefer to collect the specimen at home, you must deliver it to the lab within 3 hours after collection. Don't expose the specimen to extreme temperatures or to direct sunlight (which can also increase its temperature). Ideally, the specimen should remain at body temperature until liquefaction is complete (about 20 minutes). To deliver a semen specimen to the lab during cold weather, carry the specimen in an inside pocket.
- Alternatives to collection by masturbation include coitus interruptus or the use of a condom. For collection by coitus interruptus, you should withdraw immediately before ejaculation, and deposit the se-

Semen identification: A tool for investigating crime

Sperm cells (or their fragments) can live in the vagina for more than 72 hours after sexual intercourse. This allows detection and positive identification of semen from vaginal smears or from stains on clothing, other fabrics, skin, or hair. Identification is often necessary for legal purposes, usually in connection with rape or homicide investigations. Sperm taken from the vagina of an exhumed body that has been properly embalmed and remains reasonably intact can also be identified.

Gathering the evidence

To decide which stains or fluids require further investigation, clothing or other fabrics can be scanned with ultraviolet light to detect the typical green-white fluorescence of semen. Semen and sperm can be collected by soaking samples of clothing, fabric, or hair in saline solution. Suspect deposits

of dried semen can be gently sponged from the victim's skin.

How forensic scientists identify semen

The two most common tests to identify semen are acid phosphatase concentration (the more sensitive test) and microscopic examination for the presence of sperm. Acid phosphatase appears in semen in significantly greater concentrations than in any other body fluid. In microscopic examination, sperm cells or their head fragments can be identified on stained smears prepared directly from vaginal scrapings or aspirates, or from the concentrated sediment of material rinsed from clothing or the vagina.

Semen analysis can demonstrate that the semen of a suspect in a rape or homicide investigation is different from or consistent with semen found in or on the victim's body.

men in a specimen container. For collection by condom, first wash the condom with soap and water, rinse it thoroughly, and allow it to dry completely. (Powders or lubricants applied to the condom may be spermicidal.) After collection, tie the condom, place it in a glass jar, and promptly deliver it to the lab.

Evaluation of fertility in women

• Fertility may also be determined by collecting semen from the woman after intercourse. This method measures the sperm's ability to penetrate the cervical mucus and remain active.

• For the postcoital cervical mucus test, you report for examination during the ovulatory phase of your menstrual cycle, as determined by basal temperature records, and as soon as possible after sexual intercourse (within 8 hours).

• You're put in the same position as for a Pap smear and the doctor inserts a speculum into your vagina to collect the specimen. You may feel some pressure but no pain during this procedure, which takes only a few minutes.

Semen collection from a rape victim

- You'll be asked to empty your bladder just before the test, but don't wipe the vulva afterward because this may remove semen.
- The examiner tries to obtain a semen specimen from your vagina.
- You're put into the same position as if you were having a Pap test.
- If the doctor is using vaginal lavage to rinse out a specimen, you should expect a cold sensation when the saline solution is introduced.

What are the normal results?

Normal semen volume ranges from 0.7 to 6.5 milliliters and is slightly alkaline with a pH of 7.3 to 7.9. Paradoxically, the semen volume of men in infertile couples is frequently increased. Continence for 1 week or more progressively increases semen volume (sperm counts increase with abstinence up to 10 days, sperm motility decreases, and sperm condition stays the same).

Other normal characteristics of semen are that it coagulates immediately and liquefies within 20 minutes. Normal sperm count ranges from 20 to 150 million per milliliter. At least 40% of sperm cells appear normal, and at least 20% of sperm cells show motility (the ability to swim) within 4 hours of collection.

What do abnormal results mean?

Abnormal semen does *not* mean infertility. Only one viable sperm cell is needed to fertilize an egg. Although a normal sperm count is more than 20 million per milliliter, many men with sperm counts below 1 million per milliliter have fathered normal children.

Only men who can't deliver *any* viable sperm in their ejaculate during sexual intercourse are absolutely sterile. Nevertheless, subnormal sperm counts, decreased sperm motility, and abnormal morphology are usually associated with decreased fertility. Other tests may be necessary to evaluate the person's general health, metabolic status, or the function of specific endocrine glands (pituitary, thyroid, adrenal, or gonadal).

Abnormal semen does not mean infertility. Only one viable sperm cell is needed to fertilize an egg.

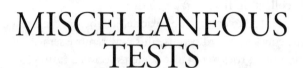

MISCELLANEOUS TESTS

SPINAL CORD FLUID

This test, which doctors commonly call *cerebrospinal fluid analysis,* analyzes the fluid within the spinal cord. For qualitative analysis, spinal fluid is most commonly obtained by lumbar puncture (usually taken from between the third and fourth lumbar vertebrae in the lower spine). A sample of this fluid for lab analysis is frequently obtained during other neurologic tests such as myelography.

Why is this test done?
The analysis of spinal fluid may be performed for the following reasons:
- To measure spinal fluid pressure, which helps the doctor detect obstruction of its circulation
- To aid the diagnosis of viral or bacterial meningitis, cranial hemorrhage, tumors, and brain abscesses
- To aid the diagnosis of neurosyphilis and chronic central nervous system infections.

What should you know before the test?
- You won't need to change your diet before the test.
- A doctor will perform the procedure, and it usually takes at least 15 minutes. You'll receive a local anesthetic.
- A headache is the most common side effect of a lumbar puncture, but your cooperation during the test helps minimize this effect.
- You'll be asked to sign a consent form.

What happens during the test?
- You lie on your side at the edge of the bed, with your knees drawn up to your abdomen and your chin on your chest.
- If the sitting position is preferred, you sit up and bend your chest and head toward your knees. The nurse helps you maintain this position throughout the procedure.

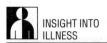 INSIGHT INTO
ILLNESS

Spinal fluid test results

TEST	ABNORMAL RESULTS	WHAT ABNORMAL RESULTS IMPLY
Fluid pressure	Above normal	Hemorrhage, tumor, or fluid accumulation caused by injury
	Below normal	Spinal obstruction above test puncture site
Appearance (normally clear)	Cloudy	Infection or various microorganisms
	Bloody	Hemorrhage, spinal cord obstruction, or injury from the test
	Brown, orange	or yellow
Protein level	Well above normal	Tumors, injury, hemorrhage, diabetes, polyneuritis, or blood in spinal fluid
	Well below normal	Rapid spinal fluid production
Gamma globulin level	Above normal	Multiple sclerosis or similar disease, neurosyphilis, Guillain-Barré syndrome
Glucose level	Above normal	High blood sugar
	Below normal	Low blood sugar, infection, meningitis, mumps, hemorrhage
White blood cell count	More than five white blood cells	Meningitis, acute infection, onset of chronic illness, tumor, abscess, infarction, multiple sclerosis or similar disease
Red blood cell count	Red blood cells present	Hemorrhage or injury from the test
Venereal disease research lab test or other blood tests	Positive	Neurosyphilis
Chloride level	Below normal	Tuberculosis, meningitis, or similar infection
Gram stain test	Infective organisms present	Bacterial meningitis

- After the skin is prepared for injection, the area is draped. You may experience a transient burning sensation when the local anesthetic is injected.
- When the doctor inserts the spinal needle between the vertebrae of the lower spine, you may feel some transient local pain.
- You should report any pain or sensations that differ from or continue after this expected discomfort because such sensations may indicate irritation or puncture of a nerve root, requiring repositioning of the needle.

- You should remain still and breathe normally; movement and hyperventilation can alter pressure readings or cause injury.

What happens after the test?

- After the specimen is collected, you'll probably be told to lie flat for 8 hours. Although you must not raise your head, you can turn from side to side.
- You'll be encouraged to drink fluids through a flexible straw.

What are the normal results?

Normally, spinal fluid pressure is recorded and the appearance of the specimen is checked. Three tubes are collected routinely and are sent to the lab for analysis of protein, sugar, and cells as well as for serologic testing, such as the Venereal Disease Research Laboratory Test for Neurosyphilis. A separate specimen is also sent to the lab for culture and sensitivity testing. Electrolyte analysis and Gram stain may be ordered as supplementary tests. (For a summary of possible findings in spinal fluid analysis, see *Spinal fluid test results,* page 667.)

JOINT FLUID

This test, which doctors call *synovial fluid analysis*, helps determine the cause of joint inflammation and swelling and also helps relieve your pain. In synovial fluid aspiration, or arthrocentesis, a sterile needle is inserted into a joint space — most commonly the knee — to obtain a fluid specimen for analysis.

Why is this test done?

Synovial fluid analysis may be performed for the following reasons:
- To help the doctor diagnose arthritis
- To identify the cause and nature of joint effusion
- To relieve the pain and distention resulting from accumulation of fluid within the joint
- To administer a drug locally (usually a corticosteroid).

What should you know before the test?

- You'll be told to fast for 6 to 12 hours before the test if glucose testing of synovial fluid is ordered. Otherwise, you won't need to change your diet before the test.
- You'll be told that you'll receive a local anesthetic. You may still feel transient pain when the needle penetrates the joint capsule.
- You'll be asked to sign a consent form.
- The doctor or nurse may ask if you're taking any medications that might interfere with the test. When possible, administration of such medications will be discontinued before the test.

What happens during the test?

- After the local anesthetic is administered, the aspirating needle is quickly inserted through the skin, tissue under the skin, and synovial membrane into the joint space.
- As much fluid as possible is withdrawn into the syringe.
- The joint (except for the area around the puncture site) may be wrapped with an elastic bandage to compress the free fluid into this portion of the sac, ensuring collection of the most fluid.
- If a corticosteroid is being injected, a nurse applies pressure to the puncture site for about 2 minutes to prevent bleeding and then applies a sterile dressing.
- If synovial fluid glucose levels are being measured, the examiner takes a blood sample.

Most people can enjoy their usual activities immediately after this test is completed.

What happens after the test?

- You'll apply ice or cold packs to the affected joint for 24 to 36 hours after aspiration to decrease pain and swelling. Use pillows for support. If a large quantity of fluid was aspirated, you'll use an elastic bandage to stabilize the joint.
- If your condition permits, you may resume your normal diet and normal activity immediately after the procedure. However, avoid excessive use of the joint for a few days after the test, even if pain and swelling subside.

What are the normal results?

Examination of synovial fluid in the lab can take many forms. Routine examination includes gross analysis for color, clarity, quantity, viscosity, pH, and the presence of a mucin clot as well as microscopic analysis for white blood cell count and differential. Special examination includes microbiological analysis for formed elements (including crystals) and bacteria, serologic analysis, and chemical analysis for such components as glucose, protein, and enzymes.

What do abnormal results mean?

Examination of synovial fluid may reveal various joint diseases, including noninflammatory disease (traumatic arthritis and osteoarthritis), inflammatory disease (lupus, rheumatic fever, pseudogout, gout, and rheumatoid arthritis), and septic disease (tuberculous and septic arthritis).

FLUID AROUND THE HEART

This test, which doctors call *pericardial fluid analysis*, detects excessive fluid around your heart. It also helps the doctor determine the cause of excess fluid and plan appropriate therapy.

The fluid examined during the test is withdrawn from inside the pericardial sac of the heart. (See *The sac that guards your heart.*) Testing is usually performed on people with pericardial effusion (an accumulation of excess pericardial fluid), which may result from inflammation (as in pericarditis), rupture, or penetrating injury. Obtaining a specimen for analysis requires needle aspiration of pericardial fluid, a procedure called *pericardiocentesis*.

Why is this test done?

Pericardial fluid analysis may be performed to help the doctor identify the cause of pericardial effusion and to help determine appropriate therapy.

What should you know before the test?

- You won't need to change your diet before the test.
- This test takes 10 to 20 minutes.
- You'll be given a local anesthetic before the aspiration needle is inserted to relieve any discomfort.
- Although fluid aspiration isn't painful, you may experience pressure upon insertion of the needle into the pericardial sac.
- You may be asked to briefly hold your breath to aid needle insertion and placement.

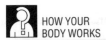

HOW YOUR
BODY WORKS

The sac that guards your heart

The pericardium, a fluid-filled sac, surrounds the heart wall. It consists of two layers. The *visceral pericardium* (also called the *epicardium*) serves as the pericardium's inner wall and the heart wall's outer layer. The *parietal pericardium*, a smooth, translucent membrane, serves as the pericardium's outer wall. The cavity between the parietal and visceral pericardium contains 20 to 50 milliliters of lymphlike lubricating fluid.

The important functions of the pericardium
Besides lubricating and isolating the beating heart, the pericardium also:
- holds the heart in a fixed position
- prevents the great vessels from kinking
- restrains ventricular dilation during exertion, preventing overstretching of the myocardium, a layer of the heart wall.

PERICARDIUM

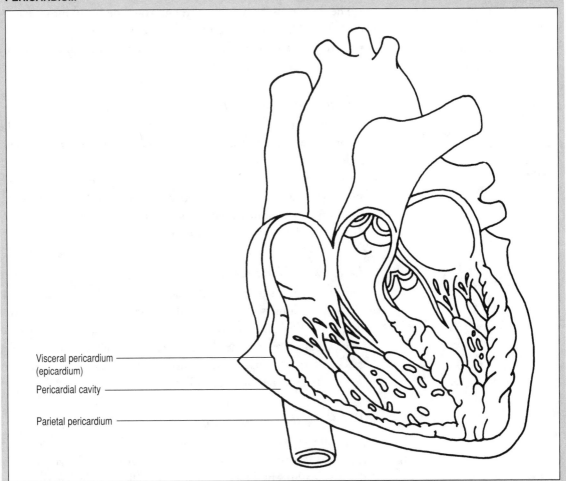

Visceral pericardium
(epicardium)

Pericardial cavity

Parietal pericardium

Once you're comfortable and well-supported, you remain still during the procedure.

• An intravenous line will be started at a slow rate in case medications need to be administered.
• Your vital signs, including pulse and blood pressure, will be monitored after the procedure.
• The doctor or nurse will ask about the use any drugs that might interfere with obtaining accurate test results.
• You'll be asked to sign a consent form.

What happens during the test?

• You lie down with your chest elevated 60 degrees.
• Once you're comfortable and well-supported, you remain still during the procedure.
• You're given a local anesthetic.
• The doctor inserts a needle through your chest wall into the pericardial sac. Fluid is gently aspirated into the syringe.
• During needle insertion, your heart rate and rhythm are carefully monitored on an electrocardiograph.

What happens after the test?

• When the needle is withdrawn, a nurse will apply pressure to the site with sterile gauze pads for 3 to 5 minutes and then apply a bandage.
• The nurse will check blood pressure readings, pulse, respiration, and heart sounds every 15 minutes until you're stable and then every half hour for 2 hours, every hour for 4 hours, and every 4 hours thereafter. This monitoring is routine.

Does the test have risks?

Pericardiocentesis must be performed cautiously because of the risk of complications, such as myocardial or coronary artery laceration, ventricular fibrillation or vasovagal arrest, pleural infection, or accidental puncture of the lung, liver, or stomach. If possible, echocardiography may be performed before pericardiocentesis. This helps minimize the risk of complications.

What are the normal results?

Normally, 10 to 50 milliliters of sterile fluid are present in the pericardium. Pericardial fluid is clear and straw-colored, without evidence of pathogens, blood, or malignant cells.

What do abnormal results mean?

Generally, pericardial effusions are classified as transudates or exudates. Transudates are protein-poor effusions that are usually caused by mechanical problems. They may be related to the presence of a tumor. Most exudates are caused by inflammation and contain large amounts of protein. If the test reveals exudate effusions, it may signal pericarditis, cancer, heart attack, tuberculosis, rheumatoid disease, or lupus.

The doctor will also look for such problems as turbid or milky liquid caused by the accumulation of lymph or pus in the pericardial sac or from tuberculosis or rheumatoid disease.

Bloody pericardial fluid may indicate a long list of problems, from a heart attack to cancer.

SWEAT TEST

Also called *iontophoresis*, this test is a quantitative measurement of electrolyte concentrations (primarily sodium and chloride) in sweat and is usually performed using a drug that makes the person sweat. It involves putting electrodes on the body and is used almost exclusively in children to confirm cystic fibrosis.

Why is this test done?

The sweat test may be performed to confirm cystic fibrosis.

What should you know before the test?

- A doctor or nurse will explain the test to the child (if the child is old enough to understand) and, if necessary, will clarify this explanation using clear, simple terms.
- The child won't need to change his or her diet, medications, or activity before the test.
- This test takes 20 to 45 minutes (depending on the equipment used).
- The child may feel a slight tickling sensation during the procedure but won't feel any pain.
- A child's parents are usually encouraged to assist with preparations and to stay with the child during the test. Your presence will minimize the child's anxiety.

This test may tickle a bit.

What happens during the test?

- The doctor washes the area that will undergo the sweat test with distilled water and dries it. (The right forearm is commonly used or, when the child's arm is too small to secure electrodes, the right thigh.)
- The doctor applies two electrodes to the area to be measured and secures them with straps. Lead wires to the analyzer are given a mild electric current for 15 to 20 seconds. The test continues at 15- to 20-second intervals for 5 minutes.
- You may want to distract the child with a book, a toy, or another diversion if he or she becomes nervous or frightened during the test.
- The doctor collects the sweat in a special container to send to the lab.

What happens after the test?

- The nurse will wash the area that was tested with soap and water and dry it thoroughly. If the area looks red, the nurse will reassure the child that this is normal and will disappear within a few hours.
- The child may resume his or her usual activities.

Does the test have risks?

The examiner will stop the test immediately if the child complains of a burning sensation, which usually indicates that the positive electrode is exposed or positioned improperly. The examiner then will adjust the electrode and continue the test.

What are the normal results?

Normal sodium values in sweat range from 10 to 30 milliequivalents per liter. Normal chloride values range from 10 to 35 milliequivalents per liter.

What do abnormal results mean?

Concentrations of sodium and chloride greater than 60 milliequivalents per liter, along with typical symptoms of cystic fibrosis, confirm the diagnosis.

PARASITES IN THE URINARY TRACT

This test is performed to identify the cause of infection in the urinary tract and the reproductive system. Samples of urine or vaginal, urethral, or prostatic secretions are examined under a microscope to detect infection by protozoan parasites called *Trichomonas vaginalis.* These parasites are usually transmitted sexually. This test is performed more often on women than men, since women show symptoms more often.

Why is this test done?

The test may be done to confirm trichomoniasis.

What should you know before the test?

- For a woman, the test requires a specimen of vaginal secretions or urethral discharge. You'll be asked not to douche before the test.
- For a man, the test requires a specimen of urethral or prostatic secretions.

What happens during the test?

Vaginal secretion

- You lie on your back, draped, on an exam table, as you would for a Pap test, with your feet in stirrups. (Shoes may make that more comfortable.)
- The examiner inserts an unlubricated speculum into your vagina and collects any discharge with a cotton swab, which is placed in a container and sent to the lab.

Prostatic material

The examiner massages the prostate to produce secretions. The secretions are collected with a cotton swab, which is placed in a container and sent to the lab.

Urethral discharge

The examiner collects the discharge with a cotton swab, which is placed in a container and sent to the lab.

Urine

You void once into a special container, taking care to collect the first portion of the urine stream. The container is then taken to the lab.

What are the normal results?

Trichomonads are normally absent from the urogenital tract.

What do abnormal results mean?

The presence of trichomonads in any of the samples confirms trichomoniasis. In approximately 25% of women and in most infected men, trichomonads may be present without any harmful results.

INDEX

Note: t indicates table; i indicates illustration.

Note: t indicates table; i indicates illustration.

Note: t indicates table; i indicates illustration.

Note: t indicates table; i indicates illustration.

Note: t indicates table; i indicates illustration.

Note: t indicates table; i indicates illustration.

Note: t indicates table; i indicates illustration.

Note: t indicates table; i indicates illustration.

Note: t indicates table; i indicates illustration.

Note: t indicates table; i indicates illustration.

Note: t indicates table; i indicates illustration.

Note: t indicates table; i indicates illustration.

Note: t indicates table; i indicates illustration.